Surgery of the

BILIARY TRACT, PANCREAS *and* SPLEEN

A HANDBOOK OF OPERATIVE SURGERY

Surgery of the
BILIARY TRACT, PANCREAS & SPLEEN

by

CHARLES B. PUESTOW, M.D., Ph.D. (Surg.)

Clinical Professor of Surgery, College of Medicine and Graduate College, University of Illinois; Attending Surgeon, University of Illinois Research and Educational Hospitals; Chief, Surgical Service, Veterans Administration Hospital, Hines, Ill.; Senior Surgeon, Henrotin Hospital, Chicago; Attending Surgeon, Presbyterian-St. Lukes Hospital, Chicago

Illustrated by JESSIE W. PHILLIPS

THIRD EDITION

429 ILLUSTRATIONS

YEAR BOOK MEDICAL PUBLISHERS • INC.
35 EAST WACKER DRIVE • CHICAGO

Second Edition, 1957
Third Edition, 1964

Library of Congress Catalog Card Number: 64-12577

PRINTED IN U.S.A.

Dedicated

to

LORRAINE

Preface to the Third Edition

SINCE PUBLICATION of the second edition of this book, much progress has been made in surgery of the pancreas. Benign pancreatic disease and especially chronic relapsing pancreatitis responded poorly to both medical and surgical therapy a decade ago. Even surgery designed for symptomatic relief, especially of pain, gave poor results. In recent years this has changed and we now have methods of surgical therapy for chronic relapsing pancreatitis which give gratifying relief of pain and also restore pancreatic function in a high percentage of patients. This edition includes extensive revision in pancreatic surgery. I am indebted to my longtime friend and associate, Dr. William J. Gillesby, who has collaborated with me in this field of surgery and research.

Additions have been made in the sections on biliary tract surgery, especially in factors contributing to the postcholecystectomy syndrome. I wish to thank my many friends who have given valuable advice on phases of this text which are out of the realm of surgical technic. I am also most grateful to Dr. Max S. Sadove who has contributed much valuable information in the field of anesthesiology.

—CHARLES B. PUESTOW.

Preface to the First Edition

SURGERY IS an important part of the therapeutic armamentarium of the medical profession and benefits many thousands of patients every year. It is one of the important factors in the gradually increasing longevity of our race. It has contributed much to the increased comfort and happiness of patients with benign diseases and has cured many thousands of cancer patients. Properly executed by skilled hands, surgery offers a great deal to mankind. Every surgeon should feel the responsibility of disseminating his knowledge, skill and judgment to his fellow surgeons. A handbook of surgery is an excellent educational medium because it offers to the adequately trained and competent surgeon a source of information for therapeutic procedures with which he is unfamiliar or has had minimal experience. It serves as a guide to methods of technic and preoperative and postoperative care which may improve his results. Such a book is not for the untrained and inexperienced physician who may wish to attempt surgical procedures for which he is not as yet adequately prepared. I was asked to prepare a book which would also serve as a guide to surgical residents who will receive competent training but who will occasionally need guidance in certain special procedures. It is with this aim that I attempt to present knowledge which I have acquired over a period of many years.

This book does not include all operations recommended for surgical therapy of the biliary tract, pancreas and spleen. It has been designed to include those procedures which I have performed and which have proved satisfactory. I have been guided not only by my own experience but by that of my associates and the medical literature. If there is questionable doubt of the value of certain described procedures, these uncertainties are mentioned in the text.

No one person can be an authority even in a limited field of surgery. I have called freely upon my surgical associates for aid and advice and they have given their services willingly. I wish to express my sincere gratitude to my surgical associates and residents. I do wish to thank Dr. Lyle A. Baker, Chief, Medical Service, Veterans' Administration Hospital, Hines, Ill., for his aid in the chapter on liver physiology and jaundice. Dr. Louis R. Limarzi, Associate Professor of Medicine, University of Illinois, has contributed a great deal to the section on surgical diseases of the spleen.

This book does not contain a bibliography, nor does the author claim to be the originator of any described surgical procedure. Any reader desiring further information has access to an adequate bibliography. Names have been attached to certain operations when common usage has justified such association.

All drawings are original. I am most grateful to Miss Jessie W. Phillips for the quality of her illustrations and for the time and effort spent in creating many and in verifying accuracy.

Table of Contents

List of Illustrations

SECTION I

The Liver

CHAPTER 1

General Considerations

Diseases of very few organs or systems of the human body respond as completely and satisfactorily to correct surgical therapy as do those of the biliary system. The great majority of patients for whom surgery of the biliary tract is indicated can be relieved of symptoms and restored to health with the liver and bile ducts capable of functioning adequately for normal physiologic comfort and longevity. Unfortunately, such good results are obtained far less frequently than our scientific information justifies. Reports of poor results of biliary tract surgery deter the patient and the referring physician from seeking surgical therapy in the early stages of biliary disease. As a result, the disease process, which usually begins in a focus that can be completely eradicated, spreads and becomes so extensive that no form of treatment can promise a complete cure or produces secondary conditions not amenable to surgery. A number of factors contribute to poor surgical results and must be avoided if operative therapy is to be of maximal value.

The surgeon must have a thorough knowledge of the anatomy, physiology and bio-chemistry of the biliary system. This information is essential to the diagnosis of the diseases of these structures and to an understanding of the principles upon which surgical therapy is based. It is fundamental that sound preoperative care should be initiated not the night before an operation but days or weeks in advance. It is as important as the postoperative care of the patient, especially when biliary physiology has been disturbed. Failure to heed or be cognizant of the importance of these basic principles may be responsible for poor surgical results.

An accurate diagnosis is essential in the treatment of biliary tract disease. Organic or functional disturbances of many other structures may produce symptoms simulating those of diseases of the biliary tract. A carefully taken history usually gives the most valuable diagnostic information. Detailed interrogation of the patient and alert attention to the chronological sequence and nature of his complaints are the most accurate means of establishing a diagnosis. The greatest single factor responsible for poor results of biliary tract surgery is an error in diagnosis. A thorough physical examination is essential and often will reveal valuable information.

Information obtained by laboratory and x-ray examination may be extremely valuable in corroborating and at times in helping to establish a diagnosis. However, this does not substitute for knowledge obtained by the five senses combined with the scientific knowledge and judgment of the surgeon. Results of these examinations may establish the existence of biliary tract disease but cannot coordinate the disease with the symptomatology of the patient. Biliary disease may be asymptomatic but coexist with other abnormalities producing similar symptoms. Knowledge and experience in this field of surgery are the surgeon's greatest assets.

Errors in surgical technic are also responsible for poor results. Biliary tract surgery is not simple and should not be attempted by a surgeon with inadequate knowledge or training. Damage to the biliary system including its ducts and blood vessels may be tragic. When such damage occurs, it is often irreparable.

Although this book is primarily a handbook of surgical technic, it is the belief of the author that the surgeon must be not only a good technician but also a diagnostician with adequate knowledge of the basic fundamentals of medical care. For this reason a few factors other than technic are included, in the hope that they may aid the surgeon in obtaining a high percentage of successful results.

CHAPTER 2

Anatomy and Physiology of the Liver

ANATOMY

THE LIVER IS the largest glandular organ in the body, weighing in the adult 3 lb. or more and constituting about 1/50 of the body weight. It is a highly vascular organ which is reddish brown in color, soft to touch and very easily lacerated or traumatized. Its external appearance is one of uniform consistency, but a cut section appears granular due to its composition of hepatic lobules. The liver is located in the abdominal cavity under the diaphragm with its greater bulk to the right of the midline. The anterior inferior edge lies approximately parallel to and behind the right costal margin and most of its substance is protected by the lower portion of the thoracic cage. This position makes the liver less vulnerable to trauma but also less accessible to the surgeon for operative procedures. The liver maintains its position under the diaphragm by the attachments of a number of ligaments, including the falciform, the coronary, the right and left triangular and the round ligament. Anatomically, the liver is composed of a large right lobe and a smaller left lobe, which are demarcated by the falciform ligament, and two smaller lobes, the quadrate and caudate. In certain animal species the lobes of the liver are more discrete and can be removed separately. Remarkable regenerative powers of the liver have been demonstrated in dogs, in which total regeneration has occurred in from six to eight weeks after removal of large portions of the liver.

A.—An anterior view of the biliary system and functionally related organs is illustrated. The intrahepatic venous system is shown diagrammatically for simplification and clarity. The liver has a dual blood supply, arterial blood reaching it through the hepatic arterial system, and venous blood from the gastrointestinal tract, pancreas and spleen entering through the portal vein. The extrahepatic relationship of these vessels to each other and to the bile ducts is of vital interest to the surgeon and is discussed in the section on the extrahepatic biliary system, in particular in Chapter 6. From the standpoint of blood supply, the liver is divided into a right and left portion of relatively equal size. The right hepatic artery which may enter the liver in one or more divisions is most susceptible to surgical injury, the sequelae of which will depend upon the amount of liver tissue supplied by the injured branch. The left hepatic artery likewise may enter as a single or branched vessel.

B.—On the inferior surface of the liver are seen the porta hepatis and the relative positions of the hepatic ducts and arteries and the portal vein and its branches. The portal vein divides into a right and left branch at the hilus of the liver. The right branch carries blood chiefly from the superior mesenteric vein, whereas the left branch receives its largest proportion of blood from the splenic and inferior mesenteric veins. The distribution of venous blood may determine in which portion of the liver blood-borne metastatic cells will be deposited and develop into tumors. The portion affected may in turn indicate the site of the primary tumor. All blood vessels and ducts enter the liver at the hilus or porta hepatis in close relation to each other. The portal vein and its branches lie posterior to the arteries and ducts.

Histologically, the liver consists of hepatic cells which carry on the main function of this organ, cells which make up the various ducts, sinusoids and vessels and Kupffer cells which are a part of the reticuloendothelial system.

PLATE 1

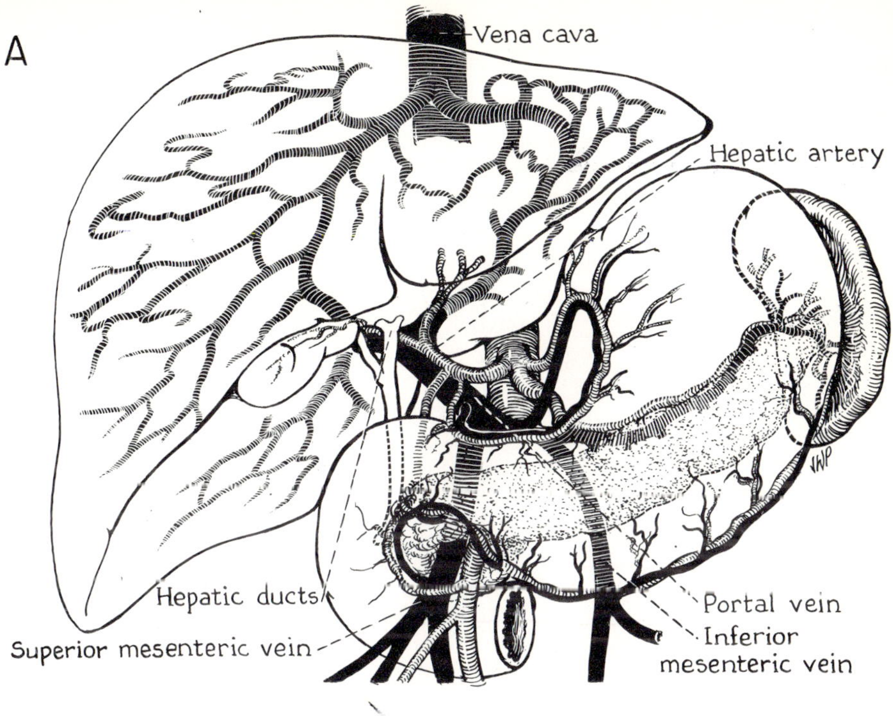
A
Vena cava
Hepatic artery
Hepatic ducts
Superior mesenteric vein
Portal vein
Inferior mesenteric vein
VWP

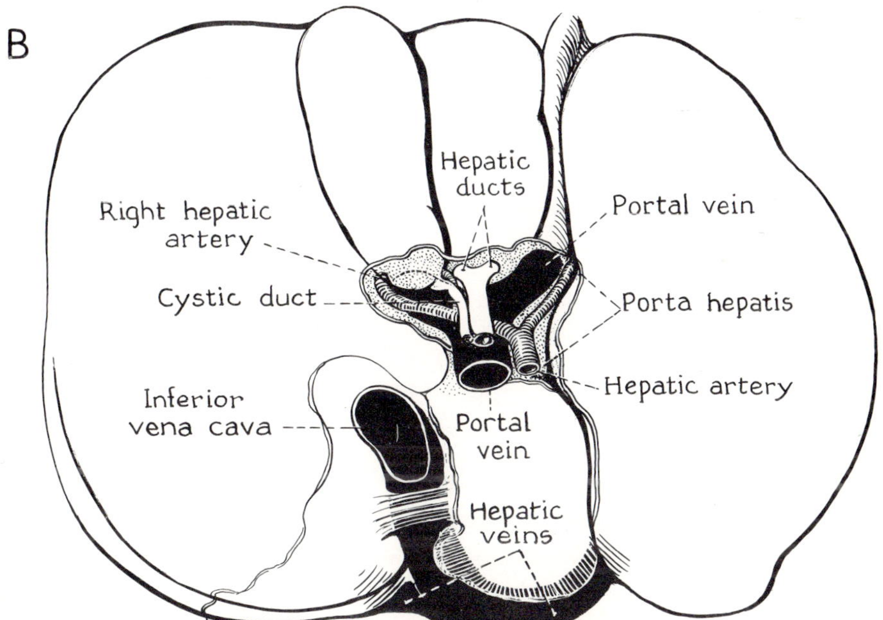
B
Hepatic ducts
Right hepatic artery
Portal vein
Cystic duct
Porta hepatis
Hepatic artery
Inferior vena cava
Portal vein
Hepatic veins

PHYSIOLOGY

The belief of the ancients that the liver is the seat of life has considerable merit. This organ performs many functions essential to life. At its own expense it protects the rest of the body from damage which might be inflicted by toxic products absorbed from the gastro-intestinal tract or from other internal or external sources. Were it not that a healthy liver has nearly five times the functional ability needed for its normal activities and were it not that this organ has greater power of regeneration than any other organ of the body, the incidence of hepatic insufficiency would be much higher.

Liver Functions

The functions of the liver have been variously classified. Those dealing with the interchange of activity between the hepatic cells and the blood stream have been called functions of internal secretion. Those concerned with the formation and discharge of bile have been termed functions of external secretion.

Metabolic functions.—The functions of the liver include a number of important metabolic activities.

1. Carbohydrate metabolism. The manufacture and storage of glycogen and its conversion into glucose as this is needed by the body all take place in the liver. This organ serves as an "automatic stoker" for the maintenance of an adequate level of blood sugar.

2. Protein metabolism. The liver carries on several important functions related to protein metabolism. Amino acids not required by the body are deaminized and urea is synthesized within this organ. The liver plays an important role in the formation of uric acid and in the synthesis of hippuric acid. It manufactures many important proteins, including fibrinogen, prothrombin, albumin and some globulin, and serves as a storehouse for proteins.

3. Fat metabolism. The liver is active in the breaking down of fatty acids and in the formation of ketone bodies. The manufacture of bile salts and their secretion into the intestine is essential to the emulsification and absorption of ingested fats.

4. Relation to vitamins. Carotene is converted to vitamin A in the liver, which also stores vitamins A, B, D and K. The absorption of fat-soluble vitamins from the intestinal tract is dependent upon the bile salts normally existent there by secretion from the liver.

5. Relation to minerals. The liver serves as a reservoir for iron and copper.

Functions related to the cardiovascular system.—The distensibility of the liver provides protection to the right heart. The loss of this protection, as is seen in cirrhosis, may be followed by cardiac damage. In the embryo, blood is formed within the liver. In the adult this organ stores an antianemic principle. Coagulation of blood is dependent upon hepatic synthesis of several essential factors such as fibrinogen, prothrombin, accelerator globulin, proconvertin, and plasma thromboplastin component. These are often reduced in cases of hepatic failure and return to normal upon recovery.

Detoxifying powers.—Many toxins, heavy metals and drugs which could produce tissue damage in other parts of the body are removed from the blood by the liver. Other toxic agents are eliminated or destroyed by the liver by conjugation, by oxidation and by the action of the reticuloendothelial system. Bacteria are removed from the blood stream by this organ. The liver serves as a detoxifying organ in all types of surgery. In the presence of liver disease of sufficient severity to interfere with this function, the risk of all surgery is greatly increased.

Functions of external secretions.—The constant destruction of red blood cells liberates hemoglobin which is converted into unconjugated protein-bound bilirubin. This gives an indirect reaction with the van den Bergh test. The unconjugated bilirubin is carried to the liver where, in passing through the liver cells to be excreted into the biliary canaliculi, it is conjugated with glucuronic acid into di- and monoglucuronides of bilirubin which react directly with van den Bergh reagent. From the biliary canaliculi the bilirubin salts pass along the bile passages into the intestine where they are converted into urobilinogen and stercobilin. Some of the urobilinogen is reabsorbed, flows back to the liver and is re-excreted in the bile and some is excreted into the urine. The absence of urobilinogen in the urine means that no bile is entering the gastrointestinal tract and jaundice is complete. An excess of urobilinogen in the urine in the presence of choluric jaundice indicates either rapid excessive hemolysis or damaged liver parenchyma. Complete jaundice is usually obstructive; jaundice with increased urine urobilinogen is usually hepatocellular. Bile salts and cholesterol are manufactured and secreted by the liver.

Liver Function Tests

No single test can give an accurate estimation of the functional capacity of the liver because of the multiplicity of functions of this organ. Many tests have been devised to determine the ability of the liver to carry on some of its various activities, but several related tests may estimate the same hepatic function. An accurate measure of the functional capacity would aid in the differential diagnosis of certain diseases of the biliary system and would be of inestimable value in determining the risk involved in surgical procedures. It must be remembered, however, that the tremendous reserve of liver tissue enables this organ to carry on normal function despite extensive damage. Functional insufficiency becomes detectable only after this reservoir is exceeded. The demonstration of impaired liver function by laboratory tests usually indicates serious damage to this organ and demands most careful pre- and postoperative management. The absence of laboratory evidence of impaired liver function is not a guarantee that the patient has a normal liver. When surgery is contemplated in the presence of biliary tract disease, it is well to assume that considerable liver damage exists despite normal function tests and to treat the patient accordingly. If laboratory evidence of liver dysfunction exists, the greatest possible precautions must be taken.

In addition to their use in the evaluation of the functional capacity of the liver, certain liver function tests are of considerable diagnostic value. This is particularly true in the jaundiced patient. It is not within the scope of this book to discuss the subject of jaundice. However, differentiation between medical and surgical jaundice is essential to correct management. Jaundice due to obstruction of the extrahepatic biliary tract or its larger radicles if unrelieved by surgery can produce progressive liver damage that is as malicious when produced by stone as when produced by cancer. However, when a patient is operated on for jaundice of hepatocellular origin, the toxic effects of certain anesthetic agents and the trauma of an operative procedure may be definitely harmful.

The differentiation of jaundice of intrahepatic and extrahepatic etiology is often difficult. Although in most cases the clinical features, such as age, history of exposure to the etiologic agent, mode of onset, the color of the patient, the condition of the liver, gallbladder and spleen on physical examination, evidences of scratch marks, palmar erythema, spider angioma or a right upper abdominal scar and demonstration of the completeness of the jaundice, lead to a diagnostic profile, in some cases the picture is completed only by corroborative evidence derived from laboratory tests. Generalized pruritus is a frequent and often early accompaniment of obstructive jaundice but is not a common symptom of hepatocellular jaundice especially in early stages. One should distinguish the saffron color of hepatitis from the olive green of long-standing obstruction. Persistent absence of bile in the intestinal tract is indicative of obstructive jaundice, whereas in liver disease some bile usually can be demonstrated in the duodenum or stools. In hepatocellular disease, the patient usually is toxic, febrile and acutely ill; most cases reach a fastigium and then recede. In obstruction due to stones the jaundice may be intermittent with or without Charcot's intermittent hepatic fever, and in obstruction due to malignancy the degree is usually total. As the duration and severity of jaundice increase, the differentiation between the two types may become less striking and diagnosis more difficult to establish. Under such circumstances, liver function tests used in conjunction with the patient's history and the clinical findings may be helpful. Jaundice is seldom a surgical emergency and time can usually be taken to establish a diagnosis.

In discussing the use of liver function tests in the differential diagnosis of jaundice, it must be emphasized that their value is always relative to other information obtained from the history and physical findings. In this discussion the use of liver function tests is limited to those tests most commonly available and those which are believed to give the greatest information. No attempt is made to analyze exhaustively all the procedures recommended as aids to the differential diagnosis of jaundice.

The scheme illustrated on page 27 presents a suggested procedure for the use of such tests when one is confronted with a jaundiced patient. It is obvious that the separation of prehepatic (hemolytic) jaundice from hepatocellular and obstructive jaundice is comparatively simple and reliable. After the former condition is eliminated, the next step is to separate hepatocellular from obstructive jaundice. When the jaundice is relatively recent, the laboratory procedures indicated are quite informative. The longer the jaundice has been present, the less reliable are the tests. This is also true when derangement of the liver is due to substances such as arsphenamine, chlorpromazine or testosterone, as well as in the presence of fatty infiltration. The clinical history of primary insult to the liver together with an enlarged tender organ suggests intrahepatic disease. The results of tests for hepatocellular function—particularly the flocculation test, the tests for cholesterol esters and more recently the enzyme tests, especially the SGLT, SGPT and LDH tests—are of great value in determining the presence and degree of hepatocellular damage and in confirming the diagnosis of medical jaundice. The prothrombin time is not only a link in the chain of differential diagnostic evidence but is also of considerable prognostic value.

The greatest diagnostic difficulty is encountered when an attempt is made to differentiate obstruction of the intrahepatic ducts (cholangiolitic hepatitis, biliary cirrhosis) from extrahepatic or surgical jaundice. The jaundice in both instances is truly obstructive, and therefore the results of the various tests for obstructive jaundice tend to be positive. As indicated in the chart, intrahepatic obstruction tends to be associated with more abnormality of hepatocellular function than does pure extrahepatic jaundice. Further, if there is deep jaundice due to extrahepatic obstruction the alkaline phosphatase value usually is high, whereas in intrahepatic obstruction the elevation of alkaline phosphatase lags behind the level of jaundice. Rarely does it rise to the high levels seen in extrahepatic obstruction, and a value over 15 Bodansky units is unusual even in the presence of deep jaundice unless the jaundice is of long duration. Intrahepatic metastatic malignancies producing jaundice may give unusually high alkaline phosphatase levels. On the other hand, the alkaline phosphatase level may be moderately elevated in the presence of only mild icterus in cholangiolitic involvement. It is in this particular group that liver biopsy may be helpful. Most physicians do not recommend cholecystography in the presence of jaundice. If, however, cholecystograms have been obtained and reveal a normally functioning gallbladder, extrahepatic obstruction is unlikely. An equivocal history and physical findings, inconclusive and overlapping results of laboratory tests and persistent, complete jaundice may require abdominal exploration to establish a diagnosis.

As indicated previously, in the presence of long standing extrahepatic obstruction or of such obstruction superimposed on primary liver disease, the results of liver function tests are likely to be con-

Laboratory Tests in Differential Diagnosis of Jaundice

Results	Laboratory Tests	Results
Dark brown ←	Color of gross stool	→ Pale
Increased ←	2 hr. urinary urobilinogen	→ Normal or low
Increased ←	Fecal urobilinogen	→ Normal or low
Positive ←	For increased hemolysis	→ Normal
Elevated ←	Reticulocyte count	→ Normal
Elevated ←	Indirect van den Bergh	→ Alteration slight
Indicate ↓ PREHEPATIC (HEMOLYTIC) JAUNDICE		*Indicate* ↓ Obstructive or Hepatocellular Jaundice

Obstructive or Hepatocellular Jaundice ↓

Results	Laboratory Tests	Results
Slight or no abnorm. ←	Flocculation tests	→ Abnormal
Elevated ←	Cholesterol and esters	→ Low
Elevated ←	Alkaline phosphatase	→ Normal or slightly elevated
Alteration slight ←	A/G ratio	→ Abnormal
Limited abnormality ←	Prothrombin time	→ Greater abnormality
Good ←	Response to vitamin K	→ Poor
Limited abnormality ←	Transaminases	→ Elevated
Indicate ↓ Obstructive Jaundice–Intrahepatic or Extrahepatic		*Indicate* ↓ HEPATOCELLULAR JAUNDICE

Obstructive Jaundice–Intrahepatic or Extrahepatic ↓

Results	Laboratory Tests	Results
Abnormal ←	1. For hepatocellular function	→ Normal
Abnormal (under 15 units) ←	2. Alkaline phosphatase	→ Markedly abnormal
Mild elevation ←	3. Direct van den Bergh	→ Higher elevation
Absent ←	Correlation, tests 2 and 3 values	→ Present
Indicate ↓ INTRAHEPATIC OBSTRUCTION		*Indicate* ↓ EXTRAHEPATIC OBSTRUCTION

When liver function tests are not definitive, liver biopsy and/or exploration may be indicated.

Long-standing extrahepatic obstruction or obstruction superimposed on liver disease gives poor differentiating results due to liver cell damage and may indicate exploration.

fusing. In general, in extrahepatic obstruction without infection there tends to be little evidence of impaired hepatocellular function. However, since in a considerable percentage of jaundiced patients infection is present at some time, hepatocellular derangement may be very definite. It must therefore be conceded that in long-standing jaundice of extrahepatic origin liver function tests are of little diagnostic aid. Deep jaundice with pruritus and little evidence of general toxemia is probably due to extrahepatic obstruction.

From a prognostic standpoint, in patients who show a depression of serum albumin, a lowering of cholesterol esters and a prolonged prothrombin time which does not respond to vitamin K, surgical procedures should be approached with caution.

Liver Biopsy

Needle biopsy of the liver has been employed in recent years with increasing frequency. It is used to diagnose the presence and nature of liver disease and to determine the existence and degree of hepatic cell damage. Efforts have been made to correlate the results of liver function tests with the histologic picture as shown by needle biopsy. Information available at present does not justify an estimation of the functional capacity of the liver by biopsy alone. Used in conjunction with liver function tests, liver biopsy may give a better picture of the severity or progress of the disease and permit a more accurate prognosis. In diffuse liver disease, a fairly accurate histologic picture of the entire organ may be obtained. When disease of the liver is localized or varies in severity in different portions of the organ, an accurate diagnosis may not be obtained by biopsy.

Repeated biopsies of the liver used in conjunction with other studies should increase our knowledge of nonsurgical diseases and should give a better understanding of their treatment. Rare and unsuspected diseases of the liver occasionally are diagnosed by biopsy. Knowledge so obtained may save the patient from undergoing an exploratory operation if the condition cannot be benefited by surgery. In the early stages of jaundice of questionable etiology, a histologic picture of the liver may help differentiate between hepatogenous disease and surgical jaundice. When jaundice is long standing, information gained by biopsy may be of little value. Negative results of biopsies may be inconclusive if the disease is not diffuse, because the tissue obtained may not be from the diseased portions of the organ.

Tumors of the liver may be diagnosed by liver biopsy if the specimen is obtained at the site of the tumor. The diagnosis of cancer of the liver by biopsy should not always serve as a contraindication to surgical exploration. The advancement of surgery of the liver now permits quite extensive resections of this organ with minimal danger. Cancer can be removed from many portions of the organ. Thus, surgery offers a possibility for cure or prolongation of life in a disease which otherwise has a hopeless prognosis.

Dangers of liver biopsy.—Needle biopsy of the liver is not without danger. Hemorrhage is the greatest hazard and has been responsible for a number of deaths. Before the procedure is attempted, careful studies should be made to rule out any hemorrhagic tendency or disease. Vitamin K should be given to all patients before and after the procedure to minimize bleeding. Perforation of structures adjacent to the liver must be avoided. Collapse of the right lung has followed the intercostal approach to the liver, and perforation of a hollow viscus of the abdomen, particularly the gallbladder and colon, has complicated the abdominal approach. The transthoracic approach should not be used if a pleural infection is present or has recently existed. The subcostal approach should not be used in the presence of intraperitoneal infection. The procedure is hazardous in the presence of suppurative disease of the liver.

Technics.—Needle biopsy of the liver should be considered a hospital procedure, and the patient should remain hospitalized for at least two days to permit recognition and treatment of possible complications. Aseptic technic should be judiciously followed. Biopsy needles utilize two main principles. In one, a needle and stilet are introduced into the liver, the stilet is removed and the needle which has a cutting edge is pushed forward with a circular motion. An aspirating syringe is attached to the needle and suction is applied to hold the plug of liver in the needle, which is then removed (Plate 2, *A*). In the other, the needle contains a longitudinally divided stilet (Silverman needle). After introducing the needle into the liver, the stilet is pushed beyond the end of the needle into the liver substance, the points spreading to grasp a portion of liver. The sheath is then pushed forward over the end of the forked stilet and both are removed together (Plate 2, *C*).

Postbiopsy care.—The patient should be kept quiet for at least 24 hours after liver biopsy. Pain frequently follows this procedure and may result from local bleeding. If internal hemorrhage results, the pain will become intensified and will spread. Signs and symptoms of internal hemorrhage will indicate gross bleeding. Pain in the right chest and right shoulder sometimes follows the intercostal approach. If clinical evidence of severe bleeding or injury to a viscus follows biopsy, abdominal exploration may be indicated.

A.—The subcostal technic of needle biopsy of the liver is the most satisfactory approach when hepatomegaly exists. The site for insertion of the needle should be fairly close to the midline and just below the costal margin. The skin and subcutaneous tissues are infiltrated with local anesthesia. A small skin incision is made sufficiently long to permit easy passage of the needle and stilet. The needle is directed posteriorly and superiorly toward the right axilla. It is pushed forward into the liver. The stilet is then removed and the needle pushed forward with a circular motion so that its cutting edge will incise a cylinder of liver tissue. An aspirating syringe is attached to the needle and suction applied to hold the biopsy specimen within the needle while it is being removed. If a tumor of the liver is suspected, a biopsy specimen may be taken from any palpable nodule below the costal margin. Damage to the capsule by the needle because of respiratory excursion is less apt to occur with the subcostal than with the intercostal approach.

B.—If the liver is not enlarged and does not extend below the costal margin, biopsy through an intercostal approach is safer. The ninth right intercostal space in the midaxillary or anterior axillary line is a satisfactory location for introduction of the needle. The needle should be directed medially and slightly upward. Before introduction of the needle, the patient should be told to exhale and then to hold his breath until the procedure is completed. Respiratory excursions are likely to cause tearing of the capsule of the liver and to produce bleeding. The needle and its stilet are passed through the chest wall and diaphragm and for a short distance into the liver. The stilet is then removed, the biopsy stilet or cutting needle introduced and a specimen obtained as rapidly as possible. A section of liver 1 or 2 cm. long is desirable for histologic study.

C.—The Silverman type of needle, introduced into the liver by an intercostal approach, is shown.

PLATE 2

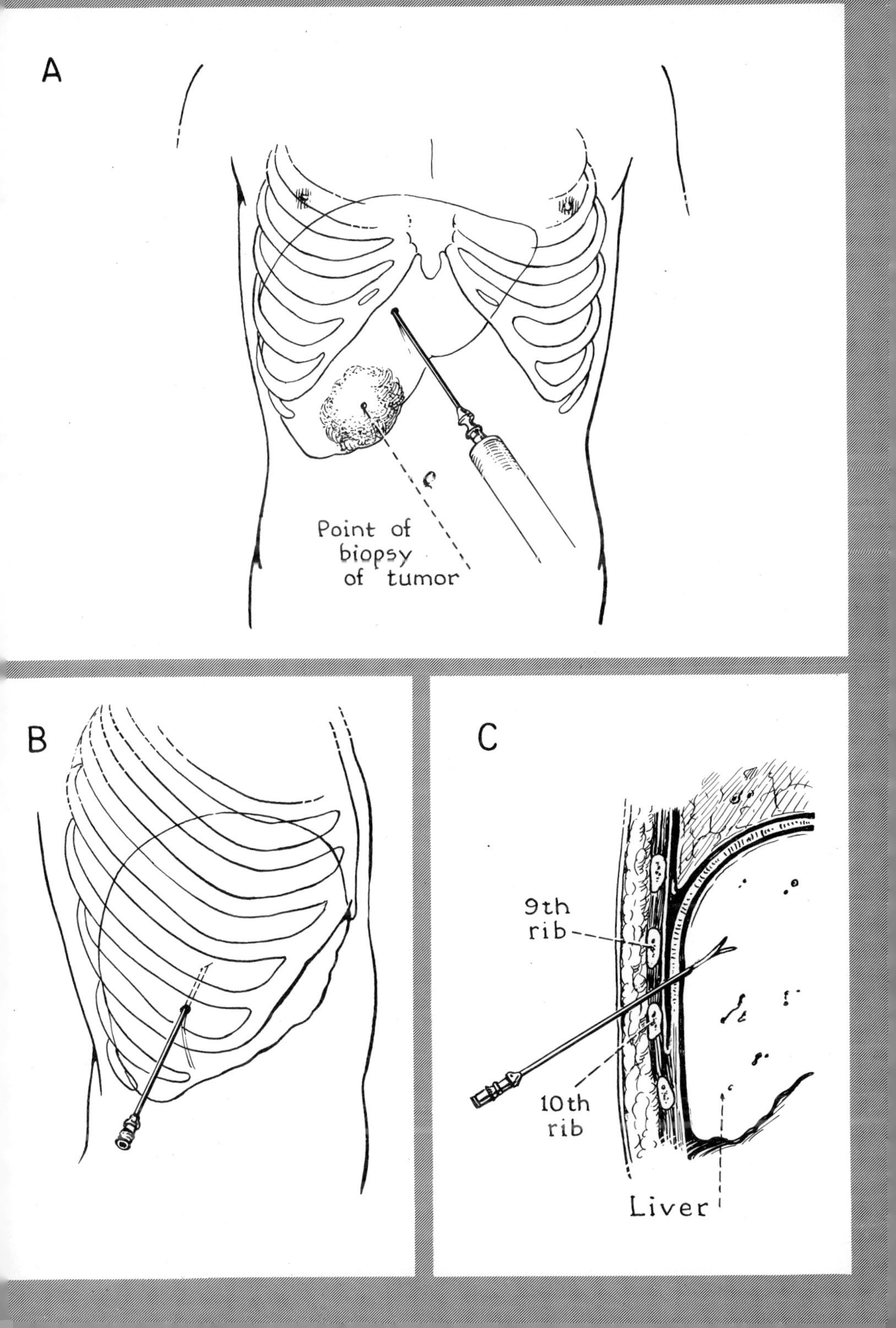

CHAPTER 3

Surgical Diseases of the Liver

THE GREAT IMPORTANCE of the liver to human existence and the inability to live without its physiologic activity make it fortunate that the liver is an infrequent site for surgical therapy. There are many physical properties of the liver which make it a difficult field for operative procedures. It is extremely vascular, very friable and easily traumatized. Sutures cannot be satisfactorily placed within its substance and, to be effective, they must include the capsule which is thin and easily torn. Cut surfaces of the liver tend to secrete bile which produces a highly irritating form of peritonitis if there is not adequate external drainage. Care must be taken not to occlude main bile ducts which could defunctionalize large segments of liver.

The commonest conditions of the liver for which surgical therapy is indicated are traumatic lacerations and abscesses. These often are difficult to diagnose and localize preoperatively. Less common diseases of the liver include cirrhosis, which produces portal hypertension with resultant ascites and bleeding varicosities, and metastatic tumors. More than 50 per cent of patients who die of carcinoma have metastatic involvement of the liver. Few of these cases are amenable to surgical therapy, but occasionally there is a solitary tumor of the liver which can be excised. Other rare surgical diseases of the liver include benign tumors, congenital cysts and some of the more unusual hepatic infections.

Great progress has been made in surgery of the liver in the past few years. Large portions can be resected, intrahepatic ducts can be isolated or anastomosed to the intestine to alleviate total obstruction of the extrahepatic biliary system, and shunt operations can divert large quantities of portal blood from passing through the liver. Surgery has little to offer, however, for hepatic cell disease which is not secondary to bile duct obstruction.

INJURIES

Rupture of the liver.—Rupture of the liver may result from a severe blow to the overlying structures, the lower right chest wall or the upper right abdomen. Such violence can result from a fall or a crushing injury. Automobile accidents in which the victim's body is thrown forcibly against some firm object, such as a steering wheel or the side of a car, occasionally are the cause of a ruptured liver. Injury may involve the free peritoneal surface of the liver, the dome of the liver or may be entirely intracapsular. Associated injuries may include fracture of the overlying ribs, tearing of the diaphragm and injury to adjacent structures.

Symptomatology.—The history and evidences of a severe injury to the right lower chest or right upper abdomen should suggest possible trauma to the liver. Fracture of one or more ribs is not uncommonly associated with injury to the liver, but there may be no external evidence of injury. The principal symptoms of rupture of the liver depend upon the presence and amount of associated hemorrhage. If the capsule is torn, bleeding may be profuse and produce peritoneal reaction. This will be accompanied by right upper quadrant pain, tenderness and rigidity of the overlying abdominal muscles. If the bleeding continues there will be symptoms of spreading peritonitis. The area of tenderness, pain and rigidity gradually increases to include the entire right abdomen. With progressive bleeding, the symptoms may spread to the left lower abdomen and finally to the entire abdominal area. In such cases, shock ensues. If bleeding occurs from the dome of the liver, the blood may accumulate in one of the subdiaphragmatic spaces, producing an elevation of the diaphragm and sometimes a depression of the liver. If the diaphragm is torn, blood may accumulate in the right pleural cavity.

Roentgenograms with the patient erect are important to determine the position of the diaphragm, the possibility of blood in the chest and evidence of injury to the overlying ribs.

A.—Injuries to the liver which damage the capsule may produce linear tears or a partial avulsion of liver substance with its overlying capsule.

B.—Subcapsular injury to the liver may result in hemorrhage into the bile ducts. If clots form within the common bile duct they may produce biliary colic. Occasionally such clots will obstruct the duct and jaundice will develop, but it usually is of short duration as the clots soon pass into the duodenum. Bleeding into the bile ducts and passage of blood into the duodenum may be profuse and evidenced by hematemesis or melena. Blood in the stools following an upper abdominal injury should suggest the possibility of subcapsular liver damage.

Repair of Injuries

If, when the capsule is damaged, bleeding into the peritoneal cavity occurs and is progressive, abdominal exploration is indicated. In most instances a right subcostal incision will give the most satisfactory exposure. In such an operation, the surgeon must be aware of the possibility of injury to adjacent organs and should carefully explore them.

C.—Linear tears of the liver may be closed with mattress sutures placed well back from the edges of the capsular tear and deeply inserted. The sutures should include a portion of liver capsule and should not be tied too tightly as they may cut through this friable organ. If a considerable portion of liver tissue is lacerated, some debridement may be indicated but this should be kept to a minimum. It may be advisable to remove a portion of the liver which is avulsed and attached by a fairly small pedicle. Under such circumstances, bleeding can be controlled by deeply placed mattress sutures. If these do not check the bleeding, a hemostatic agent such as Gelfoam should be tied over the raw liver surface by deeply placed interrupted sutures. Gelfoam is an excellent hemostatic agent and also serves as a barrier to bile leakage. Fibroblasts grow into it and give added protection.

D.—If the wound is large and if bleeding cannot be controlled in any other manner, the wound should be firmly packed with gauze over a layer of Gelfoam. The gauze pack should be sufficiently long to permit the end to be brought out through the abdominal wound.

[Repair of injuries *continued on page 36.*]

PLATE 3

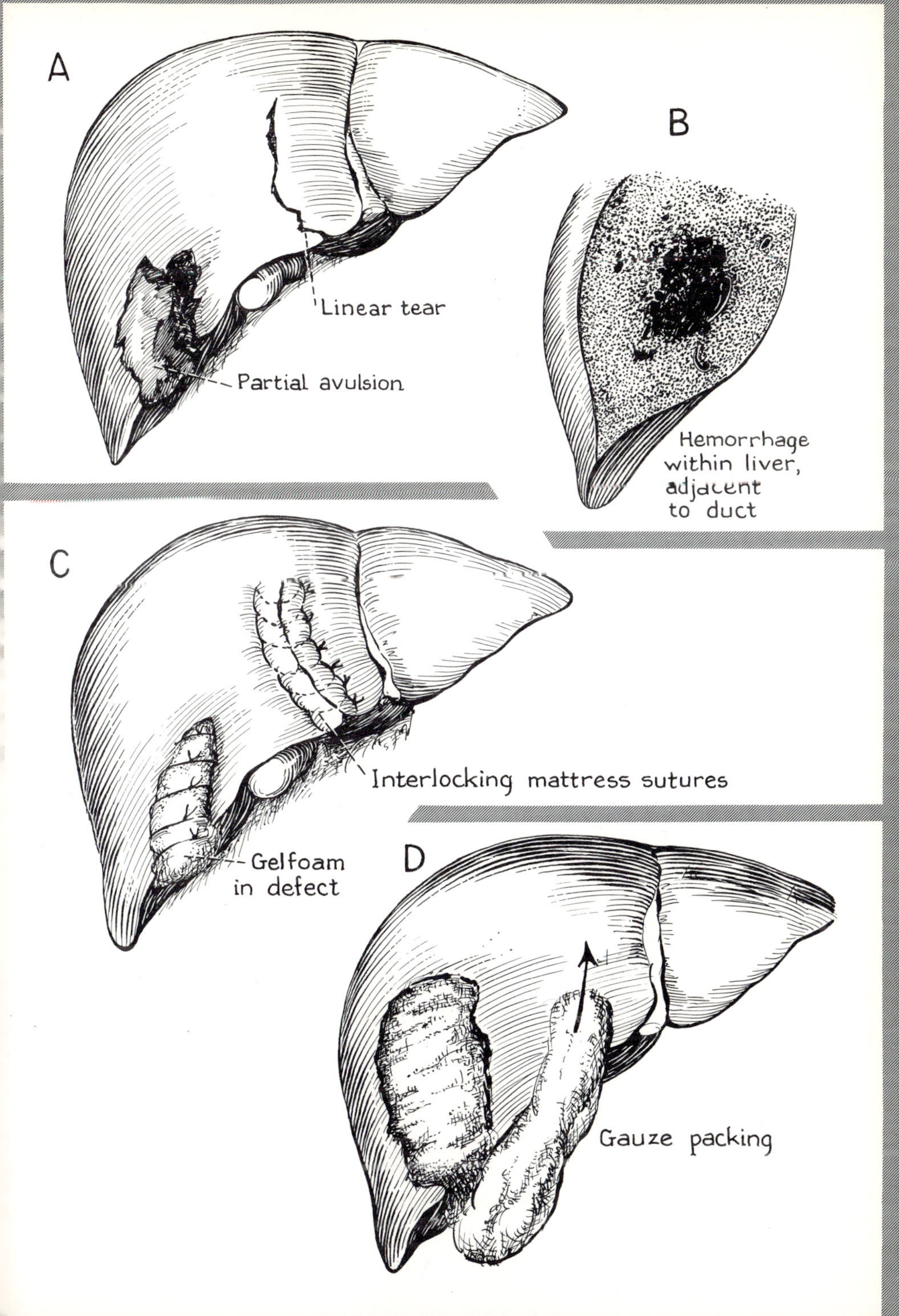
A
Linear tear
Partial avulsion
B
Hemorrhage within liver, adjacent to duct
C
Interlocking mattress sutures
Gelfoam in defect
D
Gauze packing

Persistent bleeding from injuries to the dome of the liver may require a transthoracic and transdiaphragmatic approach. An intercostal incision through the ninth or tenth right interspace or resection of a corresponding rib will give good exposure to the dome of the liver (Plate 14). A long incision extending nearly the entire length of the rib is necessary. The diaphragm is then opened and the liver treated by suture or packing. The free use of blood transfusions is indicated if hemorrhage has been profuse.

Penetrating wounds of the liver.—Stab and gunshot wounds frequently penetrate the liver. It is important to determine the course of the wound to anticipate the possibility of injury to adjacent structures. The liver partially overlies the gallbladder, bile ducts, the hepatic flexure of the colon and the right kidney, as well as the duodenum, the pyloric end of the stomach and the head of the pancreas. Penetrating wounds of these organs usually demand exploration. Stab wounds rarely have a wound of exit and the direction taken by the penetrating instrument may be difficult to determine. Bleeding from the liver due to stab wounds may not be severe enough to necessitate operation and the possibility of injury to adjacent organs may decide the advisability of exploration.

Gunshot wounds of the abdomen or lower chest usually have a wound of entrance and a wound of exit and the path of the bullet can be estimated. However, the course of the bullet through the body can vary considerably if the missile is deflected by striking a rib or other bony structure. For this reason exploration is almost invariably indicated. The incision should be long enough and should be placed to permit wide and thorough examination of the suspected course of the missile and careful examination of all involved structures. Bullets frequently carry foreign bodies with them and these may be deposited anywhere within the body. Because of this and because of the tissue destruction caused by bullet wounds, the liver should be thoroughly explored and debrided.

INFECTIONS

Hepatitis without abscess formation and without obstruction of the bile ducts is mentioned only to emphasize the dangers of anesthesia and surgery in its presence. Patients with such conditions often have severely impaired liver function and the added trauma of surgery may reduce the chance for recovery.

ABSCESSES

Abscesses of the liver are due to amebic or pyogenic infections and may be complicated by the formation of subphrenic abscesses which in turn may lead to hepatobronchial fistulas. These complications are discussed in Chapter 4.

Amebic abscesses.—Amebic infections are far more common in this country than is usually believed. The incidence has increased since the return of many soldiers who have served in foreign countries. The most common symptoms consist of fever, chills, debility and pain in the epigastrium or right upper abdomen. Diarrhea may or may not be present. It is often difficult to demonstrate the causative organism even with careful stool examination and culture. Amebic abscesses may produce enlargement of the liver at the site of the abscess, with local tenderness and fever. Frequently the diaphragm is elevated.

Treatment.—If an amebic abscess of the liver is suspected, the patient should be given a trial treatment with amebacides whether or not the organisms have been isolated from the stool. Emetine, 1 gr. intramuscularly daily for three to five days, followed by chloroquine phosphate therapy is the treatment of choice. If improvement does not follow an initial course of emetine and the drug has produced no toxic effects, it may be advisable to give a second course after a few days' rest. If this does not result in improvement or cure, careful aspiration may be done (Plate 4).

Ameboma.—Amebomas of the liver may form without central necrosis or liquefaction. They may be suspected from a history of amebic dysentery, liver enlargement and x-ray evidence of local elevation of the diaphragm. Symptoms may develop many years after an episode of amebic dysentery. Amoeba may not be found in the stools, and liver aspiration may be inconclusive. If suspected, a trial of antiamebic therapy should precede surgical intervention.

The point of insertion through the skin and the direction of the passage of the needle will depend upon the suspected location of the abscess. This may be determined by careful examination of the liver to locate its point of maximal tenderness or its area of greatest enlargement. Roentgenograms both in the anteroposterior and lateral positions are of diagnostic value, particularly for abscesses in the superior portion of the liver.

A.—Abscesses in the anterior portion of the liver may be approached from a point just below the right costal margin. It must be remembered that the inferior surface of the liver slants upward from its anterior inferior edge and, unless there is pronounced enlargement of the liver, the needle must be directed upward.

B.—In this sagittal section the aspirating needle is shown in position.

C.—Posterior liver abscesses may be approached from below the twelfth rib near the lumbocostal juncture, the needle being directed upward and forward.

D.—The posterior approach is shown in sagittal section.

E.—Abscesses in the lateral portion of the liver may be reached by inserting the aspirating needle in the intercostal space determined to be most nearly over the center of the abscess.

F.—This sagittal section shows the needle inserted through an intercostal space.

Aspiration of amebic abscesses of the liver should be carried out with sterile technic followed meticulously to prevent secondary contamination of the abscess. Constant suction should be applied to the aspirating needle to prevent its passing through the cavity and into the liver or other structures beyond. If fluid is encountered, as much as possible should be removed. The cavity may then be irrigated with an emetine solution if the abscess is of amebic origin.

PLATE 4

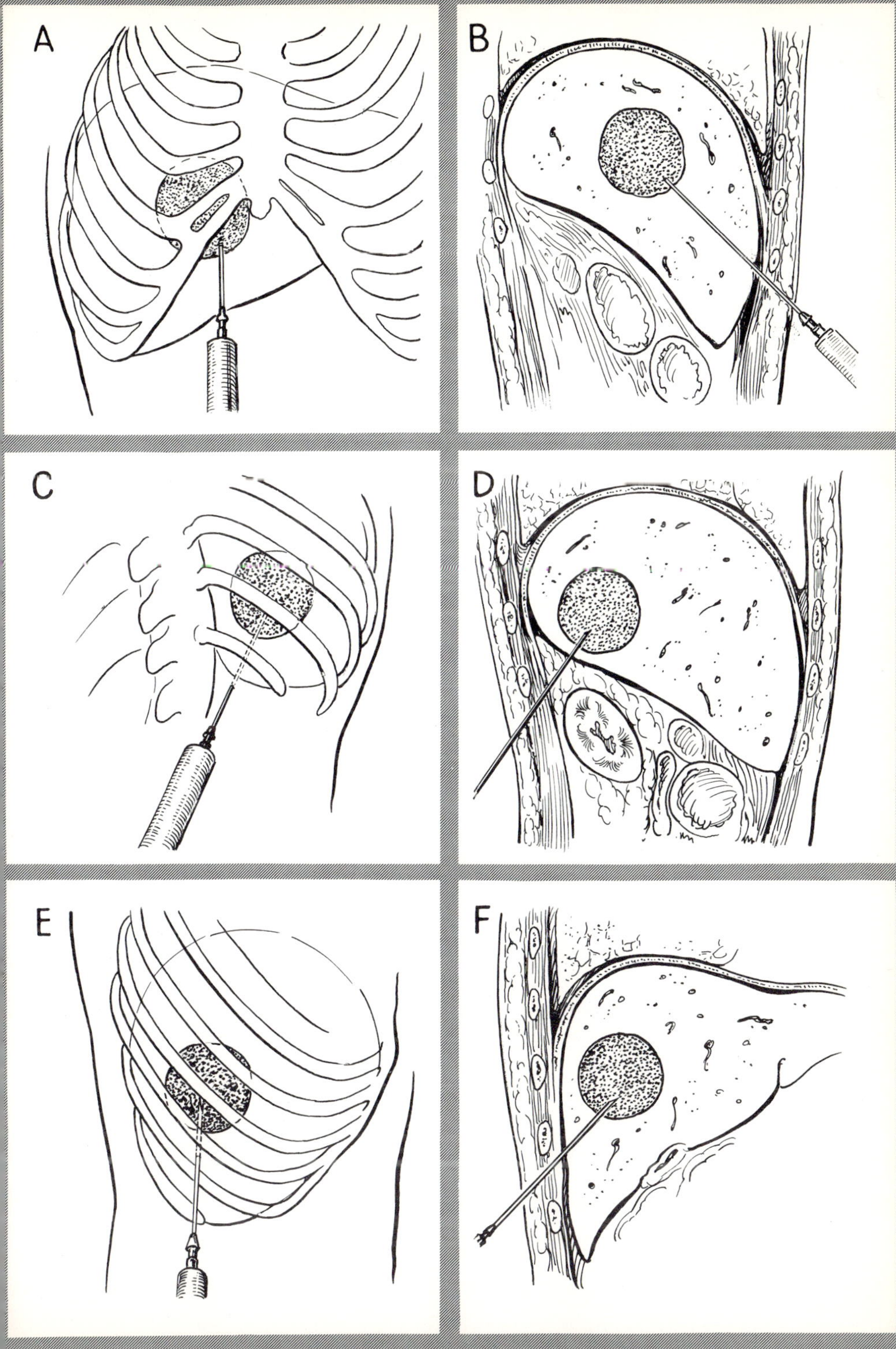

Pyogenic abscesses.—Pyogenic abscesses usually result from a suppurative process somewhere within the abdomen and frequently follow appendicitis. They may result from suppurative cholangitis, especially when partial or complete obstruction of one or more bile ducts is present. Occasionally, an intrahepatic calculus will obstruct a bile duct and abscesses will form behind it. In some instances the primary source of infection cannot be determined. Chills, fever, weakness and pain and tenderness in the region of the liver usually accompany pyogenic abscesses. Pain may radiate to the right shoulder. Nausea, vomiting and weight loss may occur. Jaundice develops in about one third of the patients.

Conservative treatment should be given a trial. Amebacides and antibiotics should be used. If these fail, surgical drainage should be established.

Drainage.—The incision should be placed so as to minimize the danger of contamination of the pleural or peritoneal cavities.

A.—If the area of bulging or tenderness is below the costal margin, a subcostal incision is made directly over this area.

B.—When the liver is exposed and packed off from the abdominal cavity to minimize gross contamination, the location of the abscess is determined by aspiration with a syringe and needle. When pus is obtained, the needle is left in place and followed down with a hemostat or blunt scissors. As the instrument enters the abscess cavity, the blades are spread to enlarge the opening. It may be necessary to increase the size of the opening by finger dissection. All pus is evacuated from the cavity, a culture is taken and Penrose drains are placed in the cavity.

C.—The Penrose drains are brought out through the skin wound.

D.—Abscesses of the posterior wall or dome of the liver can be reached by resection of the twelfth rib to enter the extrahepatic space extraperitoneally. The liver should be explored with the fingers in an effort to locate the site of the abscess. The abscess is then aspirated, opened and drained.

PLATE 5

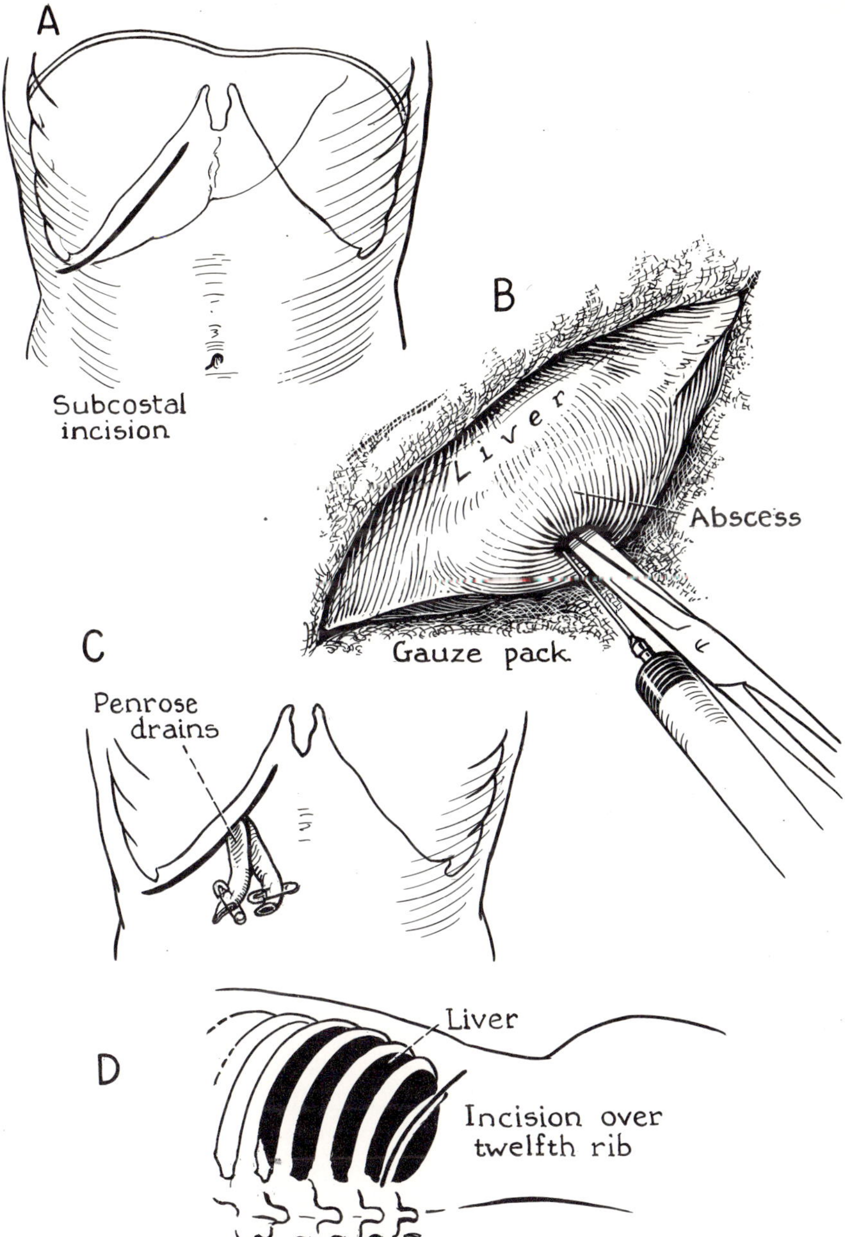
A
Subcostal incision
B
Liver
Abscess
Gauze pack
C
Penrose drains
D
Liver
Incision over twelfth rib

CYSTS OF THE LIVER

Echinococcus or hydatid cysts occasionally are seen in this country. They are produced by infestation with the tapeworm, Echinococcus granulosus. They may be single or multiple and may enlarge sufficiently to occupy almost the entire right lobe of the liver. When small, the cysts produce few, if any, symptoms. As they involve greater portions of the liver, there may be local discomfort and pain and occasionally pain in the shoulder. Other symptoms are urticaria, nausea, vomiting and constipation. Larger cysts can often be palpated below the costal margin or at the edge of the liver. Complement fixation and cutaneous tests may be of diagnostic value.

A.—Frequently the cyst wall becomes calcified as shown here.

B.—If this disease is suspected, roentgenograms of the lungs should be made, since daughter cysts frequently form in the lungs.

Treatment

Early and complete extirpation is important to remove the disease before it has spread to inaccessible parts of the body. The incision is made as nearly over the cyst as possible. As most cysts present below the right costal margin, a right subcostal incision is usual.

C.—The cyst is exposed and is packed off to prevent peritoneal implantation if leakage occurs. If the cyst wall is thick, it may be possible by gauze dissection to enucleate the intact cyst. Then, if no other cysts are found, the wound is closed, with a Penrose drain extending from the cyst cavity through the abdominal wall. If the cyst cannot be enucleated, it is aspirated to diminish the tension and a fixative solution such as Formalin injected into it. The cyst is then opened, its contents completely evacuated and all daughter cysts removed by gauze dissection. The lining is treated with Formalin.

D.—The edges of the cysts are sutured to the parietal peritoneum. A fairly large opening into the cysts is left for subsequent drainage and repeated treatment with a fixative solution.

Because of the severe and often fatal reaction which may result from contamination of the peritoneal cavity by fluid from echinococcus cysts, a two-stage operation may be advisable. The abdominal wall is opened over the cyst and a gauze pack is placed in the wound and against the cyst wall to permit sealing off of the peritoneal cavity. At a later date, the pack is removed and the cyst opened.

PLATE 6

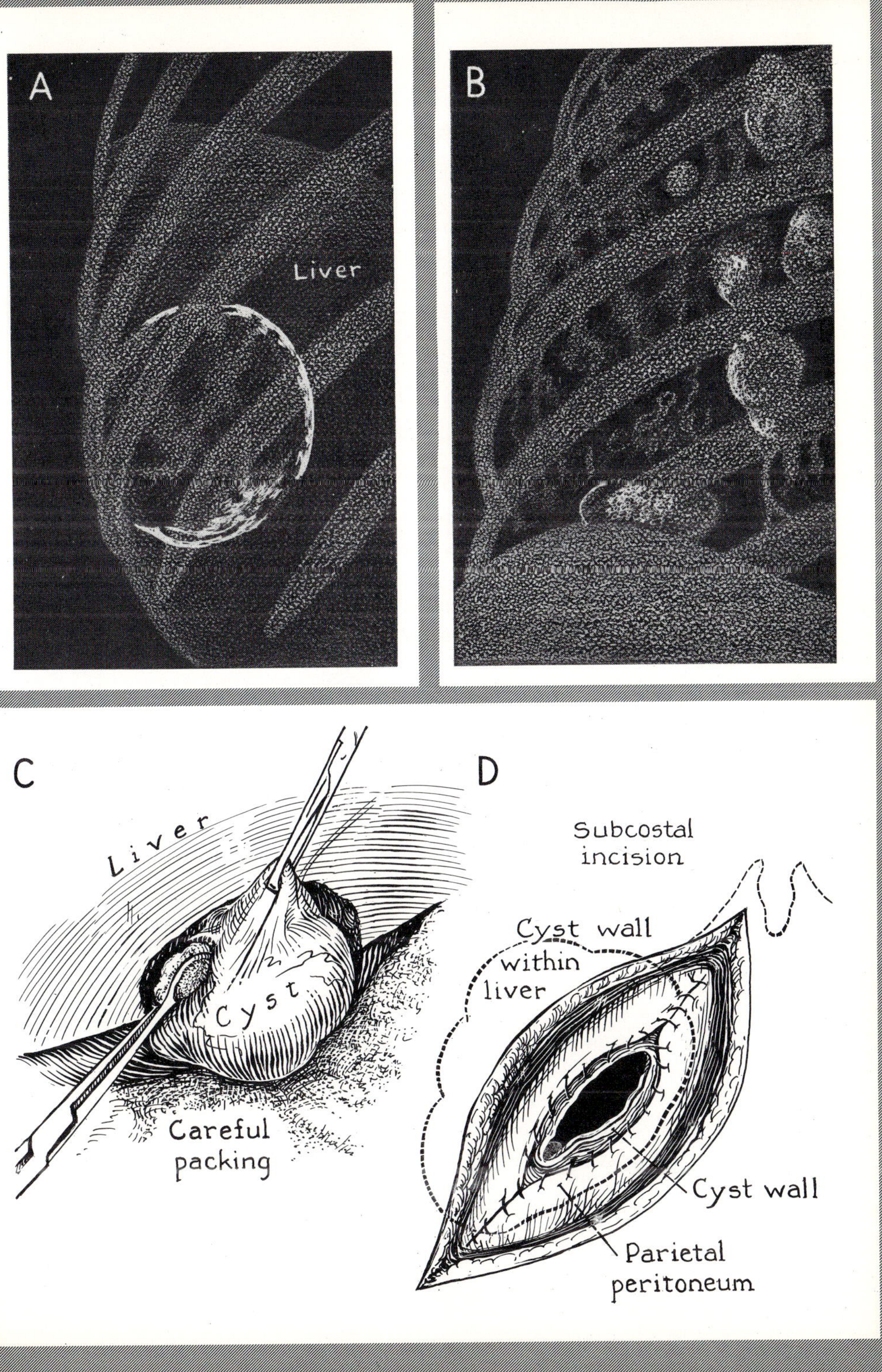
A
Liver
B
C
Liver
Cyst
Careful packing
D
Subcostal incision
Cyst wall within liver
Cyst wall
Parietal peritoneum

TUMORS OF THE LIVER

BENIGN TUMORS.—Benign tumors of the liver are rare and generally are of little surgical interest. Cavernous hemangiomas are the most common type. Lymphangiomas have been found and on some occasions have produced multiple lymphatic cysts which have so enlarged the liver that it occupied a large portion of the abdominal cavity. Partial resection of the liver for removal of much of the lymphangiomatous tissue has proved successful. Other benign tumors, including lipomas, fibromas and myomas, have been reported but are very rare.

MALIGNANT TUMORS.—Carcinomas, particularly those arising in the stomach, colon, esophagus, pancreas, gallbladder, uterus and breasts frequently metastasize to the liver. Approximately one half of all patients who die of carcinoma have liver metastases. Primary carcinoma of the liver constitutes 1–2 per cent of all carcinomas. Some of these arise from hepatic cells. Cirrhosis may be a factor in their development. They usually are multiple and growth is rapid. Others arise from the bile ducts.

TREATMENT

Advanced, multiple or deep-seated malignant lesions of the liver are not amenable to surgery or to any other known form of treatment. Solitary tumors close to the inferior edge and surface of the right lobe of the liver sometimes can be removed with a margin of adjacent liver tissue sufficiently wide to insure complete excision.

A.—After exposing the liver edge, a row of interlocking interrupted mattress sutures is placed as through-and-through stitches in the normal liver well beyond the edges of the tumor. The dotted line represents the line of incision between the tumor and the hemostatic sutures.

B.—It is seldom that the cut edges of the liver can be approximated if adequate excision of tumor and liver is made. If the interlocking mattress sutures and ligation of any bile ducts and bleeding vessels do not control bile leakage or bleeding, Gelfoam may be placed over the raw surface and tied in place with interrupted sutures.

C.—If the wedge of removed liver tissue is small, it may be possible to approximate the cut edges. Through-and-through sutures are placed behind the interlocking mattress sutures.

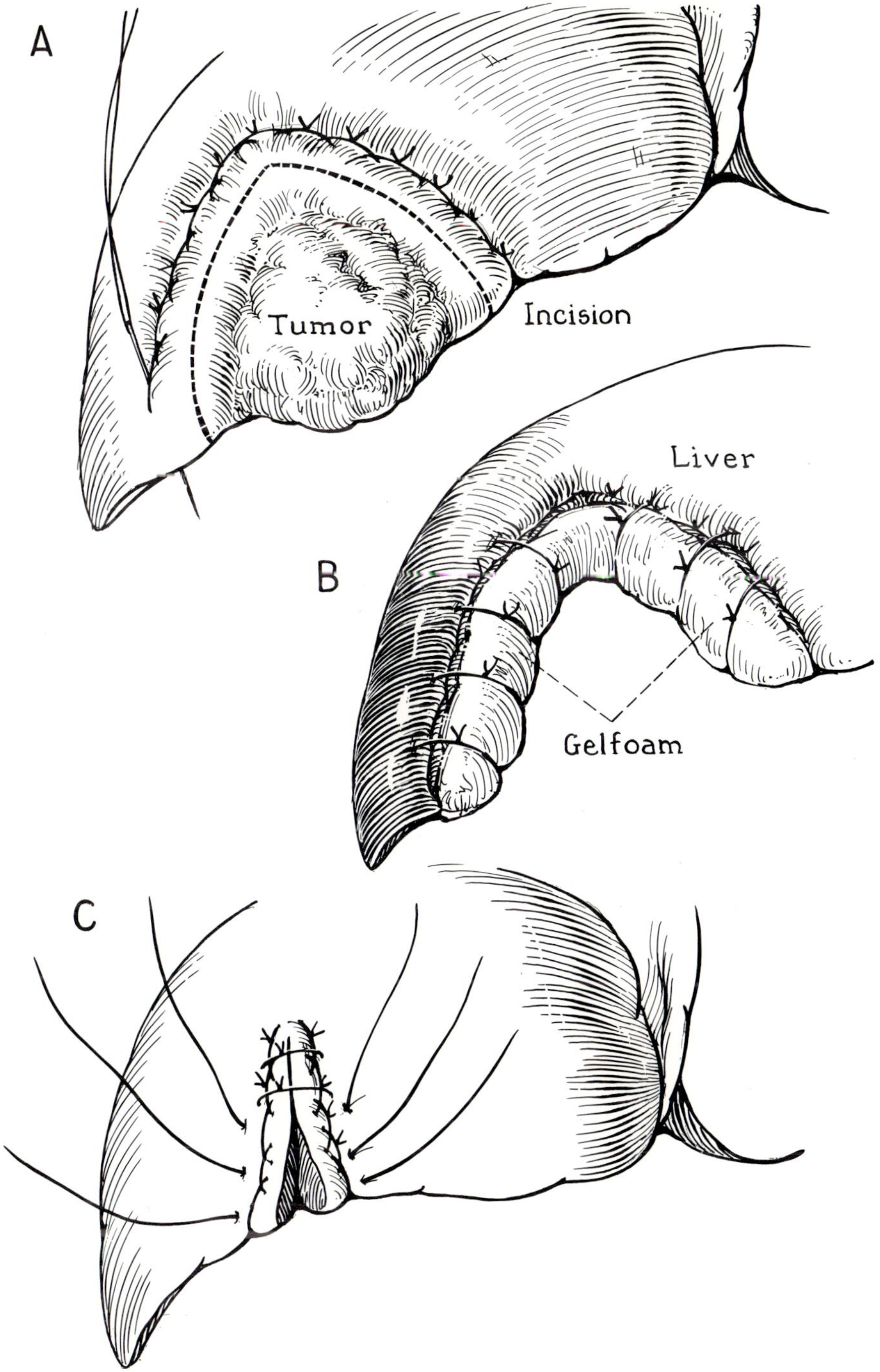
A
Tumor
Incision
Liver
B
Gelfoam
C

Excision of Left Lobe of Liver for Tumor

Almost the entire left lobe of the liver may be surgically excised to remove tumors confined to that lobe.

A.—The left lobe can be satisfactorily exposed by a high midline or a high left paramedian incision. Ready access to it also can be obtained by a left transthoracic and transdiaphragmatic approach (Plate 75).

B.—The lobe is mobilized by dividing the left triangular ligament and its lateral extension. The ligament is divided between clamps and ligated, since large veins often are encountered and will bleed profusely if not ligated.

C.—The site of resection should be selected well to the right of the tumor, if possible. Preliminary hemostasis of the lobe is obtained by overlapping interrupted mattress sutures. A long blunt needle is passed through the liver in the direction of its narrowest diameter, usually from the anterosuperior surface to the inferior and posterior surface. The needle is then passed back through the liver in the opposite direction, parallel to and about ½ in. beyond its path of introduction. Subsequent sutures placed in a similar manner form a straight line across the left lobe of the liver, each suture slightly overlapping and interlocking with the previous one.

D.—When all sutures have been placed and tied, the liver is cut across about ¼ in. to the left of the suture line. The larger vessels and ducts encountered are clamped and ligated separately. Any residual bleeding may be controlled by additional sutures or by fastening a hemostatic agent, such as Gelfoam, across the cut surface with interrupted through-and-through sutures. A straight anteroposterior transection of the lobe is advisable to avoid leaving liver tissue from which bile drainage has been interrupted by ligation of the bile ducts draining it. It is advisable to place a drain at the site of the liver resection and bring it out through the wound to permit escape of any bile which may be excreted from the cut surface. This minimizes the danger of bile peritonitis. If no bile drainage occurs, the drain is removed on the third or fourth postoperative day. In the event of bile leakage, the drain should be left in place until drainage has ceased. This acts as a safety factor and does not complicate wound healing.

Surgical removal of the right lobe has been accomplished but is a formidable and hazardous operation. It may be indicated for solitary tumors of the right lobe with no metastases or involvement of the left lobe.

PLATE 8

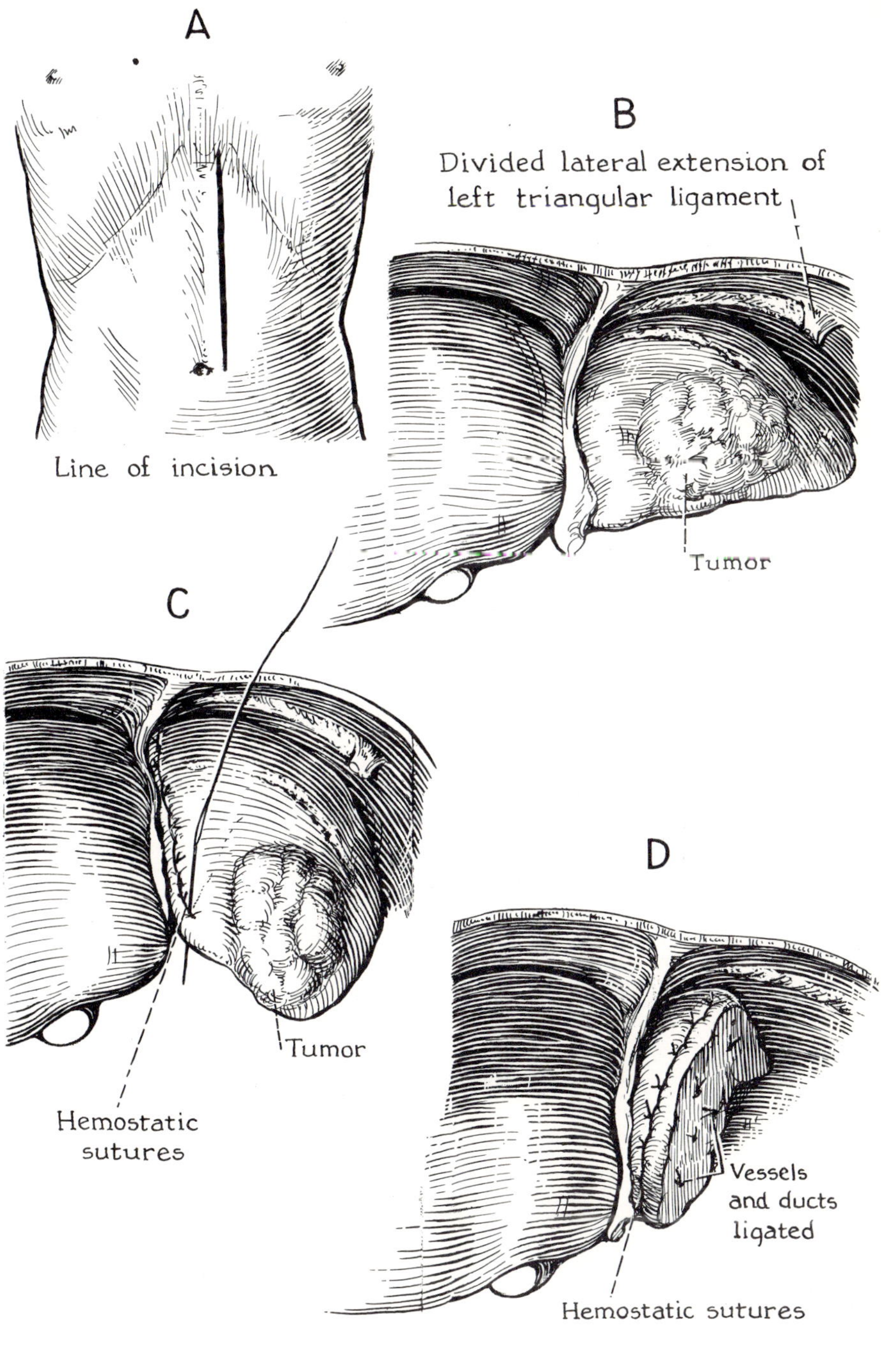
A
Line of incision
B
Divided lateral extension of left triangular ligament
Tumor
C
Tumor
Hemostatic sutures
D
Vessels and ducts ligated
Hemostatic sutures

CHAPTER 4

Complications of Liver Disease

SUBDIAPHRAGMATIC ABSCESSES OF BILIARY ORIGIN

ABSCESSES IN THE subdiaphragmatic spaces may be secondary to many diseases. The majority of these have their primary site within the abdomen and may be of either intraperitoneal or extraperitoneal origin. This discussion will be limited to subphrenic infections complicating diseases of the liver or extrahepatic biliary system. Amebic and pyogenic abscesses are the liver diseases most commonly producing this complication. Suppurative cholecystitis and cholangitis may be followed by the development of subdiaphragmatic abscesses, especially when surgery has been inadequate.

Symptomatology.—The variability of symptoms produced by subphrenic abscesses and the inaccessibility of their location to direct examination make diagnosis difficult. Onset of symptoms may be acute or considerably delayed. When the abscess is secondary to a pre-existing biliary tract disease, a history of the primary cause usually can be elicited. This history will vary with the nature of the etiologic infection.

Patients with amebic infections may give a history of a pre-existing dysentery. These infections are far more prevalent in the United States than is generally recognized and often are seen in patients who have never left the boundaries of this country. In many instances, amebic infections of the liver occur without a history of dysentery. Careful stool examinations and cultures may not demonstrate the etiologic organisms. However, a history of symptoms suggestive of liver abscess can often be obtained.

Pyogenic abscesses of the liver may be secondary to some acute infectious process within the abdomen, of either intraperitoneal or extraperitoneal location. A history of pain, tenderness and enlargement of the liver, with fever, malaise and debility, may be elicited. When the extrahepatic biliary tract is the primary source of infection, there may be a history of preceding cholecystitis, cholangitis with chills, fever and jaundice or frequent attacks of right upper quadrant pain and tenderness. Inadequate surgical treatment of such conditions frequently precedes the development of subphrenic abscesses. Inadequate drainage of a suppurative gallbladder, failure to remove stones from the common bile duct, failure to establish good drainage in the presence of suppurative cholangitis or persisting obstruction in the presence of bile duct strictures may be followed by subphrenic abscesses, particularly in the subhepatic area. Patients present a picture of sepsis with malaise, anorexia, chills and fever. Dull, aching pain in the right upper abdomen and in the right lower chest is a common complaint. Occasionally, sharp pains radiate to the neck and shoulder and are suggestive of involvement near the center of the diaphragm. Painful respiration is common. Pulmonary complications can produce the first symptoms.

Examination.—Tenderness may be elicited on deep palpation or percussion over the involved area. Percussion will reveal elevation of the diaphragm. Displacement of the liver downward is seldom seen in early stages but is often an accompaniment of well developed abscesses. Friction rubs may be heard over the right lower chest. Physical findings in the lower portion of the chest will depend upon the presence and extent of pneumonitis or pleural effusion. A respiratory lag and fulness of the intercostal spaces will be noted on the affected side.

The anatomic features of the subphrenic spaces are illustrated in Plate 9.

The subphrenic space is bounded superiorly by the diaphragm, inferiorly by the transverse colon and its mesocolon and laterally by the abdominal wall. The liver divides this area into suprahepatic and infrahepatic spaces which are further divided by the hepatic ligaments.

A.—The hand is being introduced into the right anterior superior subphrenic space.

B.—The anterior portion of the diaphragm has been cut away to show the right and left anterior suprahepatic subphrenic spaces separated by the falciform and coronary ligaments. The coronary ligament in its lateral extensions further divides each side into anterior and posterior spaces.

C.—A posterior view of the liver shows the nonperitonealized area, the right posterior superior subphrenic space and the infrahepatic subphrenic spaces.

D.—This view of the inferior surface of the liver shows the infrahepatic subphrenic spaces.

E.—The fingers are introduced through an opening in the gastrohepatic omentum to enter the left posterior inferior subphrenic space (the lesser gastric cavity).

In addition to these intraperitoneal areas there are two extraperitoneal spaces. One consists of the space between the bare area of the liver and the undersurface of the diaphragm. The other is the potential area between the diaphragm and the diaphragmatic peritoneum. Abscesses in these areas are retroperitoneal in location.

Location and spread of infection.—Infection may reach the subphrenic spaces by direct extension, lymphatic spread, hematogenous spread or direct implantation. Occasionally the suprahepatic spaces become involved by extension through the diaphragm. Subphrenic infections of hepatic origin usually are the result of direct extension, the location determined by the site of the primary infection. Abscesses in the dome of the liver may produce retroperitoneal subphrenic abscesses if they point at the nonperitonealized part of the liver. Infections reaching a peritonealized surface of the superior portion of the liver usually produce localized abscesses because the surrounding hepatic and parietal peritoneum tends to seal off the infected area. Most subphrenic abscesses of hepatic origin occur on the right because of the greater amount of liver on this side. Infrahepatic abscesses are most often found on the right side and in the

PLATE 9

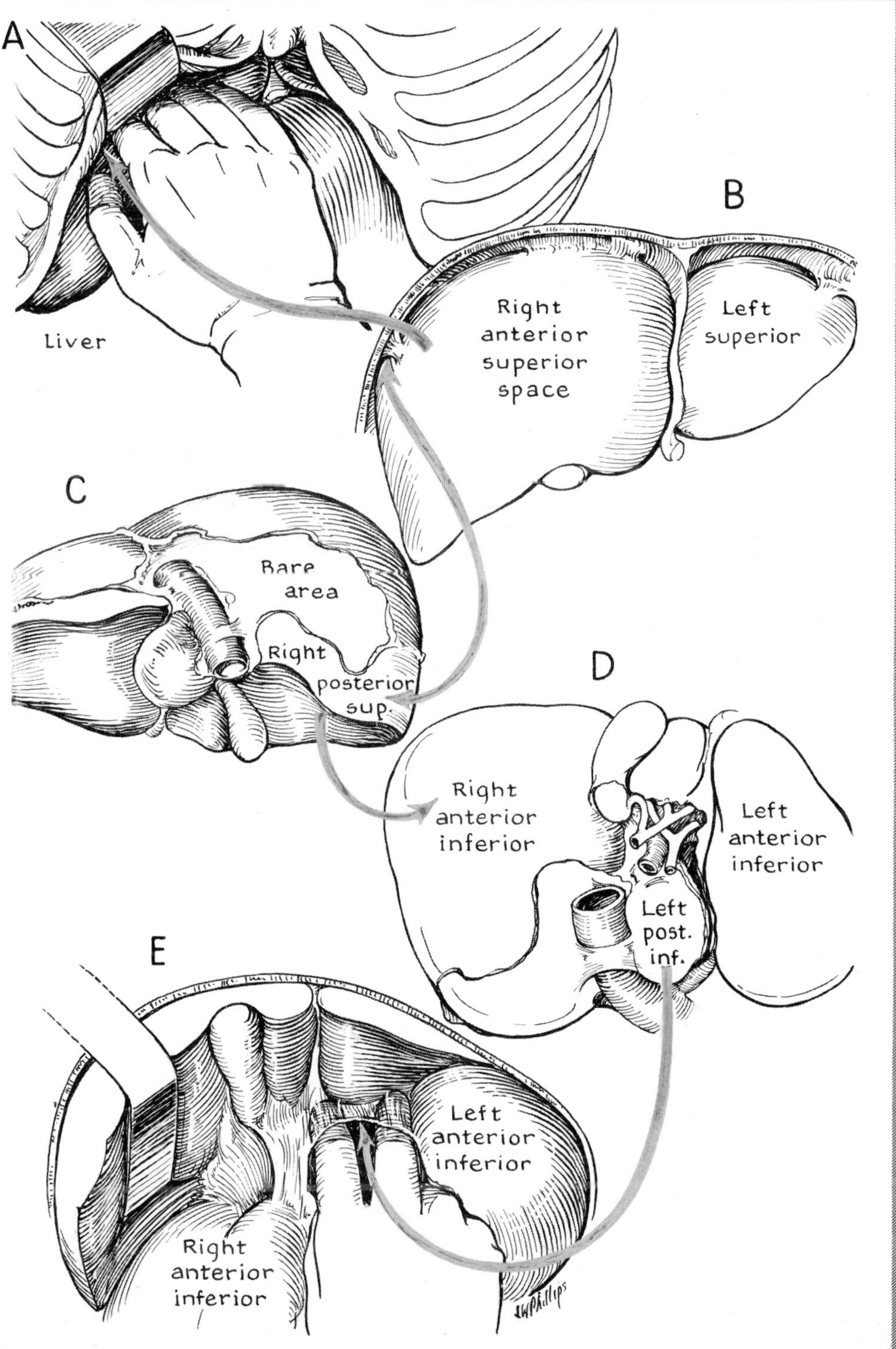
A
Liver
B
Right
anterior
superior
space
Left
superior
C
Bare
area
Right
posterior
sup.
D
Right
anterior
inferior
Left
anterior
inferior
Left
post.
inf.
E
Left
anterior
inferior
Right
anterior
inferior

vicinity of the bile ducts and gallbladder. They may communicate with the general peritoneal cavity but usually are sealed off by the omentum and adjacent organs.

Diagnosis

Roentgenographic studies.—These are of great benefit in the diagnosis of a subphrenic abscess and in the determination of its location and progress.

Early in the course of a subphrenic infection the overlying diaphragm will be elevated (*A*) and the costophrenic angle will show blunting. Frequently this will be followed by evidences of a beginning pneumonitis (*B*). Air under the diaphragm in the abscessed cavity is a late development of the disease. Roentgenograms taken in the anteroposterior (*C*), lateral (*D*) and oblique position will help to determine the location of the abscess and the best surgical approach for adequate drainage. Discoid atelectasis and an associated pneumonitis are frequent findings.

Anteroposterior views alone will not show the location of the abscess. Compare *E*, the anteroposterior view, with the lateral view shown in *F* which locates the abscess in the right anterior suprahepatic subphrenic space. Again, the anteroposterior view in *G* is similar to that shown in *E*, but the lateral view (*H*) shows the abscess to be located in the right posterior suprahepatic subphrenic space.

Left subphrenic abscesses may force the stomach downward, separating it from the diaphragm. This can be demonstrated by roentgenograms taken after the ingestion of a barium meal.

PLATE 10

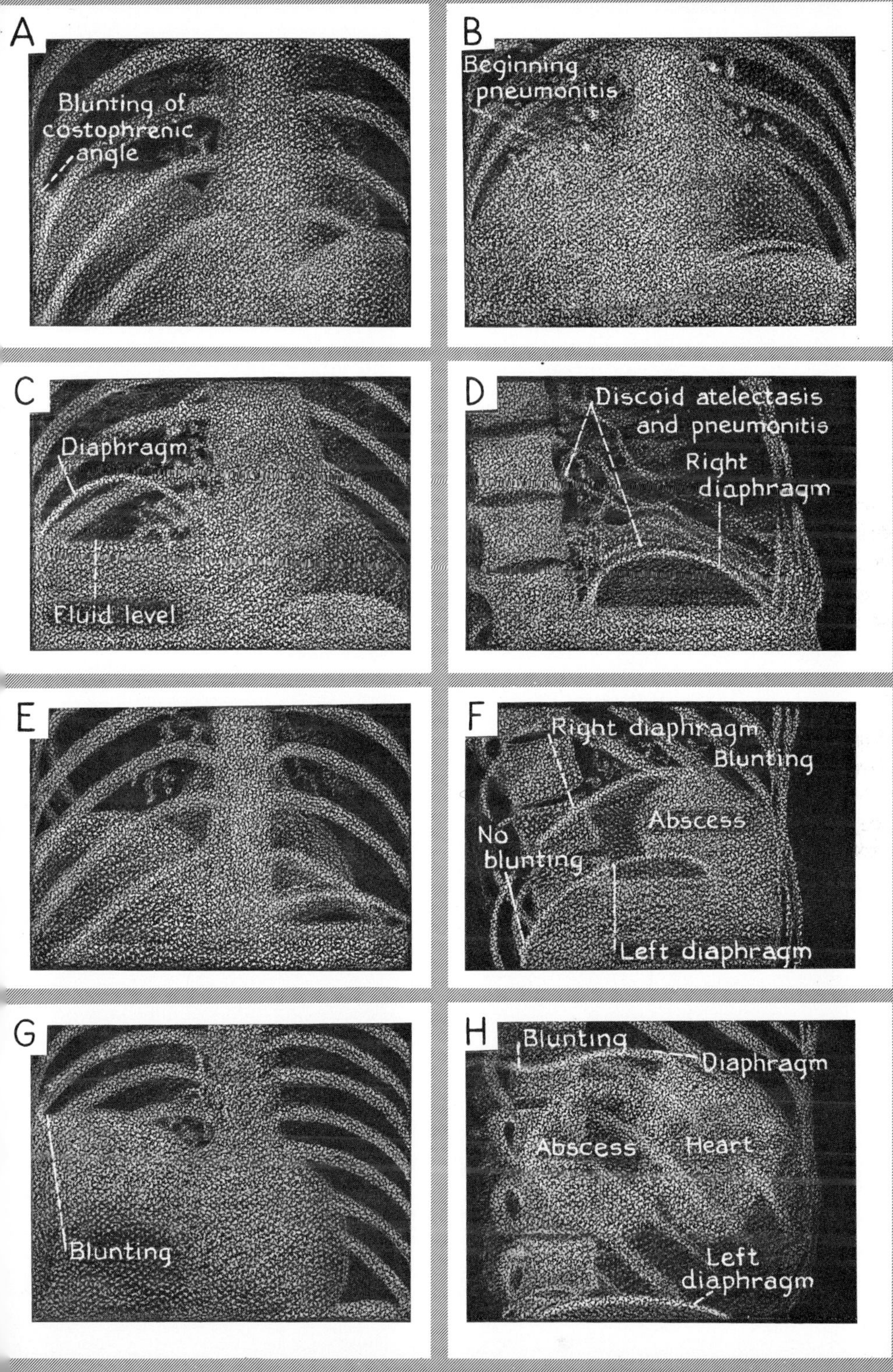
A
Blunting of costophrenic angle
B
Beginning pneumonitis
C
Diaphragm
Fluid level
D
Discoid atelectasis and pneumonitis
Right diaphragm
E
F
Right diaphragm
Blunting
Abscess
No blunting
Left diaphragm
G
Blunting
H
Blunting
Diaphragm
Abscess
Heart
Left diaphragm

Aspiration.—Aspiration of the subphrenic space for diagnostic purposes is dangerous because of the possible contamination of uninvolved portions of the pleural or peritoneal cavities. If involvement of the right posterior subphrenic space is suspected, a needle may be introduced below the twelfth right rib and passed upward and forward. Constant suction on the needle should be maintained to prevent the complete traversing of an encapsulated abscess and introduction of infection beyond it. If the diaphragm is high and the costophrenic angle obliterated, aspiration is less dangerous; nevertheless, it should be used only when the diagnosis is doubtful and the hazard of surgical exploration is great.

Thoracentesis is indicated to determine the existence and nature of pleural fluid, especially in patients in whom marked lung involvement and pleural effusion make it impossible to ascertain whether the disease is above or below the diaphragm. Sterile fluid in the pleural cavity usually indicates infection below the diaphragm. Pus is indicative of empyema, which may or may not have its origin below the diaphragm. If amebas are found in the aspirated fluid, the primary infection probably is located in the liver. If the needle pierces the diaphragm, pain in the shoulder usually is produced. If this pain occurs before pus is obtained, the abscess in all likelihood will be found below the diaphragm. Pneumoperitoneum has been recommended as a diagnostic aid but should seldom be employed. Subphrenic infections usually seal off the subdiaphragmatic space and prevent air from accumulating within it. The persistence of symptoms suggestive of subphrenic infection which cannot be diagnosed by the above-mentioned procedures justifies surgical exploration of the subphrenic area.

Treatment

Most subphrenic infections of hepatic origin will respond to conservative therapy. If an amebic infection is suspected, a trial of antiamebic therapy should be instituted. Intramuscular injection of 1 gr. of emetine daily for three to five days followed by a course of chloroquine phosphate is an accepted form of therapy. If the patient does not respond, the drug should be discontinued for a few days and then a second course given if the patient has manifested no evidence of toxic reaction. Other amebacides may be tried. True amebic abscesses usually will respond to this treatment.

Subdiaphragmatic abscesses resulting from pyogenic infections of the liver often will respond to the use of antibiotics. If the abscess is aspirated, every effort should be made to determine the identity of the causative organisms and their sensitivity to each antibiotic agent. Antibiotics should be tried before surgical therapy is instituted. Not infrequently all clinical and roentgenologic evidences of a subphrenic abscess will disappear under conservative therapy but at a later date the abscess will re-form. Therefore, it is important to keep the patient under observation for weeks or months with repeated examination to insure the permanent resolution of the abscess.

If a subphrenic abscess follows surgery on the extrahepatic biliary tract, the treatment will largely depend upon the presence or absence of an obstruction to the flow of bile. Subphrenic abscesses may follow an operation in which the continuity of the common bile duct is impaired and a resultant external biliary fistula is inadequate to afford free drainage. Varying degrees of jaundice may be present and the external fistula will drain both bile and pus. In such circumstances it is important to establish free drainage and this can often be accomplished merely by enlarging the opening through the abdominal wall. Treatment with antibiotics then can be carried out to permit subsidence of the subdiaphragmatic abscess without surgical intervention. If the abscess persists despite conservative treatment, surgical drainage and adequate treatment of the biliary disease are indicated.

[Drainage of subphrenic abscess *on page 56*.]

The surgical approach to a subphrenic abscess is determined by the location of the abscess. The approach may be transpleural, extrapleural, transperitoneal or extraperitoneal. The transpleural approach has the advantage of being the most direct, but the possible disadvantage of permitting contamination of the pleural cavity, especially when the costophrenic angle is not obliterated by the inflammatory process. If the diaphragm is high and fixed, this danger is minimal.

Transpleural Approach

A.—A one-stage transpleural procedure usually is preferable. The location of the abscess should be determined as accurately as possible so that the site of rib resection may be selected directly over it. Usually a portion of the eighth or ninth rib is removed. The skin is incised directly over the rib and a segment of rib 4 or 5 in. long is resected.

B.—The parietal pleura is then incised. If it is adherent to the diaphragmatic pleura as a result of the underlying inflammatory process, the incision may be carried through the diaphragm.

C.—If the apposing layers of pleura are not adherent and the pleural cavity has been entered, it should be sealed off by a row of sutures placed around the line of incision.

D.—The diaphragm is then incised to enter the abscess cavity. Penrose drains are placed in the abscess cavity and the wound is partially closed around them.

Two-stage procedure.—The two-stage transpleural approach has been devised to seal off the pleural cavity at the site of incision.

E.—A segment of lower rib is removed over the suspected abscess and the rib bed packed firmly with gauze to produce adhesions between the parietal and diaphragmatic pleurae. Ten or more days later the pack is removed and an incision made through the pleurae and diaphragm into the abscess cavity.

F.—The gauze pack and the induced fusion of the pleurae are shown diagrammatically.

This two-stage method imposes an added surgical procedure upon the patient and delays drainage of the abscess.

[Right posterior approach for drainage *on page* 58.]

PLATE 11

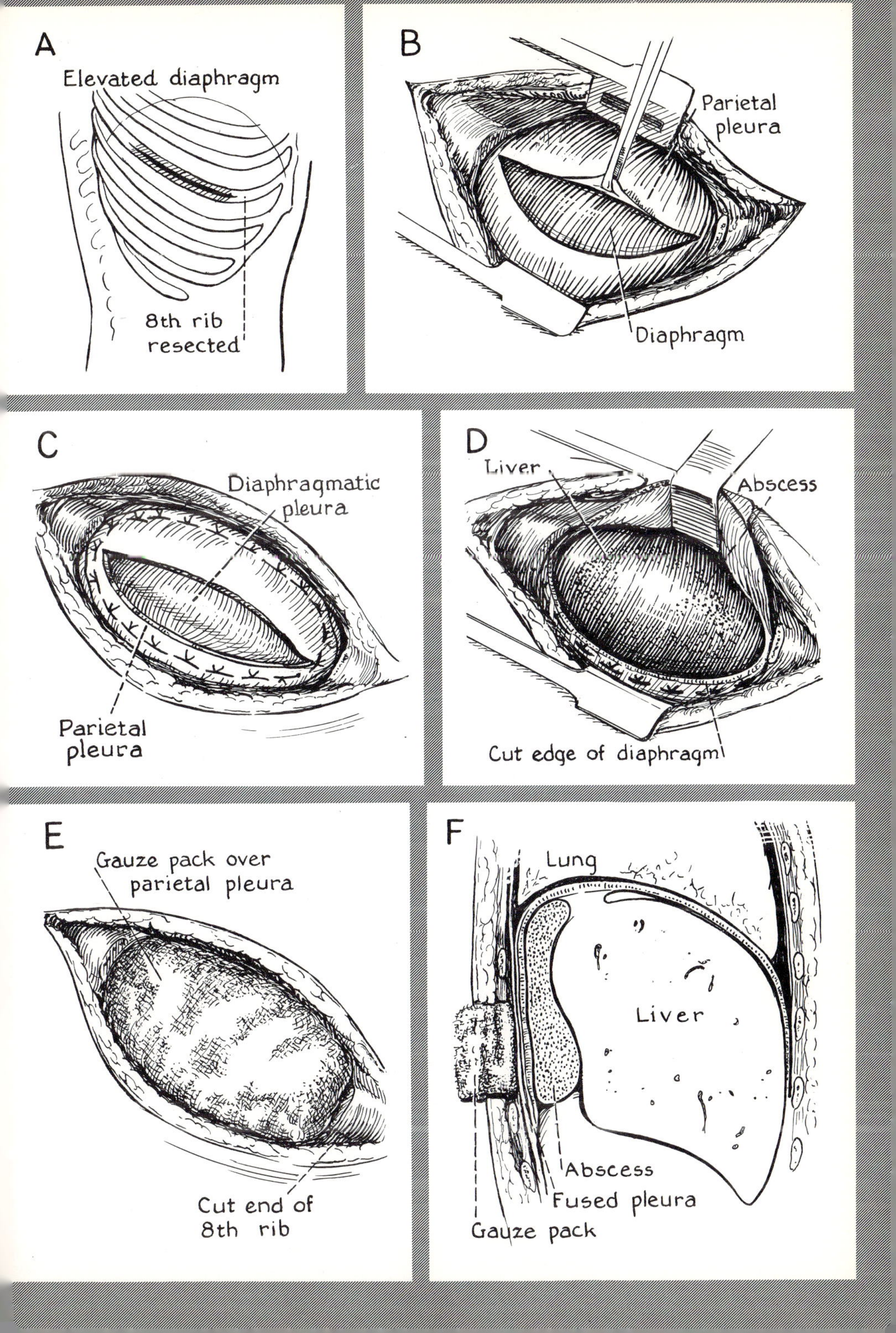

A
Elevated diaphragm
8th rib resected
B
Parietal pleura
Diaphragm
C
Diaphragmatic pleura
Parietal pleura
D
Liver
Abscess
Cut edge of diaphragm
E
Gauze pack over parietal pleura
Cut end of 8th rib
F
Lung
Liver
Abscess
Fused pleura
Gauze pack

Right Posterior Approach

The transperitoneal approach has the disadvantage of allowing contamination of the entire peritoneal cavity if it is not walled off. The right posterior extrapleural and retroperitoneal approach described by Ochsner and Graves gives excellent access to the right posterior superior subphrenic space, to the right retroperitoneal subdiaphragmatic areas and occasionally to the right anterior superior portion of the subdiaphragmatic space. It has also been recommended as an approach to the right subhepatic space.

A.—An incision is made over and down to the right twelfth rib. The entire rib is resected. Care must be taken in freeing the rib not to incise the underlying periosteum and thus to avoid opening the pleura which may lie directly below the bed of the rib.

B.—The erector spinae muscles are retracted medially and a transverse incision is made at a right angle to the spine at the level of the spinous process of the first lumbar vertebra. This will miss the costophrenic angle of the pleura which does not extend caudally to this level.

C.—The incision is carried through the muscles of the diaphragm to the renal fascia, and the kidney is displaced downward. If induration is present, aspiration to determine the presence of pus may be performed at this time.

D.—The peritoneum is now separated from the undersurface of the diaphragm by finger dissection until the abscess is reached. The cavity may be opened with the fingers. The opening should be sufficiently large to permit adequate drainage. Several soft rubber drains are placed in the cavity and brought out through the wound.

This approach has the advantage not only of avoiding contamination of body cavities but of establishing adequate dependent drainage.

[Abdominal approach for drainage *on page 60.*]

PLATE 12

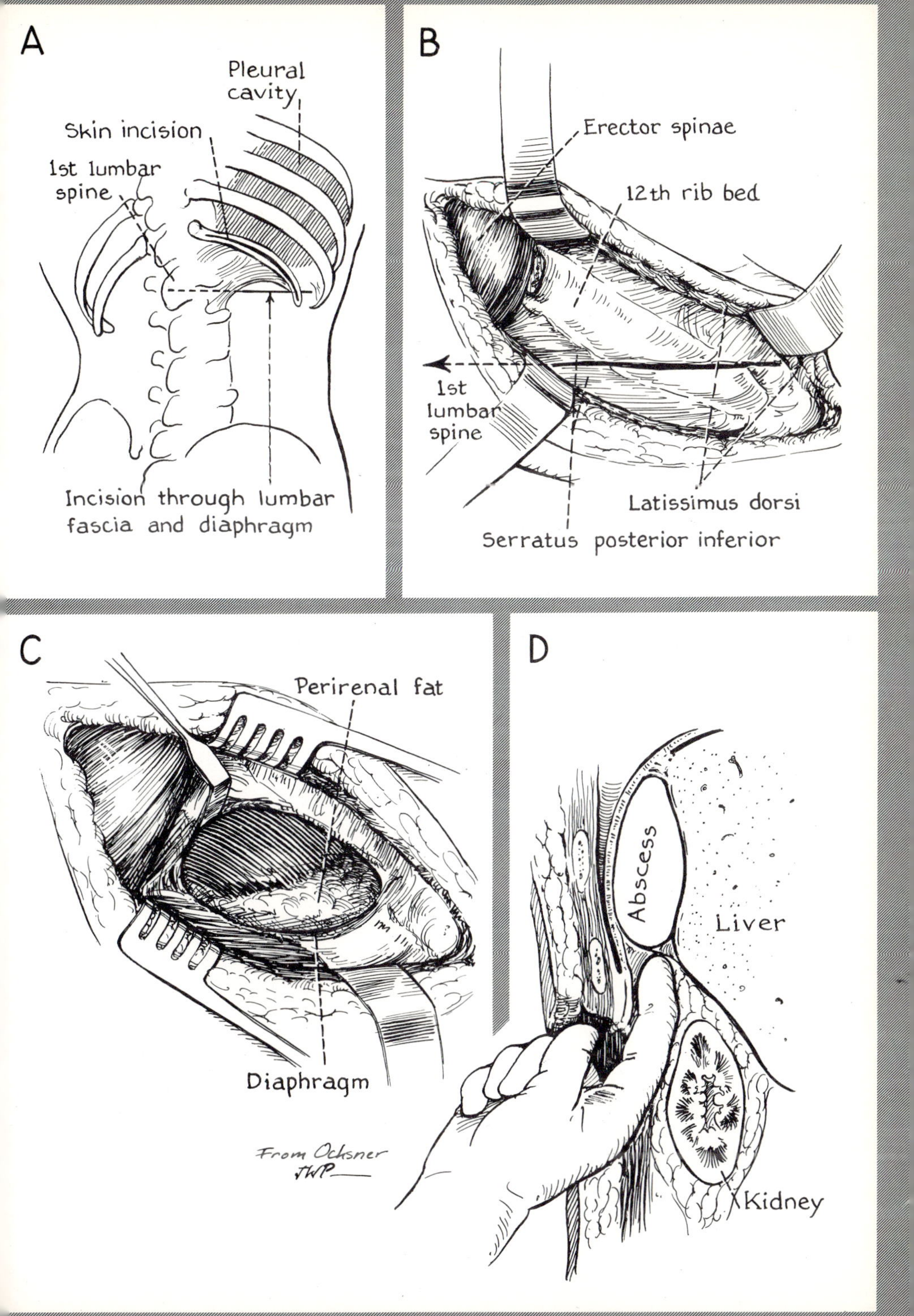

A
Pleural cavity
Skin incision
1st lumbar spine
Incision through lumbar fascia and diaphragm
B
Erector spinae
12th rib bed
1st lumbar spine
Latissimus dorsi
Serratus posterior inferior
C
Perirenal fat
Diaphragm
From Ochsner
JWP
D
Abscess
Liver
Kidney

Abdominal Approach

The anterior subdiaphragmatic spaces, both above and below the liver, are best approached through the anterior abdominal wall.

A.—If such abscesses are on the right side, a right subcostal incision is carried down through the abdominal muscles and transversalis fascia to the peritoneum.

B.—Finger dissection is continued upward, separating the parietal peritoneum from the undersurface of the diaphragm. When the abscess cavity is reached it should be opened widely by finger dissection and drains inserted. Subhepatic abscesses frequently are walled off anteriorly by the parietal peritoneum. In these instances, the abscess is opened by continuing the incision through the peritoneum.

C.—Left subphrenic abscesses can be drained through a left subcostal incision. This will give access to the areas both above and below the left lobe of the liver.

D.—This sagittal section illustrates the accessibility of the left subphrenic spaces. If an abscess has formed within the lesser peritoneal cavity, drainage can be established either through the gastrohepatic or gastrocolic omentum.

If a subhepatic abscess follows upper abdominal surgery and especially if a sinus or fistula exists, it is preferable to drain the abscess by an approach through the scar of the previous operation.

Many patients have received various antibiotics over long periods, and the causative organisms may have developed a resistance to the drugs administered. After bacteriologic studies to identify the causative organisms, it is well to determine their sensitivity to the drugs employed.

Complications of Subphrenic Abscesses

Long-standing and neglected subphrenic abscesses may lead to several types of complications. These may be systemic and are similar to those in any long-standing suppurative process. The patient may become emaciated and progressive damage to various organs of the body may develop. Abscesses occasionally rupture through the abdominal or chest walls. They may perforate through the diaphragm, producing empyema. Intra-abdominal extension may produce generalized peritonitis or may result in perforation into any of the abdominal viscera.

PLATE 13

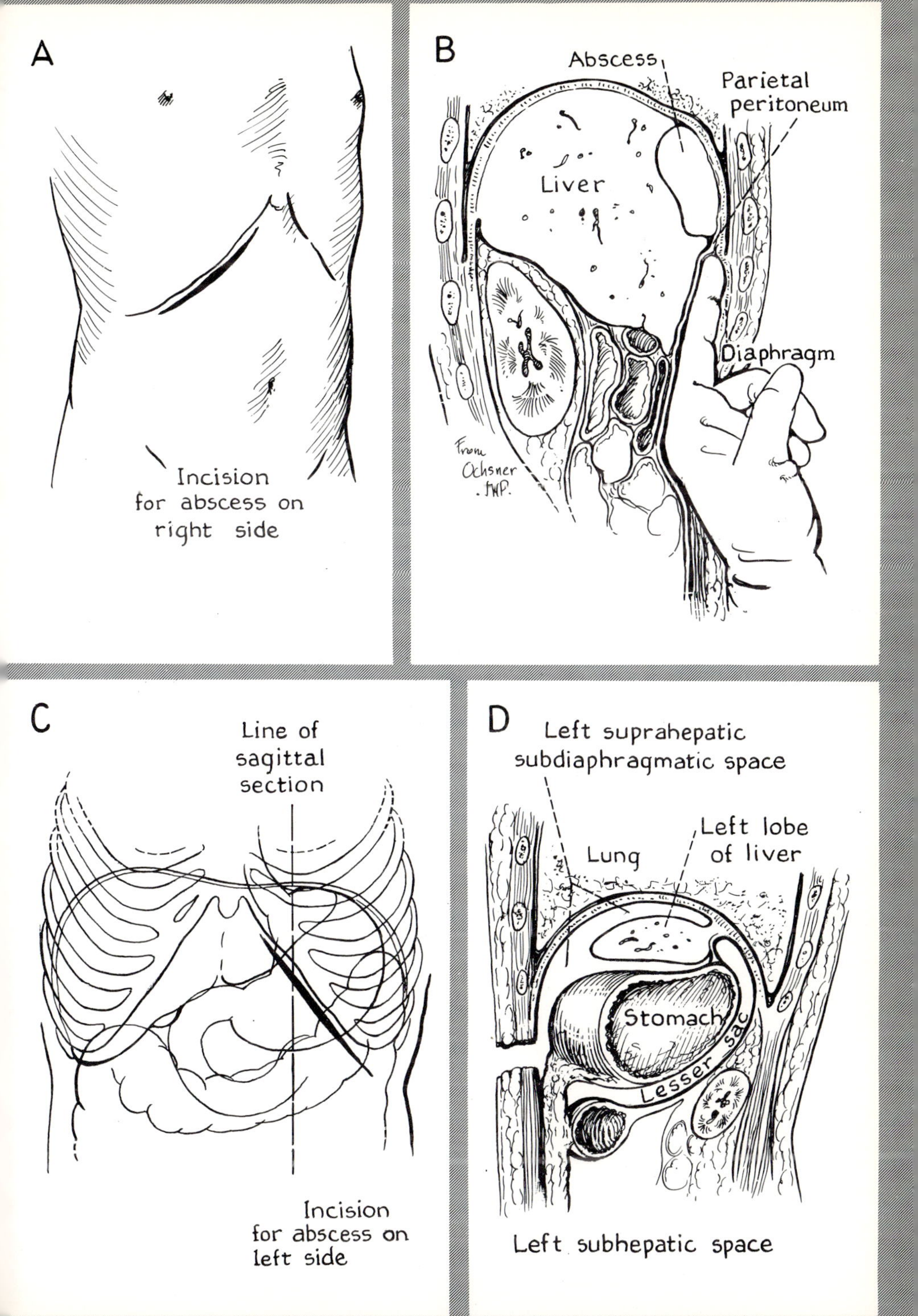
A
Incision
for abscess on
right side
B
Abscess
Parietal
peritoneum
Liver
Diaphragm
From
Ochsner
C
Line of
sagittal
section
Incision
for abscess on
left side
D
Left suprahepatic
subdiaphragmatic space
Left lobe
of liver
Lung
Stomach
Lesser sac
Left subhepatic space

Occasionally a subphrenic abscess, especially of amebic origin, will extend through the diaphragm and produce an empyema. When the lung is fixed, the infection may extend into it and eventually rupture into a bronchus. If the origin of the infection is in the liver, there may be a direct communication between the bronchial tree and the bile ducts and the patient will expectorate bile. The presence of bile in the sputum is diagnostic of hepatobronchial fistula.

A.—The diagnosis occasionally can be confirmed by bronchograms on which the opaque medium may be seen extending through the diaphragm and into the liver. The patient usually has a long history of fever and debility as a result of liver infection before the development of the fistula.

Because an amebic infection is usually the etiologic factor in the establishment of hepatobronchial fistulas, amebacides should be administered and conservative therapy attempted. Many fistulas will close spontaneously under conservative management. Occasionally, however, when the fistula is large and extensive fibrosis interferes with its closure, surgical intervention may be necessary.

B.—The fistula can be approached through the chest by resecting the right ninth or adjacent rib.

C.—The inferior surface of the lung should be separated from the diaphragm until the fistulous tract is reached. Because an empyema has preceded the establishment of the hepatobronchial fistula, the lung usually is densely adherent to the diaphragm and must be dissected from it with great care.

D.—The bronchial end of the fistula should be carefully ligated and may be oversewn. It is usually best to leave the hole in the diaphragm open to permit drainage of the hepatic abscess, especially if a subdiaphragmatic cavity can be palpated. If the tract into the liver is small and bile drainage through the extrahepatic biliary tract appears adequate, an attempt may be made to close the diaphragm.

E.—The pleural cavity should always be drained. The drain should be brought out through a separate stab wound in the most dependent intercostal space available and should be connected to a water-seal bottle.

PLATE 14

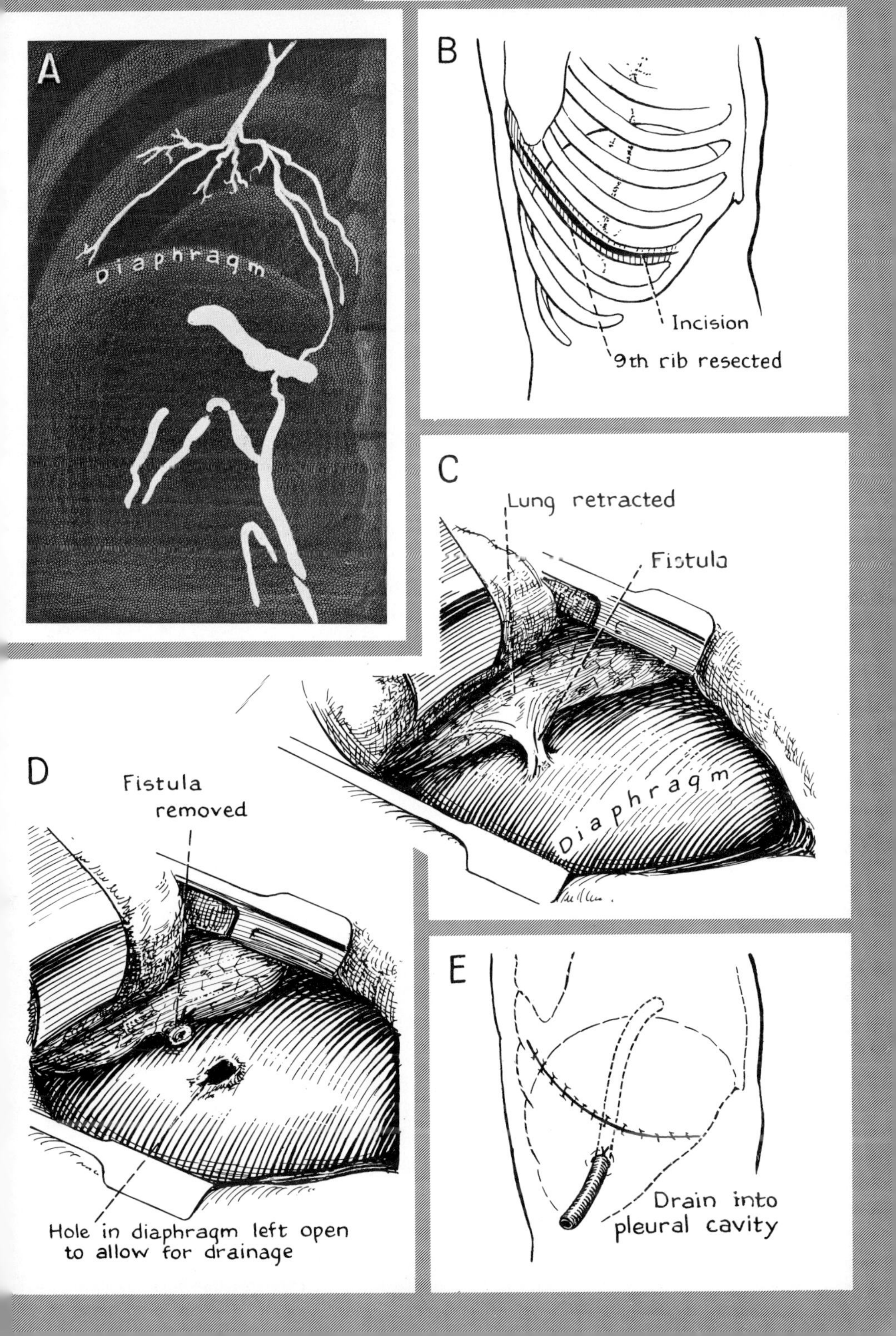

A
Diaphragm
B
Incision
9th rib resected
C
Lung retracted
Fistula
Diaphragm
D
Fistula removed
Hole in diaphragm left open to allow for drainage
E
Drain into pleural cavity

CHAPTER 5

Portal Hypertension

THE INEFFICIENCY DUE to length and resulting friction within available collateral venous channels accounts for the great rise in tension within the portal system when normal flow of blood through the portal vein or its radicles within the liver is obstructed by disease. The portal blood flow is vulnerable to obstruction at three points. The portal vein is the first point at which the circulation may be blocked effectively, and a number of processes are responsible for such obstruction.

In childhood, one such cause of portal obstruction may be an extension into the portal vein of the obliterative process which normally closes only the remnant of the umbilical vein. It is likely that this is a gradual and probably incomplete process because the symptoms of portal hypertension in the cases reported have not occurred before the age of 3 or 4 years and usually occur in later childhood. Insufficient pathologic material has been studied to establish perfectly this etiology. In later life, obstruction of the portal vein results from thrombosis secondary to intra-abdominal infection, abdominal trauma or disease states which are accompanied by a tendency to intravascular thrombosis. When the portal vein becomes blocked by thrombosis, it is probable that the process propagates by extension or embolism into the portal radicles within the liver, increasing the block. Recovery from the initial process, when it occurs, is followed by the development of severe portal hypertension. A third type of portal vein obstruction, the so-called cavernomatous degeneration, would be peculiar to the portal vein alone if it truly represents a pathologic entity. In this condition, the portal vein apparently is replaced by numerous channels and compartments. It has been suggested that this condition is a form of angioma of the vein, but it seems equally possible that it may represent a late picture of portal vein thrombosis. Recanalization of the thrombus, together with formation of adjacent collateral channels, could reasonably be responsible for the same picture.

The course of blood flow through the liver presents the second site of vulnerability to obstruction. The striking increase in fibrous tissue to which the liver is subjected mechanically increases the resistance to flow through the portal bed regardless of the primary hepatic disease.

An additional factor producing increased portal pressure is the disturbance of vascular architecture by the cirrhosis which allows transmission of arterial pressure from hepatic artery radicles to the portal system. Cirrhosis of the Laennec type is more commonly accompanied by hypertension than is biliary cirrhosis resulting from biliary tract disease and cholangitis.

The third site of obstruction productive of portal hypertension is in the hepatic veins. Thrombosis of the hepatic veins usually is fatal, but occasionally a patient survives and is left with a severe degree of portal obstruction.

Abnormal collateral circulation.—Many of the signs and the serious dangers of portal hypertension, irrespective of its cause, are manifestations of abnormal collateral circulation. Channels which are inconspicuous under normal circumstances are forced to carry greater and greater volumes of blood from the portal into the systemic system. This circulation is under a pressure which considerably exceeds ordinary venous pressure. The most important by-passes for the return of blood from the intestinal veins to the heart are the existing, normally small, communications by way of the coronary vein of the stomach and the esophageal veins to the caval system above the diaphragm. Rupture of a dilated esophageal vein under pressure may be the first sign of portal hypertension. This condition must be seriously considered in the differential diagnosis of gastrointestinal hemorrhage. Demonstration of dilated or varicosed esophageal veins by barium x-ray studies or direct esophagoscopy is at present considered pathognomonic of portal hypertension. Other available channels connecting the portal with the systemic circulation are responsible for the formation of dilated paraumbilical veins (caput medusae) and hemorrhoids so often exhibited in cirrhosis of the liver.

Ascites.—Whether portal hypertension alone can produce ascites is unknown. The role of impaired liver function and altered protein metabolism undoubtedly is important. However, under certain circumstances ascites probably results from transudation through the walls of intestinal and mesenteric veins under increased mechanical pressure plus decreased osmotic pressure. This consideration is important in determining the applicability of surgical treatment to patients in whom the major manifestation of liver disease is ascites.

Diagnosis

Demonstration of increased portal tension rarely is difficult when gastrointestinal hemorrhage is manifested by hematemesis. Roentgenographic evidence of esophageal varices (Plate 15, *A*) or direct visualization by esophagoscopy will establish the diagnosis. Such demonstration occasionally may be unobtainable if the varicose veins responsible for the hemorrhage are in the submucosa of the cardia of the stomach and the esophageal veins have not yet protruded or enlarged to a great extent. Much emphasis may be placed on splenomegaly as a clinical sign of portal hypertension. The finding of an enlarged spleen in a patient having gastrointestinal hemorrhage is indicative of esophageal varices. Differentiation must be made from blood dyscrasia with bleeding tendency and from the possible dual presence of cirrhosis and duodenal ulcer.

The final conclusion as to presence of portal hypertension may have to depend upon pressure measurements made within the portal bed at laparotomy. Such measurements are made with a saline-filled spinal manometer, suitably attached by a short rubber tube to an 18 gauge needle. The needle is introduced obliquely through the wall of a portal tributary vein and saline allowed to flow into the vein until it stabilizes at a level which fluctuates with respirations. The normal pressure is considered to be about 100 mm. of water. Elevations to 500 mm. of water may be encountered in these pathologic states.

Treatment

Two types of operative procedures are most widely accepted. They are the direct attack on varices of the lower esophagus and upper stomach (Plates 15–17) and some form of shunt operation between the portal system and the inferior vena caval system

(Plates 18 and 19). A successful shunt operation diminishes the venous pressure within the portal system by rerouting portal flow into the low pressure systemic veins.

Indications for portacaval shunt.—The single indication for portacaval shunt is hypertension within the portal system. Great care must be exercised in the selection and preparation of patients for surgery. Hemorrhage into the gastrointestinal tract may be due to the inability of the damaged liver to produce an adequate amount of prothrombin. Ascites probably is more often a result of deranged protein metabolism than of portal hypertension. It is evident, therefore, that when liver function tests and examination of the serum prothrombin give subnormal values, a period of medical management designed to improve hepatic function is essential. The decision as to whether the individual patient will benefit from an anastomosis is deferred until maximal liver function is attained. Surgery will hardly be expected to be of value in the patient whose liver cannot maintain a prothrombin level safely above the tendency to hemorrhage. At the other extreme is the patient whose liver function is within normal limits by modern methods of determination but who shows evidence of elevated portal tension. Here the dangerous factor is the hypertension producing recurring hemorrhage or ascites or both. In these patients a shunt operation is indicated. Many patients with varying degrees of damage to the liver fall between these two types. The life expectancy in the presence of cirrhosis and the danger and the debility due to repeated hemorrhage must be weighed against the risk of an operative procedure. Surgery may be offered to those whose greatest hazard lies in the complications of portal hypertension and in whom prognosis in regard to the cirrhotic process is comparatively good.

A.—The presence of esophageal varices can be demonstrated on roentgenograms.

Treatment is directed first toward the correction of blood loss and the arrest of hemorrhage in the patient with active bleeding.

Balloon Tamponade of Lower Esophagus

B.—Temporary arrest of hemorrhage may be accomplished by balloon tamponade of the lower esophagus. A multiple-lumen gastric tube has been so constructed that after introduction of the end of the tube into the stomach, a distal spherical balloon may be distended and pulled up against the esophageal hiatus. An additional balloon placed proximally on the same tube is then distended to compress the esophageal veins and points of hemorrhage.

When the bleeding has been checked or when it stops spontaneously, surgical therapy may be instituted to diminish the possibility of subsequent hemorrhage.

Gastroesophageal Resection

The scope of this book does not include the technic of resection of the lower esophagus and upper stomach. Phemister has described this procedure. Although the operation removes the bleeding vessels, it does not correct the cause for the formation of varicosities and subsequent hemorrhage may occur. However, in patients with portal hypertension in whom venous shunt operations have not been possible, gastroesophageal surgery has resulted in prolonged or permanent arrest of hemorrhage. The extent of resection is illustrated in *C*, the completed anastomosis in *D*. (For details of technic, see Johnson and Kirby's *Surgery of the Chest.*)

In our hands this operation has been very satisfactory. Even when a satisfactory splenorenal shunt is accomplished, if the operation has not taken too long and the patient is in good condition, a partial esophagogastrectomy with esophagogastrostomy will be an added safeguard against subsequent hemorrhage.

[Ligation of varices *on page 70.*]

PLATE 15

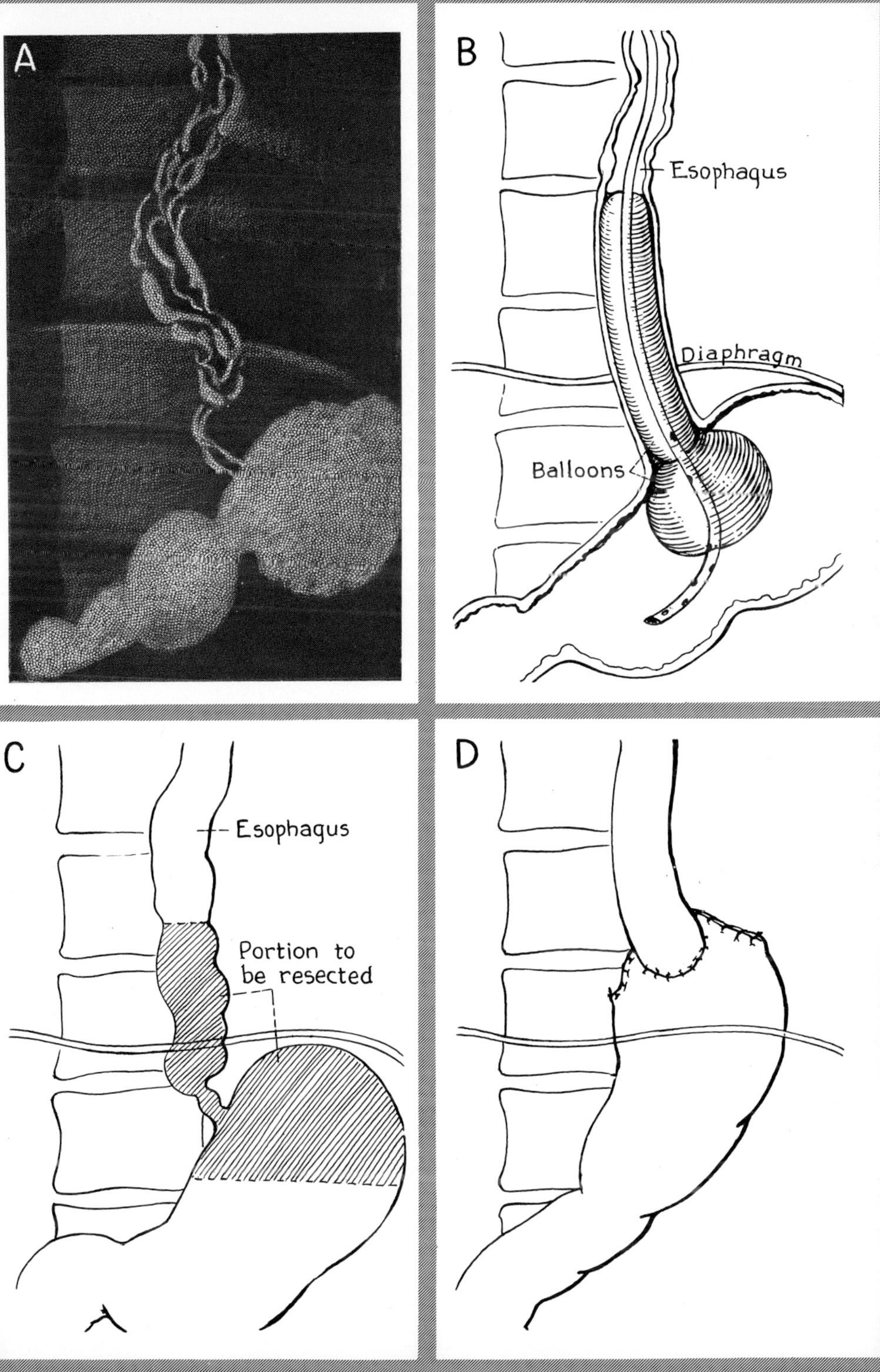
A
B
Esophagus
Diaphragm
Balloons
C
Esophagus
Portion to
be resected
D

Resection of the upper stomach and lower esophagus for the direct attack upon esophageal varices involves extensive surgery. A less formidable direct attack upon the varices, the transesophageal ligation of varices, has been quite successful in the prevention of esophageal hemorrhage. This procedure has the additional advantages of not requiring a vagotomy and of not destroying what sphincter action exists at the cardioesophageal junction. It can be performed as an independent procedure or in conjunction with a shunt operation when there is a history of esophageal hemorrhage.

A.–The left chest is opened by resection of the left seventh or eighth rib or by an intercostal incision through the seventh or eighth interspace. The left inferior pulmonary ligament is divided and the left lung elevated. The esophagus is mobilized from the diaphragm upward for 2–3 in. A longitudinal incision is made through the most accessible surface of the esophagus 1–2 in. in length and extending upward from the diaphragm.

B.–Three large varices usually present into the lumen of the esophagus.

C.–An over-and-over running stitch of chromic catgut is placed around each varix, beginning close to the stomach and continuing upward for 2–3 in. This can be accomplished by retracting on the suture as it is placed and pulling the varix into the wound.

D.–The esophagus is closed by a continuous inner row of catgut. An outer row either of continuous catgut or of interrupted cotton sutures completes the esophageal closure. This may be done in a longitudinal direction.

E.–If the esophageal incision is not more than 1 in. long, it may be closed transversely by two rows of sutures to minimize the danger of narrowing of the lumen.

[Segmental ligation of varices *on page* 72.]

PLATE 16

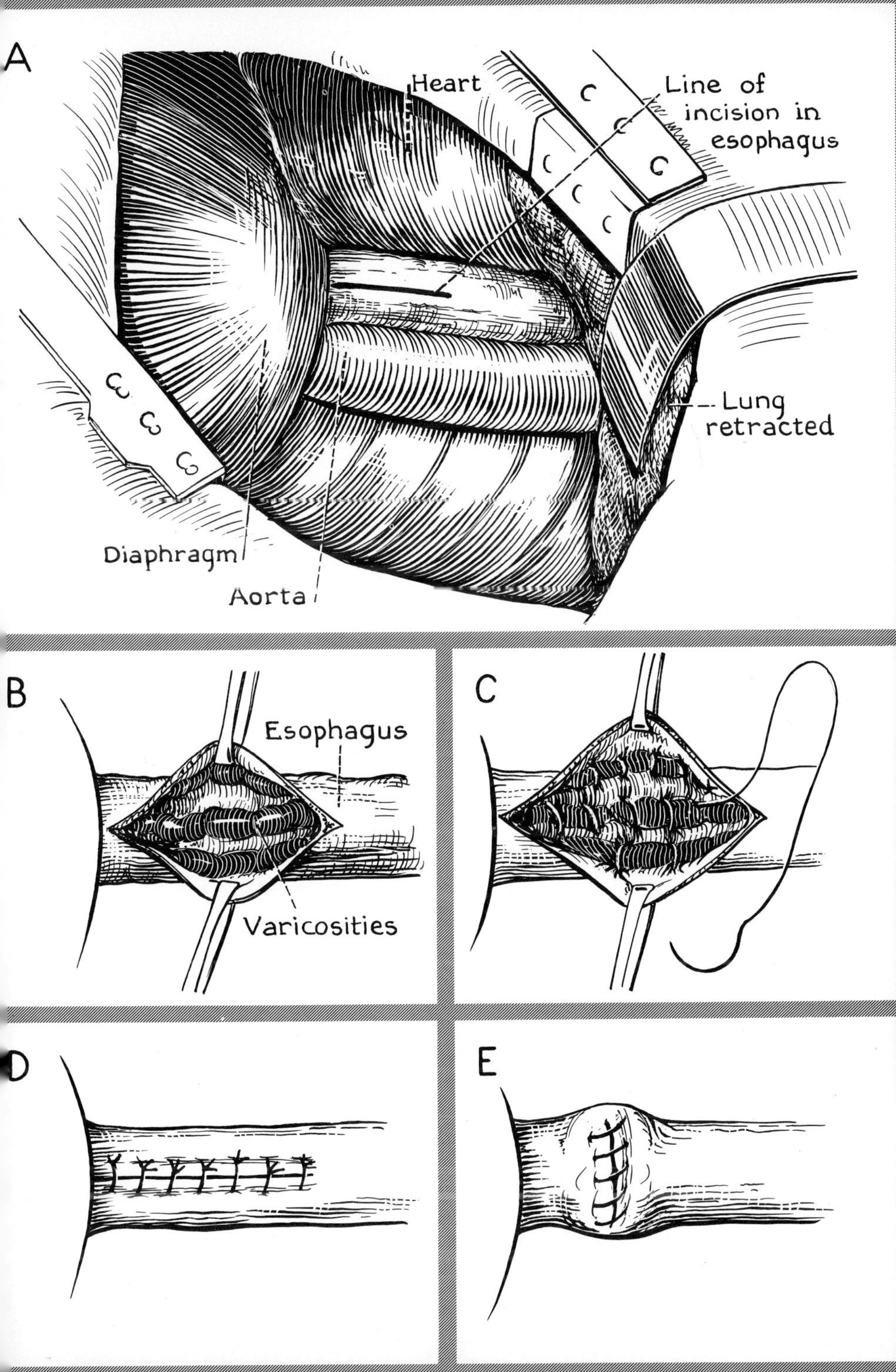
A
Heart
Line of incision in esophagus
Lung retracted
Diaphragm
Aorta
B
Esophagus
Varicosities
C
D
E

Segmental Ligation

A.—Some European surgeons have recommended incising the esophagus from the diaphragm upward for a distance of 4 or 5 in. The varices are ligated by interrupted sutures placed about ½ in. apart. A sclerosing solution is injected into the veins between the ligatures.

B.—The esophagus is then closed longitudinally.

C.—The chest wall is closed in layers. It is well to drain the left chest with a catheter drain attached to a water-seal bottle. The drain is removed after 24 hours or when it is determined that the left lung is well expanded and no fluid exists in the pleural cavity.

Before ligating esophageal varices for hemorrhage, the surgeon must be sure that the bleeding is from the esophagus and not from gastric varices. In patients in whom the possibility of gastric bleeding is suspected we explore the stomach by a transdiaphragmatic gastrotomy after ligation of the esophageal varices.

PLATE 17

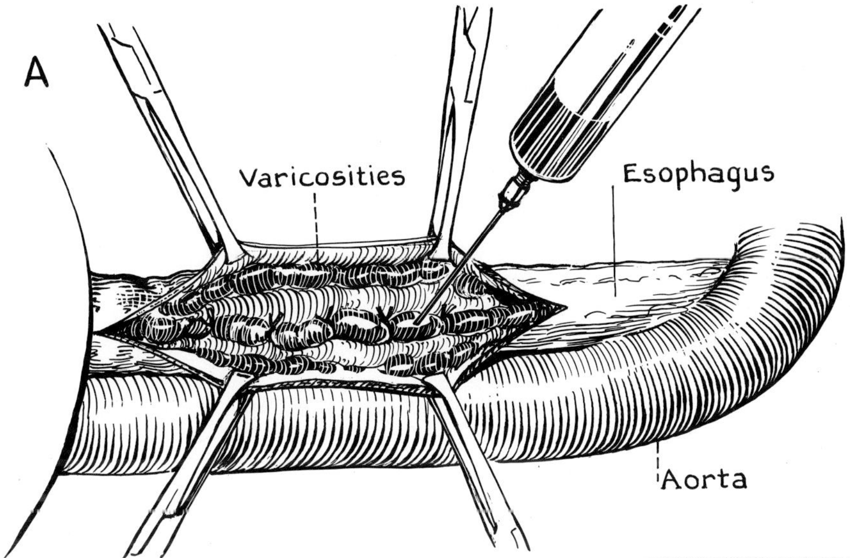

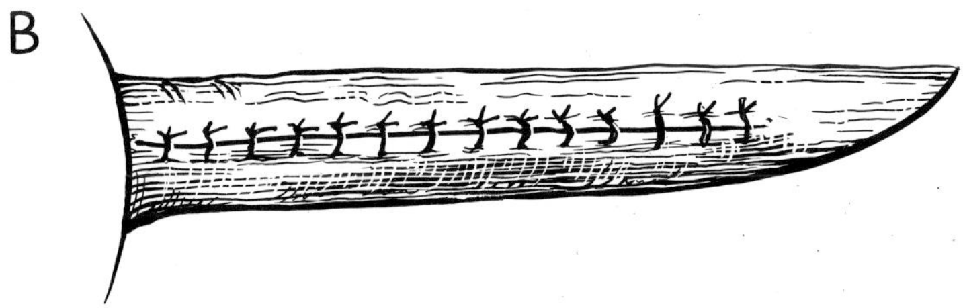

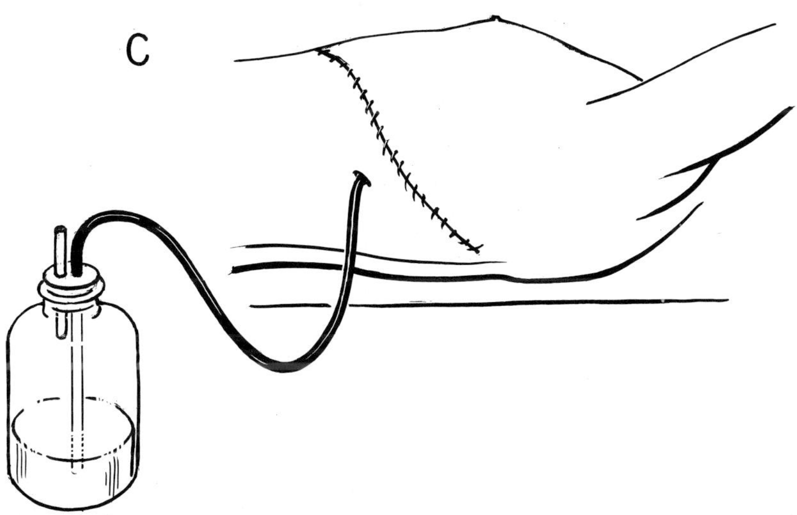

Many surgeons prefer a side-to-side anastomosis between the portal vein and the inferior vena cava which permits as much portal blood as possible to flow through the liver and the remainder to flow directly into the vena cava. Two approaches have been recommended for this anastomosis.

A.—A long incision is made through the ninth or tenth intercostal space and continued downward to or across the right rectus muscle. The ribs are spread and the diaphragm divided to permit the liver to be retracted upward into the chest cavity, increasing exposure of the vessels.

B.—The second approach is through a long, right subcostal incision which permits elevation of the liver and exposure of the right border of the hepatoduodenal ligament and its contents.

C.—Through either approach the common bile duct, hepatic artery and portal vein are freed from overlying tissues and are isolated. To expose the maximal available length of the portal vein where it crosses obliquely over the inferior vena cava the duodenum and head of the pancreas are freed posteriorly and reflected to the left. When pressure readings have demonstrated a definite portal hypertension and it is determined that the two vessels can be approximated, an anastomosis is made.

D.—The Julian modification of the Smith-Freeman clamp was devised to permit flow of blood through the portal vein to the liver during the construction of the anastomosis. This clamp constricts a portion of both the inferior vena cava and the portal vein and approximates them without completely occluding the circulation in either vessel. Two sutures are placed through the walls of both vessels at the ends of the contemplated incisions. These sutures are brought through the blades of the clamp and act as points of traction while the clamp is being applied. Parallel longitudinal incisions are then made in both vessels. The posterior wall of the anastomosis is made by an over-and-over suture of the two approximating cut edges of the vessel walls. The anterior wall is established by suturing together the remainder of the cut edges of the portal vein and vena cava.

E.—A large anastomosis is made to minimize the danger of occlusion from contraction or thrombosis. Upon completion of the anastomosis, the clamp is removed. The portal pressure should be redetermined to estimate the adequacy of the anastomosis.

PLATE 18

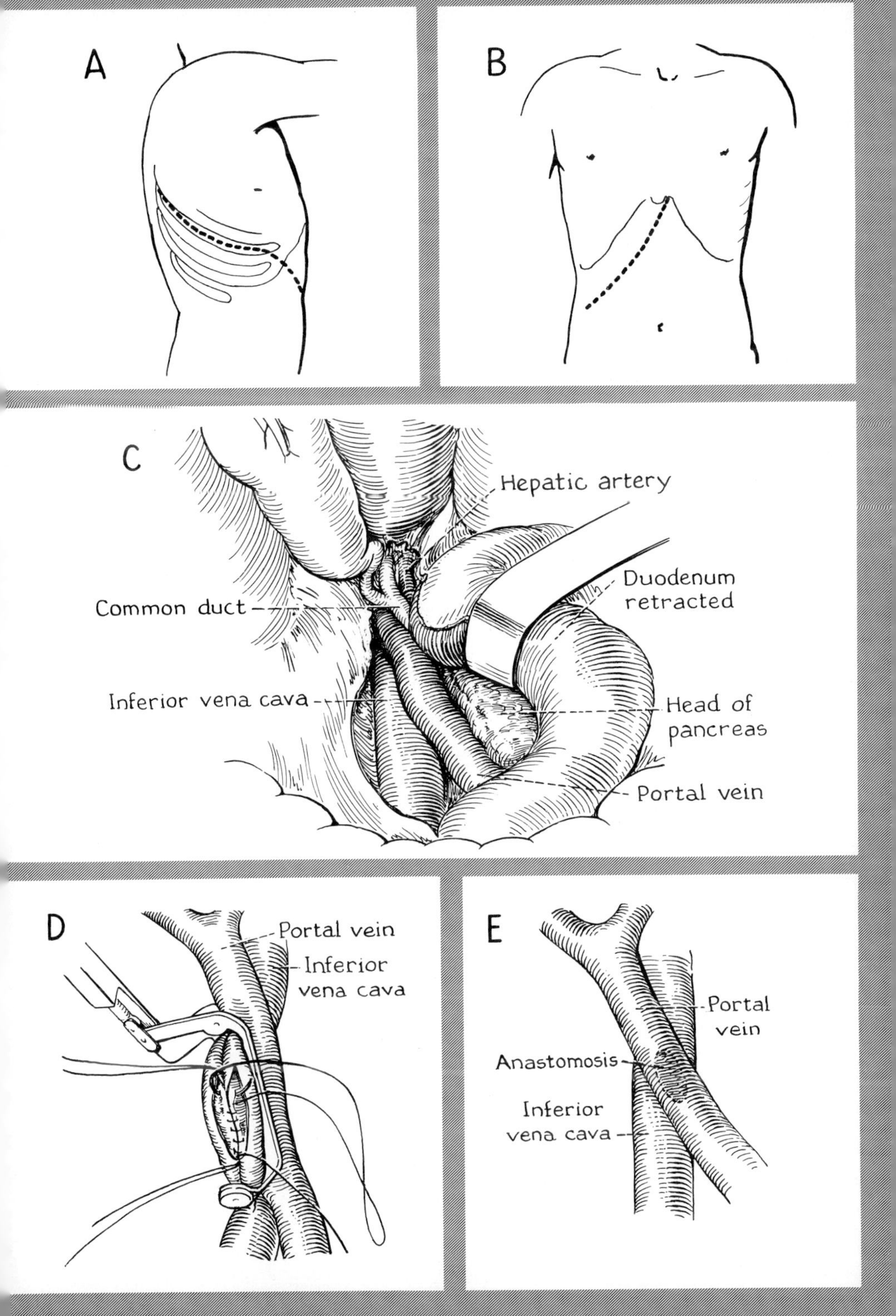

A
B
C
Hepatic artery
Duodenum retracted
Common duct
Inferior vena cava
Head of pancreas
Portal vein
D
Portal vein
Inferior vena cava
E
Portal vein
Anastomosis
Inferior vena cava

Portal hypertension may be diminished by shunting part of the blood from the portal to the systemic system by means of an anastomosis between the splenic and left renal veins. This procedure has an additional advantage in that the splanchnic inflow is further reduced by splenectomy.

A.—The patient is placed on his right side on the operating table, with the left arm extended forward and upward. Controlled intratracheal anesthesia is essential because the left pleural cavity is to be opened. A skin incision is made over the ninth intercostal space beginning close to the spine and extending downward and forward to approximately 2 in. from the midline. It is then curved downward on the abdomen over the midportion of the left rectus muscle. The incision is carried through the intercostal space and the pleura.

B.—The tenth costal cartilage is divided. The parietal pleura is incised and the lung is retracted upward. The diaphragm is opened directly beneath the thoracotomy incision, leaving a strip at the chest wall adequate to allow closure. The incision is carried downward through the midportion of the left rectus muscle and the underlying peritoneum. The spleen is mobilized by dividing the splenodiaphragmatic, splenorenal, gastrosplenic and splenocolic ligaments. The splenic pedicle is freed from the overlying peritoneum.

C.—The splenic artery is suitably ligated and divided. The greatest possible length of splenic vein is isolated for the anastomosis and clamped deep in the splenic hilus, allowing the spleen to be removed. The left renal pedicle is exposed and the renal vein carefully freed from all surrounding tissues.

D.—The stump of splenic vein is dissected from the superior and posterior surface of the pancreas for a distance sufficient to permit approximation to the renal vein without tension. An end-to-side anastomosis is accomplished between the end of the splenic vein and the anterior wall of the left renal vein in the most accessible area. The diaphragm, abdomen and chest wall incisions are closed without drainage.

PLATE 19

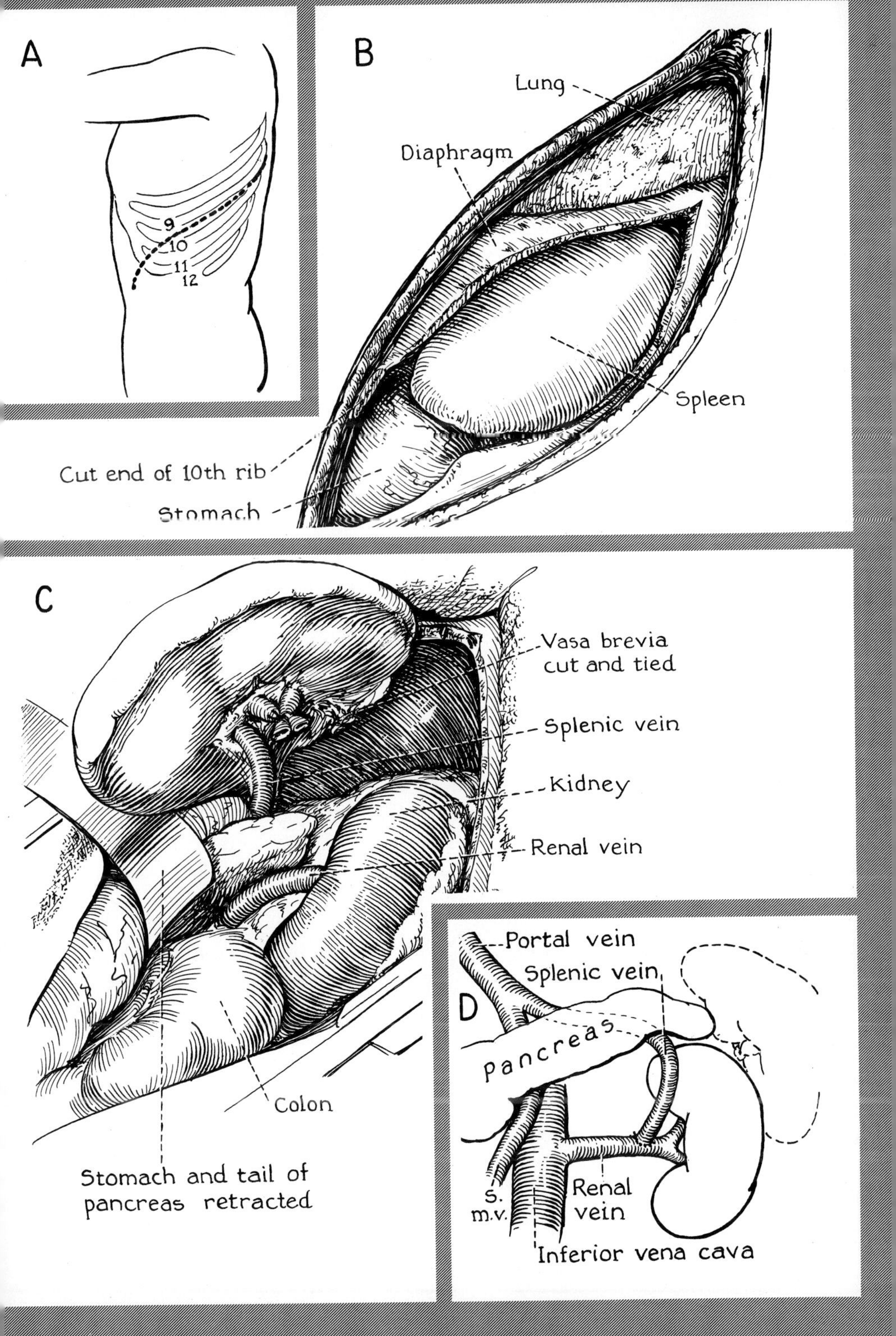
A
9
10
11
12
B
Lung
Diaphragm
Spleen
Cut end of 10th rib
Stomach
C
Vasa brevia cut and tied
Splenic vein
Kidney
Renal vein
Colon
Stomach and tail of pancreas retracted
D
Portal vein
Splenic vein
pancreas
s. m.v.
Renal vein
Inferior vena cava

Splenectomy

Splenectomy has been performed for portal hypertension to diminish the amount of portal blood by the amount normally draining from the spleen. Theoretically, this procedure should be of value in diminishing the pressure within the portal system, but in practice the results have been disappointing. Unfortunately, its previous accomplishment prevents a later splenorenal anastomosis. Therefore, splenectomy alone is not recommended as a therapeutic procedure for portal hypertension.

Ligation of Splenic Artery

Ligation of the splenic artery has been advocated to reduce portal hypertension. It is a much less formidable procedure than splenectomy in the poor risk patient and is believed by some surgeons to have the same beneficial effect. It has the same disadvantages as splenectomy and has been followed by abscess of the spleen, especially when antibiotics have not been used in conjunction with the operation.

Ligation of Common Hepatic and Splenic Arteries

In recent years ligation of the common hepatic and splenic arteries close to their origin from the celiac axis has been advocated to reduce portal hypertension. The theory of hepatic artery ligation is that, in cirrhosis of the liver, abnormal communications develop between the arterial and venous blood supply within the liver and arterial pressure tends to increase portal tension. It is known that ligation of the hepatic arteries close to the liver, especially without the protection of antibiotics, may cause death. Ligation of the hepatic artery close to the celiac axis and proximal to the origin of the gastroduodenal artery will permit an adequate anastomotic blood supply to the liver to maintain its viability. Proximal ligation of the hepatic and splenic arteries has met with encouraging results in the hands of some surgeons but has been disastrous in the hands of others. More recently the left gastric artery has been ligated in addition to the splenic and common hepatic arteries. I believe the results of these operations are too uncertain to justify a description of the technic at this time.

ASCITES

Ascites of hepatic origin is most commonly associated with cirrhosis or with primary or secondary carcinoma of the liver. Infrequently it accompanies other tumors of the liver, portal thrombosis and hepatitis. Jaundice may or may not be a symptom. The ascitic fluid of hepatic origin is usually a clear transudate unless jaundice is present, under which circumstance the fluid will be stained yellow by bile.

Ascites may result from other causes, such as cardiac decompensation, renal insufficiency or intra-abdominal disease including carcinomatosis, ovarian cysts or tumors. Intestinal obstruction, especially of the strangulation type, and inflammatory lesions may produce ascites in which the fluid frequently is bloody. Large amounts of ascitic fluid will cause abdominal distention similar to that produced by tumors and intestinal obstruction. Careful examination of the abdomen and the elicitation of a fluid wave will help establish the diagnosis.

Treatment.—Liver disease of sufficient severity to produce ascites demands all available treatment to support this organ, to diminish its functional load and to encourage recovery of function and regeneration. This includes a high protein intake, orally and often parenterally. Anemia is often a complication of liver disease and should be corrected by blood transfusion. The intravenous administration of protein hydrolysates theoretically should be of great value. These agents should be used cautiously and should be administered slowly to avoid reactions which may be detrimental to liver function. Their use is not discouraged but their value is doubtful. Intravenous use of human albumin may be beneficial but is expensive. Blood and blood plasma are the most satisfactory sources of usable protein but their origin should be investigated carefully to minimize the danger of homologous serum jaundice. Vitamin therapy is indicated, particularly the administration of vitamins B and K.

Paracentesis abdominis (Plate 20) is commonly performed in ascites of hepatic origin in which diagnosis has been established and repeated tappings are necessary. If ascites results from portal hypertension, one of the aforementioned operations for this condition should be contemplated.

Paracentesis

Paracentesis abdominis, the puncturing of the abdominal wall with a trocar and the evacuating of fluid through its cannula, is a simple procedure but is not without danger because it is done blindly and abdominal viscera may be injured.

A.—The site selected for insertion of the trocar usually is below the umbilicus, in the midline or in either lower quadrant. The insertion should not be directly above the pubis because of danger of injury to the bladder. Hemorrhage from the inferior epigastric vessels may occur if the trocar is inserted in the midportion of the rectus muscles. Paracentesis should not be done in close proximity to abdominal scars, since loops of intestine adherent to the parietal abdominal wall may be damaged or punctured by the trocar. If the patient has had multiple abdominal operations or peritonitis or other abdominal inflammatory disease, insertion of a trocar is hazardous.

Paracentesis can readily be performed under local anesthesia, a small area of skin and the underlying fascia being infiltrated with the anesthetic agent. The skin incision should be made long enough to permit easy passage of the trocar.

B.—The diagram shows the trocar introduced through the abdominal wall.

Other Operations to Establish Collateral Circulation

Efforts have been made to establish collateral circulation between some of the abdominal viscera whose venous blood drains into the portal system and the parietal peritoneum or abdominal wall in an attempt to divert some of the portal blood into the systemic system. Scarification of the parietal peritoneum and suture of the omentum to it have been recommended. Transplantation of a portion of the omentum to a prepared pocket between the parietal peritoneum and the overlying fascia or muscles has been performed.

C and *D.*—In the Talma-Morison operation, an upper midline incision is made and a pocket is formed on each side between the parietal peritoneum and the posterior rectus sheath. The omentum is split longitudinally, each half being placed in the pocket on the corresponding side. The results of this operation have not been encouraging. However, it may be of benefit when other more satisfactory procedures cannot be used.

PLATE 20

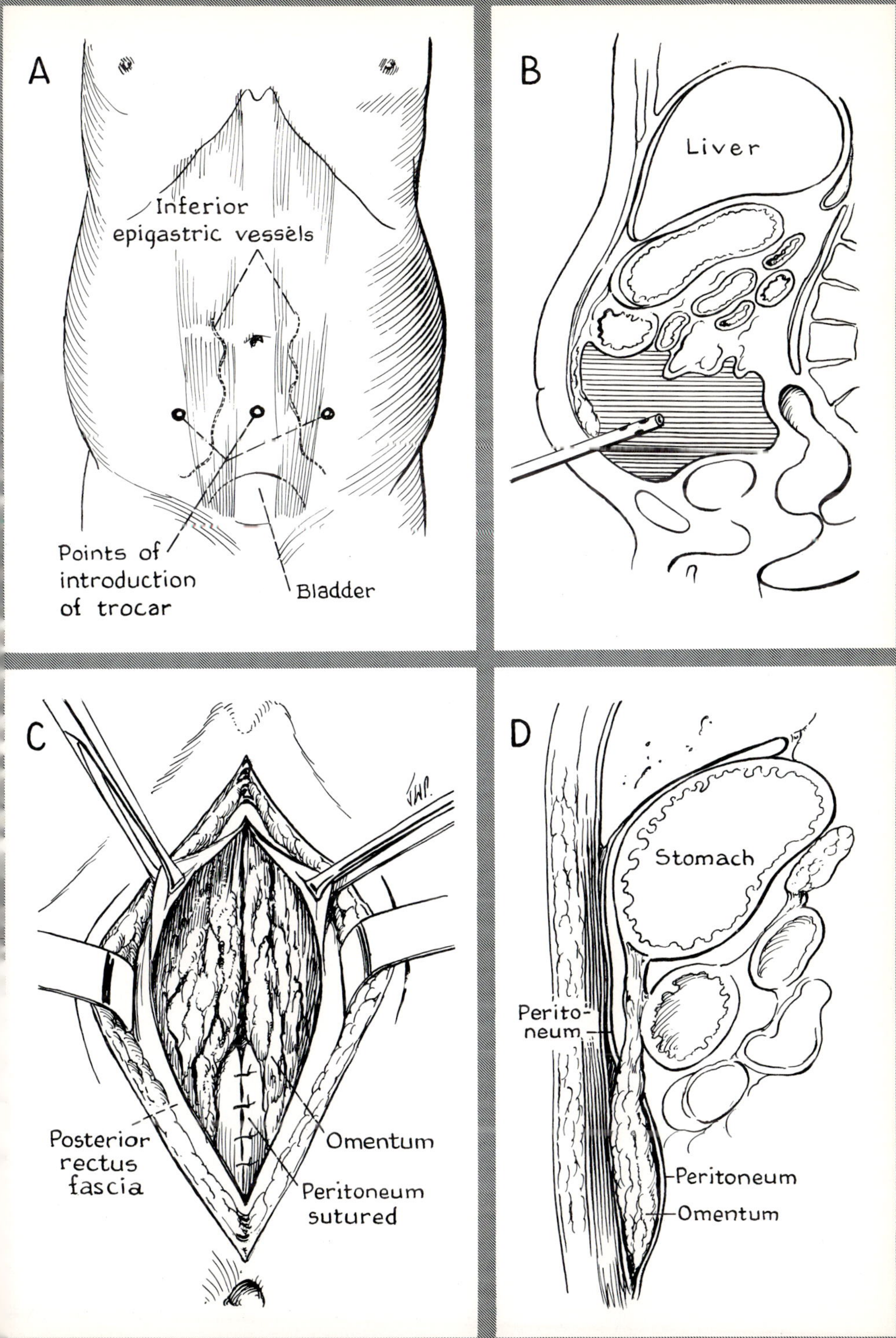
A
Inferior epigastric vessels
Points of introduction of trocar
Bladder
B
Liver
C
JWP
Posterior rectus fascia
Omentum
Peritoneum sutured
D
Stomach
Perito-neum
Peritoneum
Omentum

SECTION II

The Extrahepatic Biliary System

CHAPTER 6

Anatomy and Physiology of the Extrahepatic Biliary Tract

ANATOMY

THE EXTRAHEPATIC biliary system consists of the right and left hepatic ducts, common hepatic duct, cystic duct, gallbladder and the common bile duct (choledochus) with its termination at the ampulla of Vater. The hepatic ducts emerge from the liver at the porta hepatis where there may be two in number or where several ducts may be present to merge into the right and left hepatic ducts. They lie anterior to the portal vein and its branches. A short distance from the liver the two hepatic ducts usually merge to form the common hepatic duct. This is joined at varying distances from the liver by the cystic duct which is normally 2–3 mm. in diameter or about the size of a kitchen match and leads to the gallbladder.

The gallbladder, a pear-shaped organ with a capacity of about 35 cc., lies under the right lobe of the liver in the gallbladder fossa. It extends forward, downward and slightly to the right, with its fundus lying close to the anterior edge of the liver near the lateral border of the right rectus muscle. The undersurface is covered by peritoneum which is reflected onto it from the liver. The serous coat of the gallbladder is derived from this peritoneum which frequently invests the fundus but covers the body and neck only on the undersurface. The entire gallbladder occasionally is invested by peritoneum and may hang from the liver by a mesentery-like fold. The neck of the gallbladder may lie close to or in contact with the common bile duct. The hepatic surface of the gallbladder is firmly fixed to the liver, securely anchoring the body of the gallbladder. Thus, if the gallbladder becomes distended by obstruction of the cystic duct, the organ expands in all directions and the neck may press against the common bile duct and obstruct it by external pressure. The cystic duct extends from the neck of the gallbladder usually in an arc or curve toward the hilus of the liver to run parallel to and below the cystic artery. Although it commonly enters the hepatic duct on the right side, it may cross anteriorly or posteriorly to open into either of these surfaces or into the left side of the duct. It is important for the surgeon to be familiar with and recognize all these anatomic possibilities to perform successful gallbladder surgery.

A.—The cystic duct usually joins the common duct in the mid third of the distance between the hilus of the liver and the duodenum, most frequently on the right side of the common hepatic duct.

B.—The cystic duct may be greatly enlarged, particularly when a stone has passed from the gallbladder through it into the common bile duct. Its diameter may be greater than that of the common hepatic duct.

C.—The cystic duct may parallel and be densely adherent to the common hepatic duct for a considerable distance before their lumens unite. It is important to recognize this because stones may lodge in the distal portion of the cystic duct and may not be located even though the common duct is explored.

D.—Aberrant hepatic ducts may emerge from the liver and join the cystic duct at any point. If they are large and are ligated, drainage of bile from a portion of the liver will be obstructed.

E.—The neck of the gallbladder may be adherent to the common bile duct and the latter structure damaged unless a very careful dissection is made.

F.—The cystic duct may empty into the common duct on any surface. It may cross the hepatic duct to join it on the left side or may extend around it to empty into the posterior surface. Occasionally, aberrant hepatic ducts enter the posterior wall of the gallbladder. If these are not recognized and ligated, there may be considerable postoperative leakage of bile into the peritoneal cavity.

PLATE 21

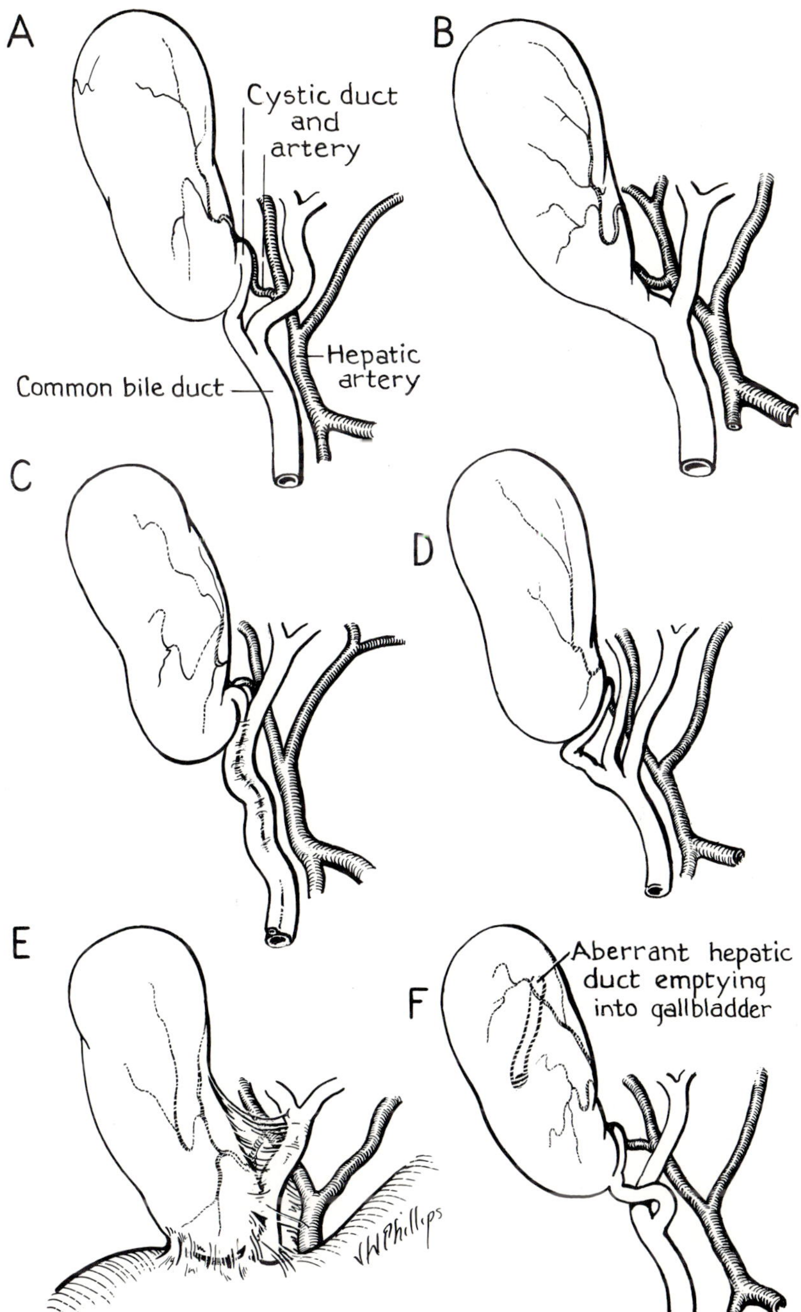
A
B
Cystic duct and artery
Hepatic artery
Common bile duct
C
D
E
F
Aberrant hepatic duct emptying into gallbladder
JWPhillips

The common bile duct passes downward posterior to the first portion of the duodenum to reach the posteromedial surface of the second portion of the duodenum. It then passes between the pancreas and the duodenum, in a groove within the pancreas or occasionally surrounded by pancreas, to enter the medial surface of the duodenum at the papilla of Vater.

A.—Occasionally the common duct will run a somewhat spiral course as it passes obliquely through the duodenal wall. This histologic section cut longitudinally through the distal choledochus and duodenal wall shows the duct cut longitudinally except in the midportion of the slide where the duct spirals and is cut transversely in two places.

B.—More frequently, the duct runs a comparatively straight course. These histologic sections show the folds of mucosa in the distal end of the duct and ampulla of Vater which exert a valve-like action and help prevent regurgitation of the intestinal contents into the biliary tract. The duodenal musculature, through which the common duct passes obliquely, is an additional protection against regurgitation into the common duct.

Relation to pancreatic duct.—There is a great deal of variation in the relationship of the common bile duct and the main pancreatic duct as they approach and enter the duodenum.

C.—The pancreatic duct may join the common bile duct proximal to the sphincter of Oddi.

D.—The common bile duct and main pancreatic duct may traverse the duodenal musculature separately but enter a single ampulla.

E.—More frequently the common bile duct and pancreatic duct have separate orifices into the duodenum which may be varying distances apart. There has been a great deal of speculation as to the importance of the anatomic relationship of these two ducts to the interrelation of pancreatic and biliary tract disease. If the ducts join proximal to the sphincter of Oddi, which is located at the base of the ampulla of Vater, it has been hypothesized that bile may regurgitate into the pancreatic ducts or pancreatic juice may regurgitate into the biliary system, producing certain pathologic changes. This is a controversial question.

PLATE 22

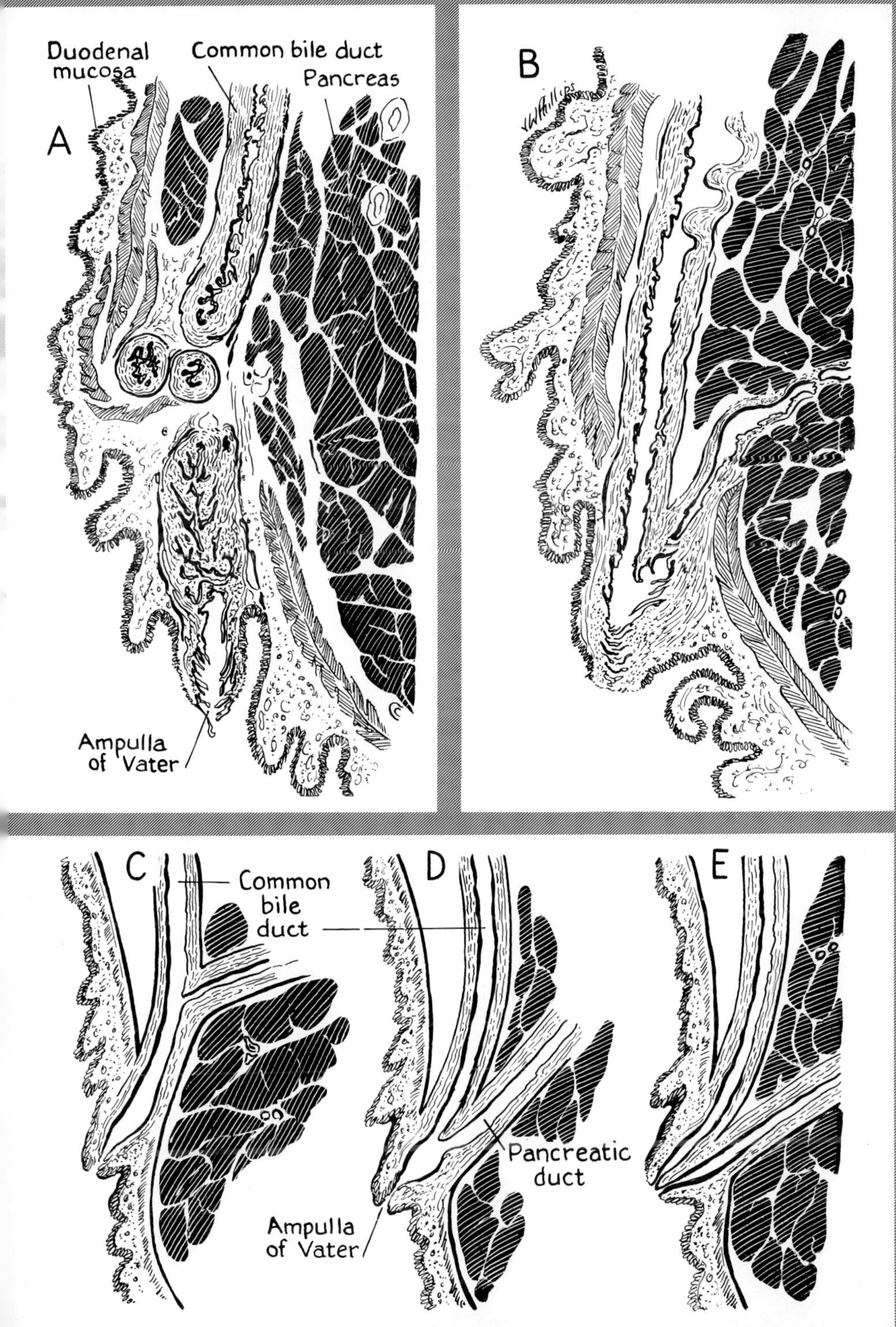

A
Duodenal mucosa
Common bile duct
Pancreas
Ampulla of Vater
B
C
Common bile duct
D
E
Pancreatic duct
Ampulla of Vater

The hepatic artery and its branches have a close relationship to the extrahepatic bile ducts which is important to the surgeon. The hepatic artery arises from the celiac axis, runs forward and to the right above the head of the pancreas to a position in the gastrohepatic ligament to the left of the common bile duct. There it courses upward to the porta hepatis. Near the liver, it divides into the right and left hepatic arteries which enter the liver as single or divided vessels.

A.—The right hepatic artery most frequently courses posterior to the common hepatic duct and gives off the cystic artery superior to the cystic duct.

Many variations in the origin, location, branching and distribution of the hepatic artery are found. Occasionally this artery may arise directly from the aorta or from the superior mesenteric artery. Anomalies in the origin of the hepatic artery usually are of little surgical significance. However, in one patient we found the hepatic artery to course between the inferior vena cava and portal vein, passing to the right of the portal vein and then to its normal position to the left of the common bile duct. This was of considerable surgical significance since it interfered with the contemplated establishment of a portacaval anastomosis. The anomalies of greatest interest to the surgeon are those occurring in the terminal branch of the hepatic artery, the left and right hepatic arteries and their branches. These vessels may have any conceivable relationship to the bile ducts.

B.—The right hepatic artery may cross anterior to the common hepatic duct where it is more vulnerable to injury.

C.—The right hepatic artery may follow along the cystic duct and be mistaken for the cystic artery.

D.—Two or more cystic arteries may arise from the right hepatic artery.

E.—The right hepatic artery may originate as a separate artery and course along the right side of the common bile duct.

F.—The gastroduodenal artery may arise from the hepatic artery not far from the hilus of the liver and course downward along the common duct where it may be injured by exposure of the common duct.

[Anatomy of arteries *continued on page* 92.]

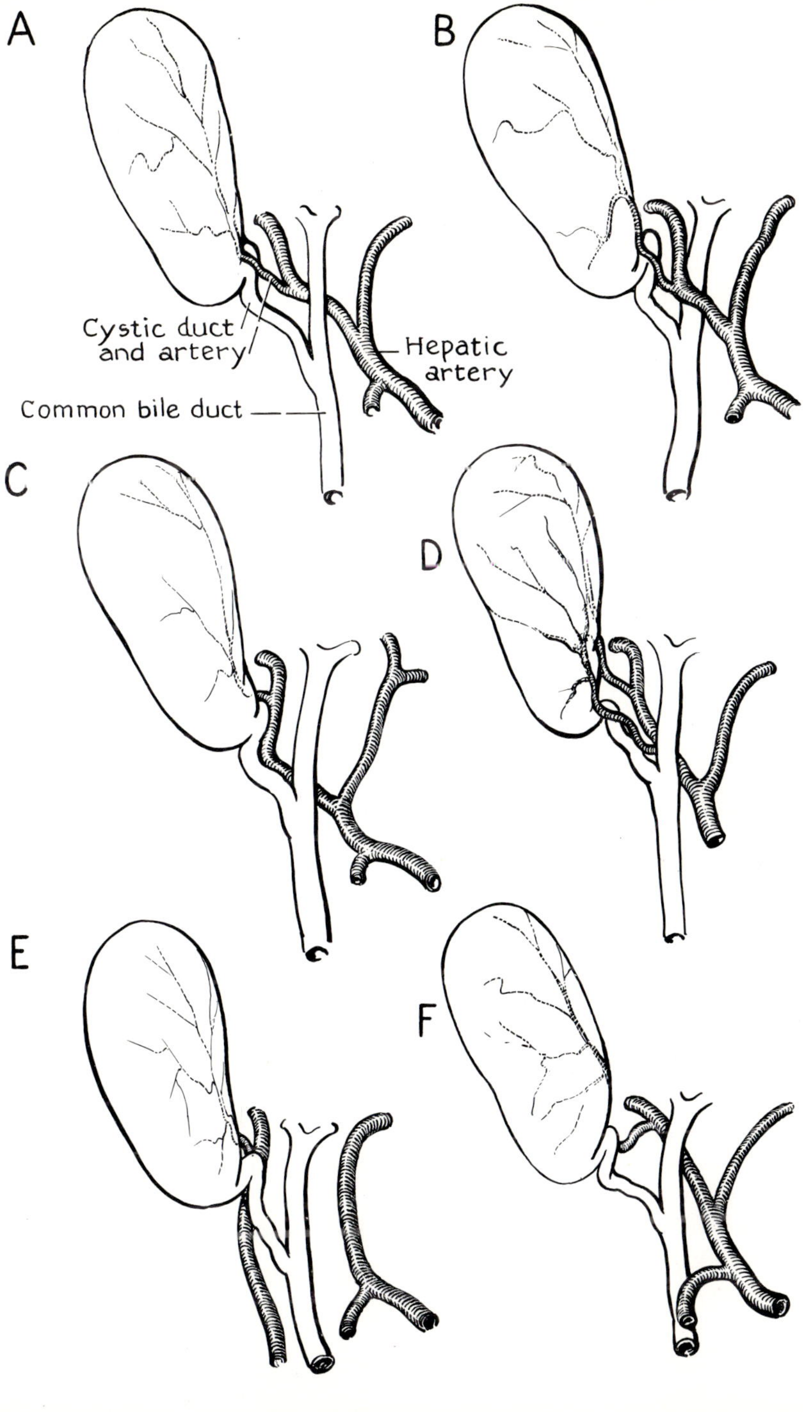
A
B
Cystic duct
and artery
Hepatic
artery
Common bile duct
C
D
E
F

Cystic arteries may arise from structures other than the right hepatic artery.

G.—The cystic artery may arise directly from the hepatic artery. In this figure, a second cystic artery is seen to arise from the right hepatic artery.

H.—Occasionally it takes its origin from the left hepatic artery.

I.—Occasionally it will arise from the gastroduodenal artery and course along the common bile duct and cystic duct to the gallbladder.

J.—One cystic artery has been found to arise from the left hepatic artery and a second from the right hepatic artery.

K.—The right hepatic artery may course along the cystic duct for a considerable distance up the bed of the gallbladder before entering the liver.

L.—Occasionally the main hepatic artery will course along the cystic duct. If this should be ligated, the arterial blood supply to the entire liver is markedly impaired and death is likely to follow.

The lesser omentum, a double layer of peritoneum, extends from the stomach and duodenum to the liver. The hepatoduodenal ligament is the portion of the lesser omentum passing from the duodenum to the liver. Within the lesser omentum between the liver and duodenum lies the common bile duct, hepatic artery, portal vein, nerves and lymphatics. The common bile duct is in the right free edge anteriorly. The hepatic artery lies to the left of the common bile duct and both structures are anterior to the portal vein. Near the hilus of the liver, the peritoneal fold also covers the cystic duct and cystic artery.

If there is any question as to the identity of the cystic artery, it is well to isolate and divide the cystic duct first and dissect it and the neck of the gallbladder upward better to expose the artery. As variations of the normal arrangement of the arteries and ducts exist in about three fourths of all patients, ample dissection must be made whenever biliary tract surgery is performed. Failure to recognize anomalies may have two serious consequences. Ligation of the right hepatic artery or of the common hepatic artery may prove fatal. Hemorrhage from an anomalous or accessory vessel which is unexpectedly divided may obscure the field and blind attempts to control the bleeding may result in damage to the bile ducts.

PLATE 23

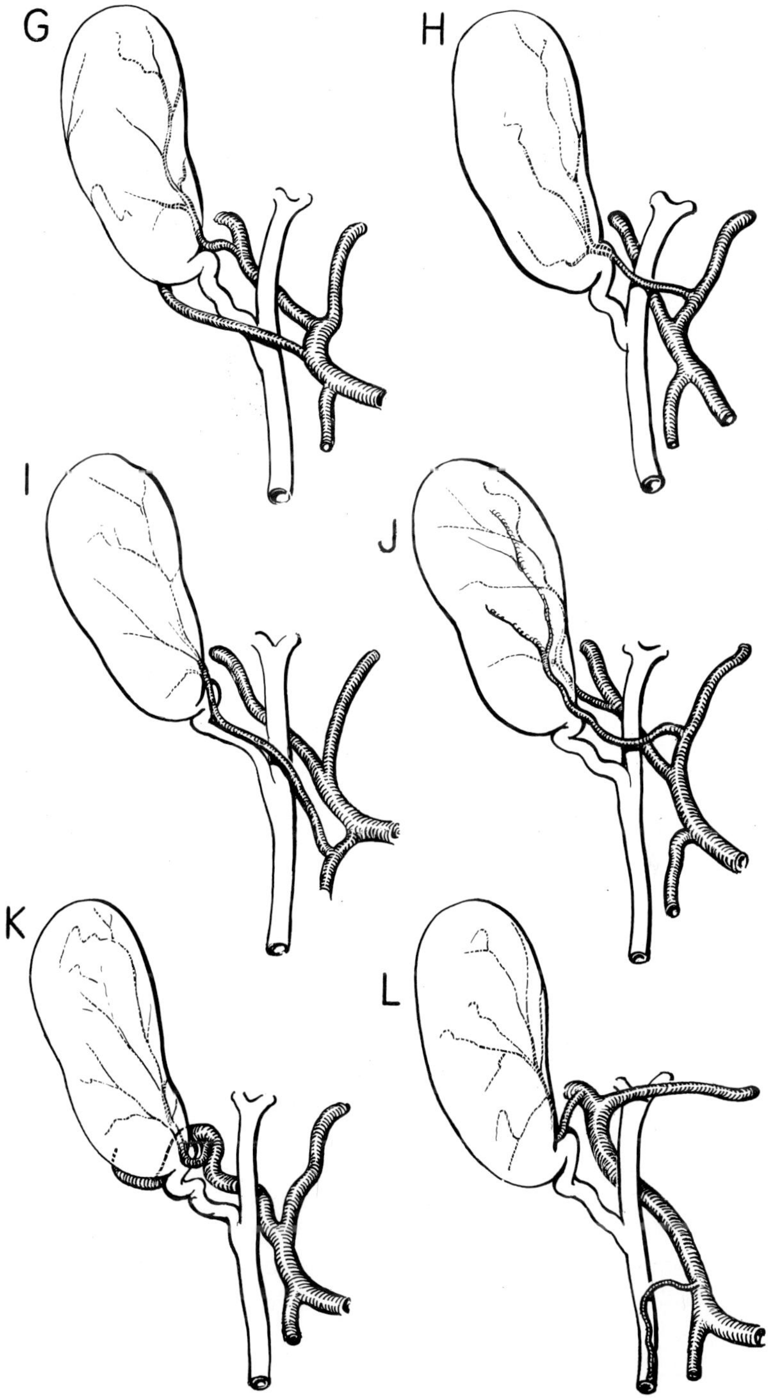

PHYSIOLOGY

The most important physiologic functions of the extrahepatic biliary tract are the transmission of bile from the liver to the intestine and the regulation of its flow. When the gallbladder and bile ducts are not diseased and are normally functioning, they respond in a fairly uniform manner in various phases of digestion. Bile is secreted continuously by the liver but in varying amounts. In the fasting state, bile is accumulated and concentrated in the gallbladder. It is forced into the gallbladder by an increased pressure within the common bile duct produced by the action of the sphincter of Oddi at its distal end. Very little, if any, bile flows into the duodenum during the fasting state. The stimulation produced by the psychic or hormonal influence of food or by the passage of gastric contents into the duodenum causes a contraction of the gallbladder with a questionable slight relaxation of the tonus of the sphincter of Oddi and results in an outpouring of bile into the duodenum. The gallbladder empties a large portion of its contents in the first few minutes after the ingestion of food. It continues to empty and its contents added to the increased amount of bile secreted by the liver are passed into the duodenum through the period of digestion when the stomach is emptying. When the stomach is emptied, duodenal peristalsis diminishes, the gallbladder relaxes, the tonus of the sphincter of Oddi increases slightly and very little, if any, bile passes into the duodenum. The diminishing amount of bile secreted by the liver is retained in the common duct and forced into the gallbladder.

The sphincter of Oddi serves to maintain an increased pressure within the common bile duct and thus to force bile into the gallbladder. It may also serve to prevent regurgitation of duodenal contents into the common bile duct. This function is not essential because, when it is not active, regurgitation is prevented by the sphincter action of the duodenal musculature through which the common duct passes and by the valvelike folds of mucosa within the ampulla of Vater and distal portion of the common duct.

Effects of cholecystectomy.—When the gallbladder is removed there is a loss of tonus of the sphincter of Oddi and the pressure within the common bile duct drops to that of intra-abdominal pressure. Bile is no longer retained in the bile ducts but may flow quite freely into the duodenum during both fasting and digestive phases. This corresponds to the physiologic activity of animals normally not provided with gallbladders. It has been demonstrated in both man and animals that the extrahepatic bile ducts dilate after cholecystectomy. This occurs despite a drop in intraductal pressure. I believe the dilatation and the loss of tonus of the sphincter of Oddi are the result of a disturbed innervation of these structures resulting from cholecystectomy.

Pathogenesis of Biliary Dyspepsia

Biliary dyspepsia consists of a feeling of fulness, indigestion and belching occurring soon after the ingestion of food. It usually accompanies gallbladder disease and is relieved by cholecystectomy. It occurs whether or not the gallbladder is infected. I believe the dyspepsia is due to an insufficient amount of bile present in the duodenum at the beginning of a meal to produce proper fat digestion. In the presence of gallbladder disease, the sphincter of Oddi may continue to function to some degree and may partially interfere with the free flow of bile into the intestine. Removal of the diseased gallbladder is accompanied by a loss of tonus of the sphincter of Oddi, and the unimpaired flow of bile into the duodenum both in the fasting state and during feeding provides an adequate amount of bile in the duodenum to permit proper digestion. This seems to be a logical explanation for relief of dyspepsia following removal of an organ which has been physiologically inactive and has not been a site of infection. The importance of the presence of an adequate amount of bile to mix with food in its passage from the stomach to prevent dyspepsia is borne out by other surgical procedures. After the Roux-Y operation for stricture of the common bile duct, food passes for a considerable distance through the small bowel before it is mixed with bile. These patients almost invariably complain of a mild form of dyspepsia similar to that produced by gallbladder disease and which can be relieved by the oral feeding of bile salts.

The foregoing hypothesis of the normal and abnormal physiology of the extrahepatic biliary tract is supported by studies in comparative anatomy and physiology. Those animals which have a functioning gallbladder have a sphincter mechanism at the distal end of the common bile duct which functions quite similarly to that of man. The animals which do not possess a gallbladder do not have a sphincter at the distal end of the bile duct, and intraductal pressure equals intra-abdominal pressure. These anatomic and physiologic variations are not determined by food habits, and certain species of animals do not possess gallbladders whereas closely allied species are normally provided with them. Removal of gallbladders in such animals as dogs, which have a sphincter mechanism at the duodenal end of the duct, is followed by loss of sphincter tonus and a drop of intraductal pressure to that of intra-abdominal tension. The normal presence or absence of a gallbladder and sphincter mechanism does not seem to be an important factor in the ability of the animal to digest its food. I believe digestive disturbances occur primarily when a sphincter mechanism is active at the duodenal end of the common duct and a gallbladder is present but unable to function. Many people who have asymptomatic gallbladder disease are free from digestive disturbances because a loss of sphincter tonus has developed in conjunction with the disturbed concentrating and contracting power of the gallbladder.

CHAPTER 7

Diseases of the Gallbladder

ACUTE CHOLECYSTITIS

ACUTE INFLAMMATION of a previously undiseased gallbladder may occur, particularly in association with certain systemic infections. In the great majority of cases, however, acute cholecystitis is an inflammatory process developing in a chronically diseased gallbladder which usually contains stones. The attack may be initiated by obstruction of the neck of the gallbladder due to a gallstone impacted within it. Infection is seldom the primary cause of the attack but may become a serious complicating factor.

Symptomatology.—Occasionally a patient may develop acute cholecystitis without a well established history of biliary pain or dyspepsia. Most patients, however, have had repeated attacks of biliary colic and indigestion. The acute attack begins with right upper quadrant or epigastric pain usually more severe than in previous colics. The pain persists and may increase in intensity. Frequently it will radiate to the back or upward into the chest or scapular region. Nausea and vomiting accompany the onset of the pain. Fever, often with chills, develops rapidly.

Examination will reveal tenderness and muscle rigidity in the upper right abdomen. Because of distention, edema and swelling, the gallbladder frequently can be palpated. Varying degrees of leukocytosis are common.

Course.—If early operation is not performed, the symptoms of the acute attack usually will subside within four to 10 days. The pain gradually diminishes but is sufficiently severe to require opiates for several days. The nausea and vomiting diminish but the irritability of the stomach makes it advisable to minimize oral feedings for several days. Fever and leukocytosis slowly subside as do the local tenderness and muscle spasm. However, if operation is performed immediately after the subsidence of all symptoms and signs, the gallbladder will be found to be subacutely inflamed and there will be considerable edema of it and of the peritoneum covering the bile ducts and blood vessels.

In a small percentage of patients, the disease will progress and lead to gangrene of the gallbladder with possible perforation. When gangrene develops, the usual subsidence of symptoms does not occur, the pain, tenderness, rigidity and fever continuing and often increasing. The gradual development of gangrene usually allows sufficient time for the omentum to become adherent to the gallbladder. If perforation occurs under such circumstances the resulting abscess will be localized to the right upper abdomen and a generalized peritonitis will not result. Occasionally perforation occurs before the walling-off process is complete, and peritonitis may result. The pain then usually increases in intensity and spreads from its localized area in the right upper abdomen to involve an increasing area of the right side and gradually to include the entire abdomen. The area of tenderness and rigidity will increase until the entire abdomen is involved. There will be increasing distention, and audible peristalsis will diminish until the abdomen becomes silent. The fever and leukocytosis will continue or increase and the patient's condition will become critical.

Treatment.—A great deal of controversy exists in the surgical literature regarding the advisability of early or late surgery for acute cholecystitis. It is generally agreed that the disease demands surgical intervention. Many authors advise surgery within the first 48 hours of the disease. Early operation has the advantage of minimizing the danger of gangrene or perforation. As the inflammation and edema at this time may not have involved the covering of bile ducts and vessels to as great a degree as they will at a later stage, the exposure and examination of these structures and their identification may be accomplished more accurately. Unfortunately, few patients with acute cholecystitis are seen by the surgeon within 48 hours of the onset of symptoms. In my own cases, those patients giving a history of previous biliary tract disease have had attacks of colic for an average of six years before onset of the acute attack. They had been treated conservatively for the previous attacks and conservative management had been instituted for the attack of acute cholecystitis. Very few were seen by a surgeon during the first two days of the disease.

When the patient is not seen shortly after the onset of acute cholecystitis and the symptoms and findings are not suggestive of gangrene or perforation, I believe operation should be delayed until the acute symptoms have subsided. Fluid and chemical balance should be restored by the intravenous administration of appropriate fluids. The fever, pain and tenderness should be permitted to subside. It is well to ambulate the patient for a few days before operation. Acute inflammation of the gallbladder is accompanied by temporary diminution of liver function. Proper conservative therapy will permit this organ to improve its physiologic activity which is important to the morbidity of biliary tract surgery. The most opportune time to operate on a patient following an attack of acute cholecystitis is from four to six weeks after the subsidence of symptoms. This delay permits the inflammation and edema to subside and aids the surgeon in the performance of an accurate and complete cholecystectomy. Unfortunately, many patients will not return to the hospital for operation when they have completely recovered and are symptom free. Operation from seven to 10 days after the subsidence of symptoms may increase the technical difficulties at operation owing to residual disease but will not be as great a hazard as the danger of recurrent attacks and their complications.

Conservative management of acute cholecystitis places a definite responsibility upon the surgeon. The patient must be hospitalized and carefully observed. If the local pain, tenderness and rigidity do not subside or if they increase, immediate operation is imperative. Gangrene or perforation with development of a localized abscess or peritonitis will be suggested by an aggravation of symptoms and an increased area of abdominal involvement. Such symptoms must be recognized at once and the patient treated as a surgical emergency. Advancement in our knowledge of the preparation of patients for surgery, their nutritional state, fluid and chemical balance, the protection of liver function and antibiotic therapy has greatly reduced the mortality of acute cholecystitis. Equally good results have been reported by various authors with conservative and emergency treatment. Each patient presents an individual problem which must be evaluated to determine the most opportune time for surgical therapy.

Cholecystectomy (Plate 31).—In acute cholecystitis, as in other types of biliary tract surgery, the completion of surgical therapy in a single operation is preferable to an incomplete operation which requires subsequent surgery. For this reason, cholecystectomy is the operation of choice. It may be technically more difficult to remove an acutely diseased gallbladder than one which is chronically diseased, and some variations in technic may be indicated. When possible, it is best to remove the gallbladder from below. Inflammation and edema of the peritoneum overlying the bile ducts and blood vessels may make it difficult to isolate and identify these structures. The increased vascularity will result in more troublesome bleeding. Isolation of the cystic duct and artery may be tedious but must be carefully performed, and the common duct and hepatic artery must be identified before any structures are clamped and divided. Fortunately, the stone obstructing the neck of the gallbladder or cystic duct usually can be palpated and used as a landmark for locating the cystic duct. It may be advisable to clamp and divide the cystic duct close to the obstructing stone to minimize the danger of damaging adjacent structures. The edema and inflammation may make it impossible to preserve a layer of peritoneum sufficient to cover the bed of the gallbladder after removing the organ. After dividing the cystic duct and the cystic artery, the gallbladder will readily shell out of its bed. An effort should be made to leave some tissue over the raw liver surface. If oozing occurs from the liver bed, this area should be packed with warm moist gauze packs until the bleeding has stopped. Coagulating agents or gauze packing should not be left in the bed of the gallbladder at the completion of the operation because there is the possibility of irritation to the common duct and subsequent development of an obliterating type of cholangitis. A rubber drain should always be placed under the edge of the liver in the region of the gallbladder bed and brought out through the wall of the abdomen to permit the escape of any bile or pus which may develop and which could produce a peritonitis if there were no access to the surface.

Some surgeons prefer to remove acutely inflamed gallbladders beginning at the fundus and dissecting to the neck (Plate 33). This procedure has the disadvantage of increased bleeding because the cystic artery has not been ligated before the dissection. Bleeding may also obscure the field after the gallbladder has been freed from its bed and the cystic artery and cystic duct are being isolated prior to division. If the gallbladder is removed from above downward, great care must be used in isolating these structures and in locating the common duct to avoid damage to it when the cystic duct is clamped. Traction on the gallbladder may angulate the common duct and endanger its inclusion in the cystic duct clamp.

Cholecystostomy (Plate 30).—Although cholecystectomy is the operation of choice for surgical treatment of acute cholecystitis, the risk of its performance may not be warranted in selected cases. This is particularly true in elderly people who are acutely ill and debilitated by the inflammation of the gallbladder or by other disease. If the gallbladder has perforated and a local abscess has formed, removal of the organ may be hazardous. Under such circumstances, cholecystostomy may be the operation of choice. It can relieve the acute emergency with a minimal risk. It can be completed more quickly than cholecystectomy, thus shortening the time of operation and the length and depth of anesthesia.

Choledochostomy (Plate 34).—Stones are found in the common bile duct in from 5 to 15 per cent of patients with acute cholecystitis. Where choledocholithiasis is suspected and it is technically feasible, the common duct should be explored. A history of jaundice may suggest common duct stones. However, jaundice can occur without stones being present in the common duct. When the gallbladder is acutely distended, its neck may press against the common duct and cause obstruction by external pressure. If this condition is found and if the cystic duct is very small and no stones can be palpated in the common duct, choledochostomy may not be indicated. Cholangitis or hepatitis may produce jaundice. In all operations for acute cholecystitis, an effort should be made to palpate the common duct and expose it if possible. Pronounced dilatation or palpable stones within the duct are indications for its exploration. If choledochostomy is performed, the duct should be drained with a T-tube.

CHRONIC NONCALCULUS CHOLECYSTITIS

A number of pathologic conditions of the gallbladder may exist without stone formation and are included in the classification of chronic noncalculus cholecystitis. Cholecystectomy is not followed by the high incidence of relief of symptoms when performed for noncalculus disease as is noted following its use for cholecystic disease with calculi. Noncalculus disease of the gallbladder does not carry with it the dangers associated with stones. Surgical therapy usually is not indicated and seldom, if ever, is urgent. Other organic or functional disorders may coexist and produce similar symptoms. This is true particularly in the presence of an indefinite or bizarre history.

Symptomatology.—Various forms of indigestion may be associated with chronic noncalculus cholecystitis. A feeling of fulness, belching, distention and heart burn are common complaints. These symptoms often come on or are aggravated by the ingestion of food. There may be qualitative food distress from some of the rougher types of vegetables and from fatty foods. Patients may also complain of quantitative food distress, that is, a greater amount of indigestion following a large meal. Pain may vary from a mild discomfort in the epigastrium or right upper quadrant to severe colics simulating those produced by calculi. The pain is likely to be brought on or aggravated by the intake of food. Some patients may complain of symptoms simulating peptic ulcer. Nervousness and emotional instability are common and may be accompanied by a feeling of weakness and debility. Constipation, "spastic colitis" and diffuse abdominal cramping or discomfort are common. Physical examination usually yields little information of value. Slight tenderness in the region of the gallbladder or over the liver is occasionally elicited.

Cholecystography.—A variety of interpretations may be obtained from cholecystograms. These may range from a nonfunctioning gallbladder to one that is interpreted to be normally functioning. Frequently the x-ray studies will indicate a poorly functioning gallbladder both as to its ability to concentrate dye and to empty. Calcification is occasionally seen in the wall of the gallbladder.

Diagnosis.—The diagnosis of chronic noncalculus cholecystitis is difficult to establish and more difficult to determine as a responsible factor in the patient's symptomatology. The patient should be thoroughly studied before any operative procedure is recommended. These studies should include gastrointestinal evaluation, care being taken to rule out esophageal lesions and esophageal hiatus hernias. Functional abnormalities of any portion of the gastrointestinal tract produce similar symptoms. Diseases of the urinary tract should be excluded. Stool studies to help eliminate pancreatic disease are important. The history should include a careful investigation for factors responsible for emotional or nervous system instability.

Treatment.—Patients in whom studies suggest chronic noncalculus cholecystitis should be treated conservatively. Operative procedures are seldom urgent and should be delayed. This is true especially when the gallbladder has some power of concentrating dye and of contracting and when pain is minimal. If abdominal exploration is eventually decided upon, all intra-abdominal organs should be carefully examined before the gallbladder is removed. Cholecystectomy is the procedure of choice if no other cause for the patient's symptoms is found, but results are likely to be unsatisfactory. Greatest relief is obtained by this operation in patients who have had severe pain of a colicky nature not attributable to other disease.

CHRONIC CALCULUS CHOLECYSTITIS

Chronically diseased gallbladders containing stones are one of the commonest pathologic conditions found in adults. They do not always produce symptoms and frequently coexist with other diseases producing symptoms similar to those of gallbladder disease. The removal of an asymptomatic, diseased gallbladder without correction of the true pathologic state accounts for a high percentage of poor results following biliary tract surgery. When a diseased gallbladder is producing symptoms and no coexisting disease is present, properly executed biliary tract surgery produces excellent results in a very high percentage of patients with a minimal risk. For this reason, it is important for the surgeon to be familiar with the symptomatology, diagnosis and differential diagnosis of biliary tract disease and to have the technical knowledge and ability to execute biliary tract surgery properly.

Symptomatology.—The symptoms produced by chronic cholecystitis and cholelithiasis may be grouped under several headings.

Dyspepsia. Digestive disturbances in chronic cholecystic disease probably are produced because there is an inadequate amount of bile available in the duodenum to mix with food immediately after its ingestion. This is the result of impaired gallbladder function. The most common complaints are a feeling of epigastric fulness and associated belching. These may occur during the ingestion of a meal or shortly after its completion. The dyspepsia frequently is associated with certain foods, the so-called qualitative food distress. Leafy and bulky vegetables and fatty or fried foods are most often indicted by patients. Distress produced by these foods does not necessarily indicate a digestive disease since many normal human digestive systems are unable to assimilate them. When these symptoms are due to cholecystic disease they may persist for years before additional symptoms develop. Perhaps even more important than qualitative food distress is quantitative food dyspepsia. Patients have their greatest degree of indigestion after the large meal of the day and are more likely to have distress after large Sunday and holiday dinners. The type of food eaten is of less importance than the amount. Patients with cholecystic disease often will eliminate one food after another, believing it to be the causative factor of their distress, until the diet is so restricted that nutritional deficiencies develop.

Pain. Pain is another accompaniment of cholecystic disease. It may consist only of an epigastric discomfort, perhaps best described as "a misery." This may occur periodically for years before severe pain develops. However, a true colic may be the first manifestation of a diseased gallbladder. There are few pains as severe as that produced by calculus cholecystitis. Onset usually occurs a short time after the ingestion of the heavy meal of the day. The commonest sites of origin are in the epigastrium and in the right upper quadrant. The pain may be localized or may radiate in various directions. It may travel around the right costal margin to the back, around both costal margins or occasionally be entirely confined to the left upper quadrant of the abdomen. Frequently it will radiate to the right scapular region. Occasionally it will radiate downward in the abdominal cavity. The pain may simulate cardiac pain in its location, and the differentiation may be difficult. Intensity of the pain often requires medication for relief. Small doses of morphine may aggravate the pain, owing to the production of a spasm of the sphincter of Oddi. Large doses of morphine usually give relief, although the pain may not subside until the patient has had an episode of nausea and vomiting. Nitroglycerin is recommended because it is supposed to relax the sphincter of Oddi. Its administration does not always produce relief.

Tenderness. Soon after the onset of pain tenderness can be elicited. It may be in the epigastrium but more often is noted in the right upper quadrant over the gallbladder area. Spasm of the right rectus muscle frequently accompanies the pain. Residual tenderness with or without muscle spasm may be detectable for one or more days after the attack. Fever and leukocytosis occur when the gallbladder becomes inflamed or acutely distended.

Jaundice. A sallowness of the skin which the patient interprets as jaundice may be noted but does not always indicate an increased icterus. A careful examination of the patient's sclera should be made to determine the presence or absence of true jaundice. Jaundice usually indicates the presence of stones in the common bile duct, but interference with the passage of bile through the common duct may result from pressure by the neck of the gallbladder against the common duct when the cystic duct is obstructed and the gallbladder becomes distended.

The behavior of patients during severe biliary colic is quite characteristic. They do not lie quietly but tend to roll around, put pressure against the upper abdomen and are restive, in contrast to patients with perforated peptic ulcer whose pain is aggravated by motion. Patients who have had repeated attacks of biliary colic often present a mottled skin in the right upper abdomen from repeated application of local heat. Occasionally a distended gallbladder can be palpated during or after a biliary colic but this is not the rule.

Diagnosis.—A good history is the most important single factor in the diagnosis of biliary tract disease. Cholelithiasis producing characteristic symptoms is seldom confused with manifestations of other diseases. In my experience the average patient gives a history of six years' duration before submitting to surgical therapy. They have had multiple attacks of biliary colic, usually increasing in frequency and severity. These have been accompanied by right upper quadrant tenderness followed by residual soreness on palpation for several days. Indigestion consisting of a feeling of fulness, belching and distention accompanies the attacks and is also present between them. Both qualitative and quantitative food factors induce indigestion, which is not periodic as it is in the patient with a typical peptic ulcer. Fever and leukocytosis may accompany the attacks. Jaundice is not common. The typical history usually does not present a diagnostic problem. Atypical symptoms demand a careful clinical investigation to eliminate diseases of other systems of the body. Much confirmatory evidence of cholecystic disease can be obtained by cholecystography.

CHOLECYSTOGRAPHY

Roentgenographic studies of the gallbladder are a most important adjunct in the diagnosis of cholecystic disease. With the development of radiopaque dyes which are secreted by the liver and concentrated in the gallbladder, visualization of the gallbladder is greatly improved and interpretation of its functional capacity as well as the determination of the presence of abnormalities within it can be made with remarkable accuracy. Used in conjunction with a careful clinical evaluation of the patient's history and other findings, cholecystography will insure better results of surgical therapy for gallbladder disease. However, mistakes will be too frequent if this aid to diagnosis is used as a substitute for careful clinical study and sound judgment on the part of the physician. Cholecystography can, with remarkable accuracy, inform us of the functional and organic status of the gallbladder. It can indicate the presence or absence of disease and often can reveal its nature. However, it cannot correlate the condition of the gallbladder with the symptomatology of the patient. Many persons have abnormal gallbladders which are asymptomatic. If these are removed on roentgenologic diagnosis alone, many patients will continue to suffer from symptoms due to other pathologic conditions. Although the percentage of errors in the interpretation of cholecystograms is small, errors occur sufficiently often to demand a careful correlation between the clinical history of the patient and radiologic evidences of disease.

Technic.—A number of technical factors in securing cholecystograms may confuse the interpretation and lead to erroneous diagnosis. It is customary to give patients an iodine-containing dye the evening before examination and to restrict the intake of fats with the evening meal. The next morning the patient should take repeated enemas to remove from the bowel gas and feces which may overlie the gallbladder and confuse the picture. One to 2 oz. of castor oil may be given to the patient the evening before administration of the dye. This aids greatly in evacuating the large intestine and avoiding confusing shadows. Some radiologists recommend the administration of castor oil on the same evening as the dye is taken. This may result in a rapid evacuation of the intestinal tract without absorption of an adequate amount of dye to give a good gallbladder shadow. X-rays of the gallbladder are taken from 12 to 18 hours after the oral ingestion of dye. A fat meal is then administered to stimulate evacuation of the gallbladder. From 10 to 20 minutes after the fat meal, additional exposures are made. The first of these are usually taken with the patient prone. Films taken with the patient in the upright, decubitus and Trendelenburg positions frequently will be helpful. Films taken in both the supine and the Trendelenburg position while pressure is being applied to the gallbladder area often will show stones which would escape detection on routine examinations.

If the gallbladder is not visualized by cholecystography, the examination should be repeated on the following day, an additional dose of dye being given the evening of the initial examination. In as many as 10 per cent of cases, the second examination will either demonstrate normal function or outline stones within the gallbladder.

[Illustrative cholangiograms *on page 108.*]

A.—This is a cholecystogram of a normally functioning gallbladder. The position may vary greatly. With increasing obesity the gallbladder will tend to assume a more horizontal position.

B.—This roentgenogram of the gallbladder in *A* was taken one hour after ingestion of a fat meal. The degree to which the shadow will diminish in size varies considerably and indicates the emptying capacity of the gallbladder.

C.—Abnormalities in the shape of the gallbladder are commonly encountered and do not necessarily indicate functional impairment of the organ. This deformity is quite common and is called a phrygian cap.

D.—The gallbladder in *C* contracted down satisfactorily after the administration of a fat meal.

E.—Septa may be located in various portions of the gallbladder and usually are congenital in origin. They may consist of a small infolding into the lumen of the gallbladder or may completely divide the structure into two separate cavities.

F.—Polypoid lesions of the gallbladder present areas of decreased density of the shadow owing to displacement of radiopaque dye within the gallbladder. They usually can be differentiated from stones because of their fixed position which does not vary with changes in position of the patient.

[Cholecystograms *continued on page 110.*]

PLATE 24

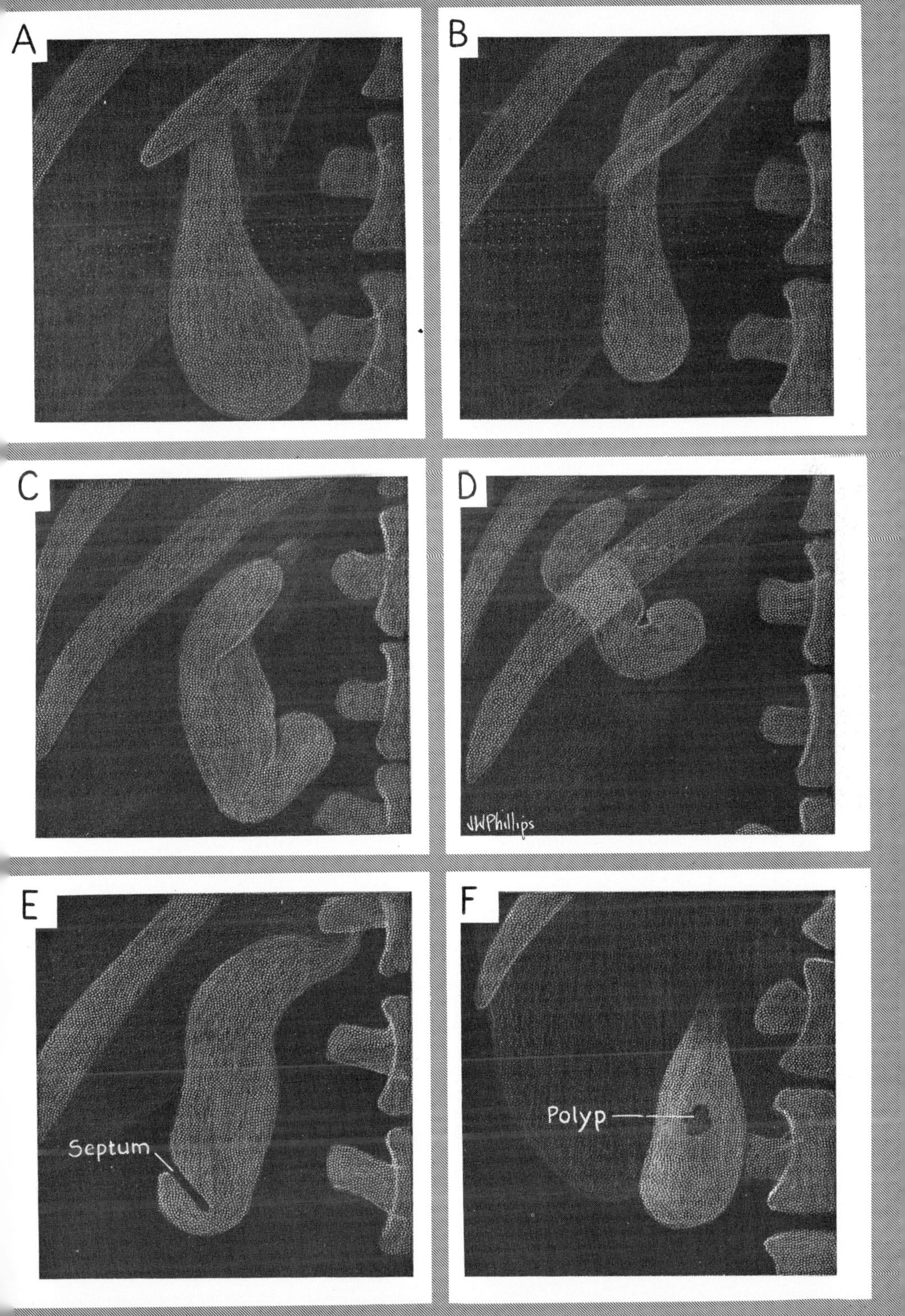

Gallstones which contain calcium are radiopaque and can be detected on x-ray films without the use of gallbladder dye. Cholesterol stones are radiolucent and are detected by negative shadows caused by displacement of radiopaque dye. If the dye does not enter the gallbladder, cholesterol stones will not be seen on roentgenograms.

G.—This shows a gallbladder containing concentrated dye with negative shadows produced by cholesterol stones.

H.—Some gallstones contain an opaque center surrounded by cholesterol and will produce contrasting shadows of stones.

I.—Amorphous calcium may be deposited in poorly functioning gallbladders and is spoken of as milk of calcium. This produces a diffuse opacity in the gallbladder, with the greatest density in the most dependent portion.

J.—Large solitary stones frequently produce a negative shadow surrounded by a circular opacity which is due to the deposition of calcium on the surface of the stone.

K.—Occasionally a gallbladder will extend down to or below the pelvic brim. This film shows such a gallbladder containing radiopaque stones, four of which are in the fundus of the gallbladder and one is lodged in the gallbladder neck.

L.—This gallbladder contains a stone blocking the neck of the gallbladder. The gallbladder is distended and contains calcium deposits. Such obstructing stones frequently are covered with a layer of calcium.

[Cholecystography *continued on page 112.*]

PLATE 24

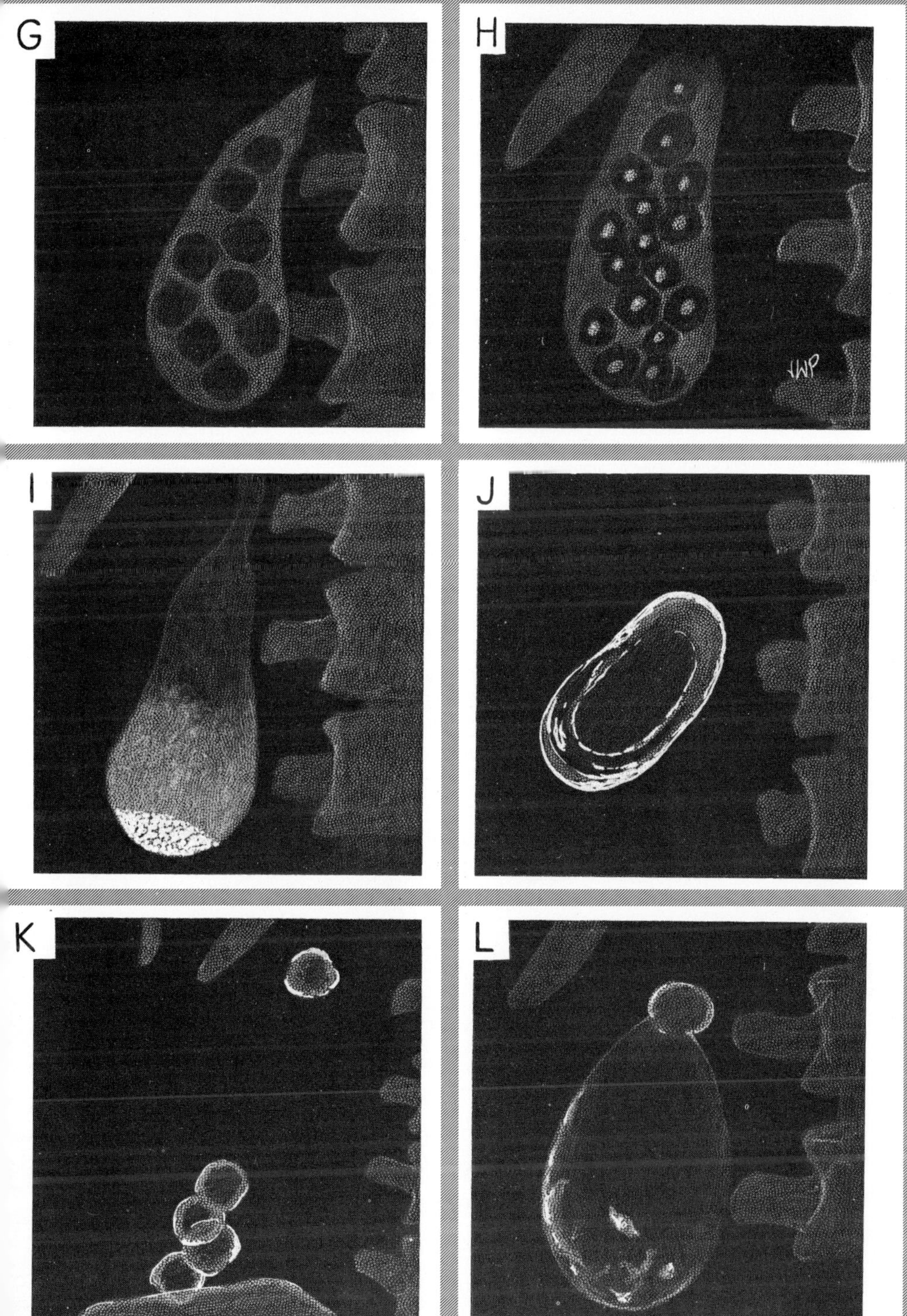

Modifications for Improved Accuracy

M.—Occasionally a functioning gallbladder may contain stones of the same opacity as the dye within the gallbladder. This will result in a homogeneous shadow suggesting a normally functioning gallbladder without stones.

N.—A plain film of the gallbladder region without dye will reveal these stones as opaque shadows. This film is of the same patient. She was given a barium meal which visualizes the stomach and duodenum. The gallbladder can be seen to contain opaque stones. This stresses the importance of taking a preliminary film of the gallbladder area the day before routine cholecystograms are made.

Occasionally a gallbladder which has diminished power of contraction will concentrate the bile within it to a thick viscid fluid. Following the ingestion of dye, additional bile will enter the gallbladder and will cast a shadow. Small stones may be present in such gallbladders and float between the layers of bile of different density.

O.—When the film is taken with the patient prone, such stones may not be visualized.

P.—A film taken with the patient in the upright position shows the layer of calculi forming a horizontal line across the gallbladder above the viscid bile.

Q.—A film taken with the patient lying on his right side again shows the stones floating between the two layers of bile and parallel to the long axis of the body. These films emphasize the importance of securing radiograms in various positions.

[Cholecystography *continued on page 114.*]

M

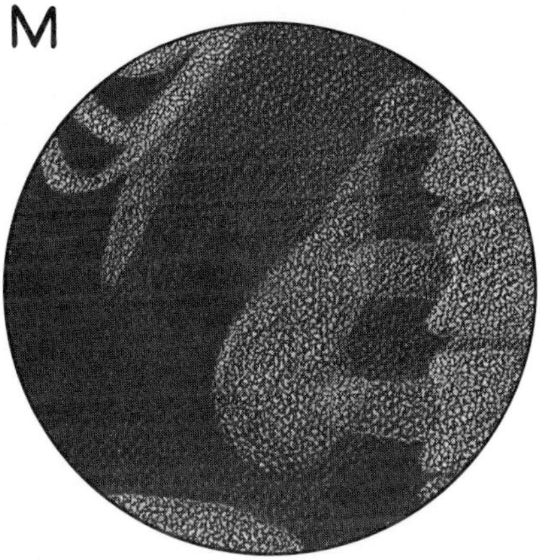

N

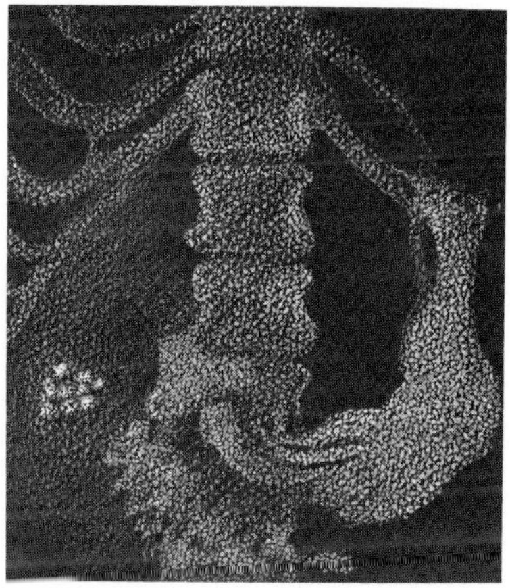

O

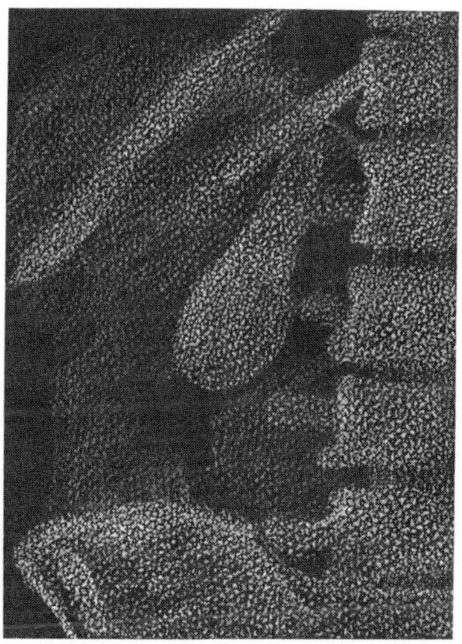

P

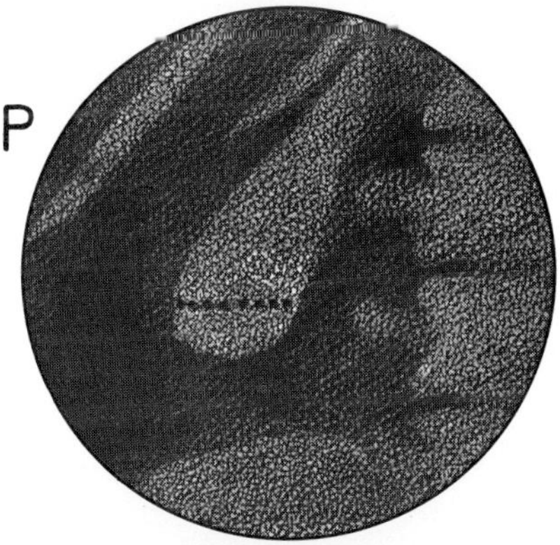

Q

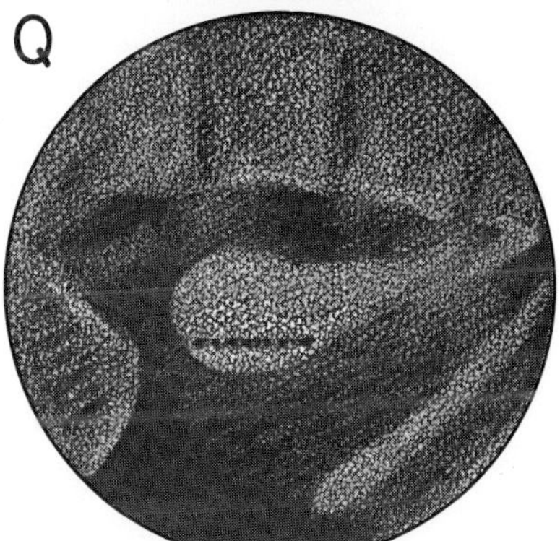

Causes of Unsatisfactory Cholecystograms

A number of factors may produce unsatisfactory cholecystograms. Failure of an adequate amount of dye to reach the liver may result from ingestion of an insufficient amount of dye, vomiting of the dye, pyloric obstruction with gastric retention or diarrhea causing inadequate absorption of the dye from the intestinal tract. Impaired liver function from various types of liver disease and from passive congestion may greatly reduce the secretion of dye.

Physiologic disturbances of the gallbladder may produce unsatisfactory cholecystograms. Gastric hyperchlorhydria or peptic ulcer can cause the gallbladder to empty rapidly. A low fat or fat-free diet may result in physiologic stasis of the gallbladder. Such diets are often prescribed or are self-selected by patients with digestive disturbances. The lack of stimulus to gallbladder emptying over a long period results in distention of the gallbladder with bile. Then when dye is administered, the dye-laden bile may enter the gallbladder but is diluted by the residual bile and the density of the cholecystogram is decreased. When a gallbladder visualizes poorly and a cholecystographic examination is to be repeated, the patient should receive a fat meal at noon on the day before examination to stimulate gallbladder contraction and to minimize the effects of stasis.

The action of certain drugs may interfere with the function of the extrahepatic biliary tract. Morphine produces spasm of the sphincter of Oddi, whereas atropine causes relaxation. Such action may interfere with gallbladder function.

The presence of air or fecal matter in the gastrointestinal tract overlying the gallbladder may make interpretation difficult. Some roentgenologists prefer to administer castor oil 24 hours before the ingestion of dye. It has been shown that castor oil does not cause the gallbladder to empty. The use of castor oil does not eliminate the use of enemas on the morning that roentgenograms are secured.

The accuracy of cholecystography makes it a most valuable adjunct in the diagnosis of chronic cholecystic disease with stones. When the interpretation of cholecystograms confirms the clinical diagnosis, the surgeon has added reassurance of the advisability of surgical therapy. Occasionally a patient will give a history of repeated attacks of typical biliary colic and dyspepsia but the radiologist will report the cholecystograms as presenting a normally functioning gallbladder without stones. Such a report should deter the surgeon from operating immediately and he should again carefully review the history and all x-ray and laboratory data. If he still is convinced that the patient's symptoms are produced by cholelithiasis, he is justified in performing a cholecystectomy. Occasionally such gallbladders will be found to contain stones which displace so little dye in the gallbladder as to be unrecognizable on the roentgenograms.

The intravenous injection of Cholografin (iodipamide) methylglucamine is useful to visualize the bile ducts in particular and at times the gallbladder or the cystic duct stump. Occasionally, when dye administered orally has failed to demonstrate the gallbladder, intravenous dye has revealed the gallbladder containing stones. Its greatest value, however, is to demonstrate the bile ducts in patients who have previously had the gallbladder removed.

The value of intravenous cholangiography varies with the functional capacity of the liver. It is not without danger, and sensitivity tests should be made before injecting the full dose of the dye. The bile ducts are best visualized in 10–15 minutes, with optimum concentration of dye in 20–25 minutes. Visualization of the gallbladder begins in about one hour, and the greatest concentration of dye within it is noted in about two hours.

A.—This is a conventional postcholecystectomy cholangiogram. It shows the common and hepatic ducts of normal diameter, with no evidence of stone.

B.—In this patient, a plain film of the abdomen revealed an opaque shadow which could have been within the common bile duct. This intravenous cholangiogram reveals a normal duct with the opaque shadow some distance away.

C.—This postcholecystectomy intravenous cholangiogram shows marked dilatation of the bile ducts, with bile flowing freely into the duodenum and with no visible evidence of stones.

D.—A postcholecystectomy cholangiogram demonstrates dilated bile ducts with a fairly large stone in the choledochus.

E.—This patient's gallbladder could not be visualized after oral administration of dye. The intravenous cholangiogram reveals normal bile ducts with a small gallbladder contracted down around one large stone.

F.—Following oral administration of dye, no gallbladder shadow was seen. Intravenous cholangiography demonstrated a gallbladder containing stones. The bile ducts appear normal.

[Intravenous cholangiography *continued on page 118.*]

PLATE 25

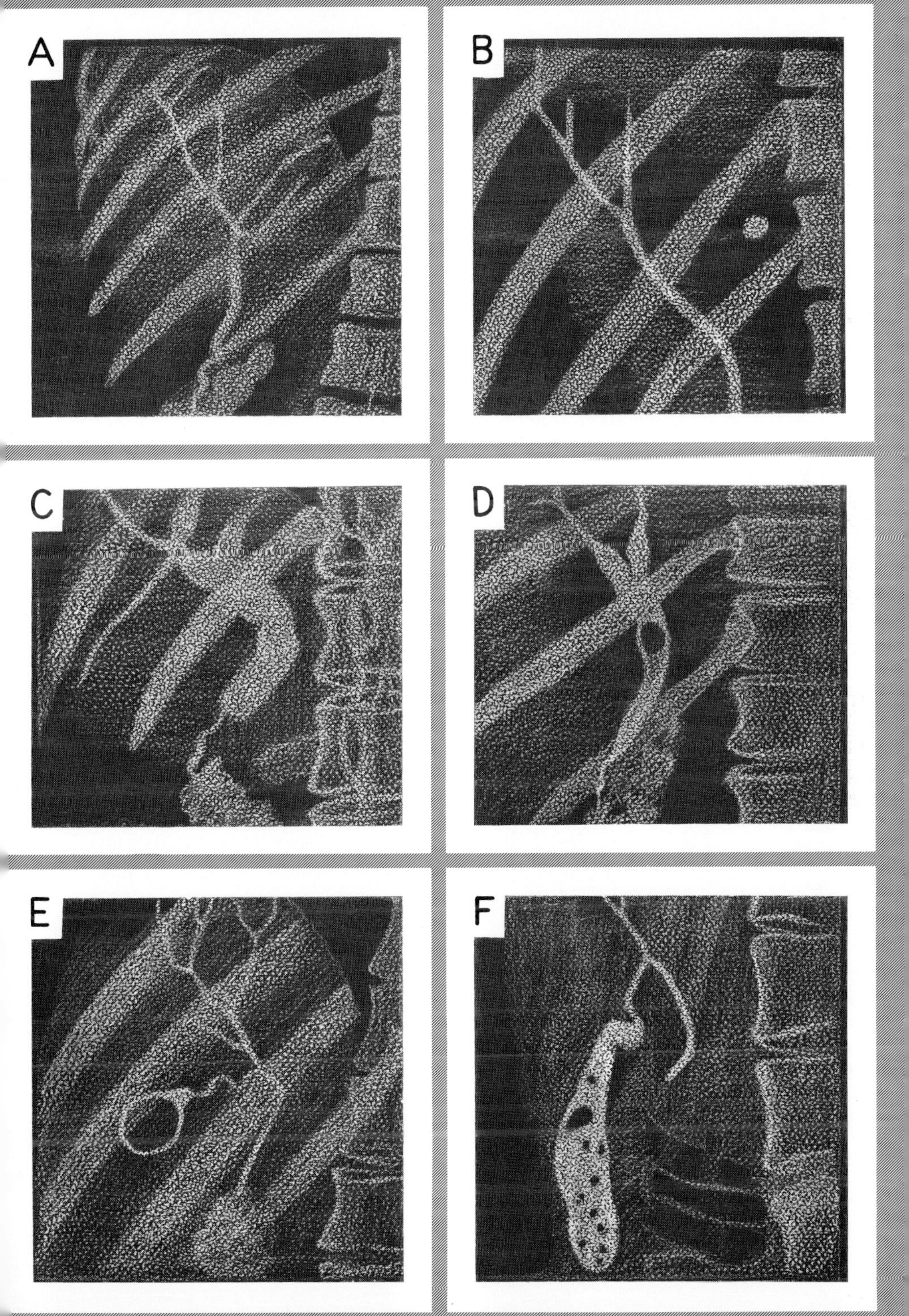

Body Section Radiography

Intravenous cholangiography frequently is unsatisfactory because of overlying shadows which may confuse interpretation of the film. These shadows may be due to gas or various other contents of the gastrointestinal tract or to dye in the pelvis of the kidney or ureter. Body section radiographs, also called laminographs, planographs, etc., frequently eliminate most extraneous shadows while visualizing the opaque medium in the bile ducts. This technic has greatly increased the value of intravenous radiography.

G.—A conventional intravenous cholangiogram faintly suggests the common duct but poorly defines it and does not demonstrate a calculus.

H.—This body section radiograph, made of the same patient after a second intravenous injection of Cholografin, clearly demonstrates the bile ducts and shows a calculus in the distal end of the common bile duct.

I.—Although this conventional cholangiogram suggests a dilated choledochus, overlying shadows make the interpretation uncertain and inaccurate.

J.—A body section radiograph was made of the same patient as that in *I.* It clearly shows a greatly dilated common duct containing two large calculi. Extraneous shadows have been quite well excluded.

K.—The use of opaque medium to visualize the extrahepatic biliary tract, whether given by mouth or vein, usually is contraindicated in the presence of jaundice. It seldom elicits information of value, especially if the level of serum bilirubin is above 5 mg. per 100 ml. Occasionally, however, some information may be gained by such studies. *K* is a body section radiograph of a jaundiced patient which demonstrates a very marked dilatation of the bile ducts with apparent obstruction at the distal end of the common duct. Conventional films of this patient had failed to show the bile ducts.

L.—This is an operative cholangiogram taken after the direct injection of dye into the common duct at the time of operation. It reveals a tremendous dilatation of the bile ducts due to obstruction of the distal choledochus.

PLATE 25

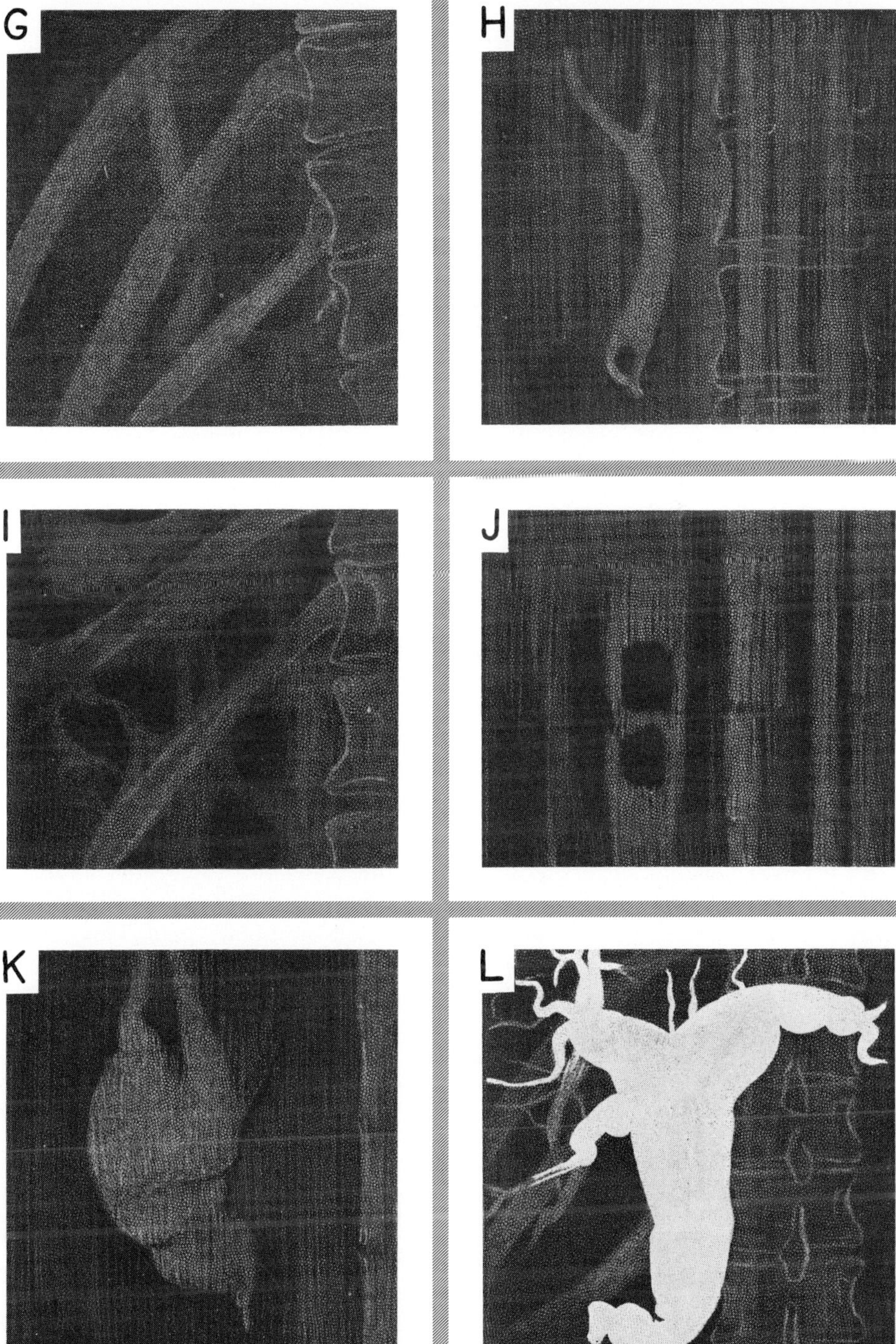

Differential Diagnosis

As errors in diagnosis are responsible for the greatest number of unsatisfactory results of biliary tract surgery, it is important that an exhaustive study of the patient be made before surgery is attempted. In the patient with typical biliary symptoms diagnosis is not difficult. However, when such symptoms do exist, coexisting diseases which are not recognized and treated may be the cause of a persistence of symptoms postoperatively. It is not within the scope of this book to give a detailed discussion of all pathologic conditions which may complicate biliary tract disease or be confused with it. However, the more common ones will be enumerated to emphasize their importance to the surgeon.

Functional disorders of the alimentary tract produce the largest and most confusing group for differential diagnosis. The symptoms closely simulate those of the more bizarre and less typical biliary tract complaints. These unfortunate patients frequently are treated over long periods by conservative management and eventually in desperation have their gallbladders removed because the organ is pathologic even though it may not be producing symptoms. The highly nervous or emotional patient with bizarre symptoms seldom is cured by cholecystectomy.

Many organic diseases may produce symptoms suggestive of biliary tract disease. Those of the alimentary tract are most frequently encountered. Esophageal hiatus hernia can produce dyspepsia with belching, a feeling of fulness and distention soon after eating. There may be pain in the epigastric or substernal region which at times is severe and hard to differentiate from biliary pain. This condition frequently coexists with cholelithiasis. The high incidence of cholecystectomy preceding the recognition and treatment of hiatus hernia attests to the confusion of these two diseases. Peptic ulcer which produces typical symptoms is not hard to differentiate from biliary disease. When its symptoms are bizarre, they may be confusing and careful study is then necessary to make an accurate diagnosis.

Inflammatory changes of the appendix may closely simulate cholecystic disease. This is especially true in a high-lying appendix. Lesions of the colon, particularly those of the cecum and ascending colon likewise may present a confusing diagnostic picture. Careful stool studies and x-rays of the colon are of great diagnostic value.

Renal calculi, particularly when located in the pelvis of the right kidney, can produce pain equally as severe and occasionally located in the same region as that produced by biliary colic. The careful study of the urinary tract usually will clarify this diagnosis.

Acute pancreatitis is very difficult to diagnose. This is attested to by the infrequency with which the diagnosis has been made preoperatively in patients in whom the existence of this condition is demonstrated on abdominal exploration. The pain, tenderness and leukocytosis may closely simulate those of cholecystitis, especially of the acute variety. An elevated blood serum amylase value is a significant finding in acute pancreatitis. Accurate diagnosis is most important because acute pancreatitis should be treated conservatively whereas acute cholecystitis may demand more urgent surgery. Pain produced by chronic pancreatitis seldom is similar to that of biliary tract disease. Chronic pancreatitis produces deep-seated pain above or slightly to the left of the umbilicus and radiating through to the lumbar area of the back. This contrasts to the right upper quadrant pain of biliary tract disease which frequently radiates around the right costal margin or to the right scapular area. When doubt of the diagnosis exists, it usually is advisable to observe the patient carefully and to use supportive therapy until the true nature of the disease can be more definitely ascertained.

Coronary artery disease may produce pain similar to that of biliary tract disease. Chronic pancreatitis produces deep-seated pain the epigastrium or to the substernal area. When doubt exists, a careful cardiac survey should be made, including electrocardiographic studies. Many physicians believe that there is a definite relation between biliary tract and cardiac disease. Biliary colic can produce electrocardiographic changes suggestive of cardiac disease. After the subsidence of the colic or following removal of a diseased gallbladder normal electrocardiograms are sometimes obtained. However, one should avoid any surgery, if possible, on a patient who has recently had a true anginal attack, and for this reason preoperative diagnostic accuracy is important.

Pneumonia can produce pain suggestive of disease of the gallbladder. Careful physical and roentgenologic examination of the chest will help determine the existence of pulmonary disease.

Asymptomatic Gallstones

Why does chronic cholecystitis or chronic cholelithiasis exist without producing clinical evidence of its presence? It is probable that symptoms are produced when the gallbladder cannot function but the sphincter of Oddi continues to maintain a high intraductal pressure and interferes with the free passage of bile into the intestinal tract. In contrast to this group, patients may lose the tonus of the sphincter of Oddi in conjunction with the loss of function of the gallbladder. This will permit a free flow of bile into the intestine and minimize or eliminate digestive disturbances of biliary origin. Absence of infection in the gallbladder is another factor in asymptomatology. Prevention of the extension of disease and of the development of complications has been used as an argument in favor of removal of the asymptomatic gallbladder. There is some difference of opinion that this is just cause for the surgeon to urge cholecystectomy. The patient should be apprised of the dangers of the disease and of the advantages of early removal of the gallbladder. If he declines surgical therapy, he should be made aware of the symptoms which herald complications, particularly the effort of small stones to pass through the cystic duct. When such symptoms occur, surgery should not be delayed.

Cholecystic disease may be a precursor to cardiac disease. This fact is not sufficiently well established to justify cholecystectomy to prevent coronary disease. Carcinoma of the gallbladder almost invariably is associated with a long-standing chronic cholecystitis and cholelithiasis. The development of carcinoma of the gallbladder, however, occurs so rarely that operation upon a diseased gallbladder hardly seems justifiable merely for the prevention of carcinoma.

Large solitary gallstones.—This condition, even though asymptomatic, I believe presents a real hazard. These stones cannot pass through the cystic duct and when they become lodged in the neck of the gallbladder often produce rapidly developing and serious complications. These may consist of an acute cholecystitis, gangrene of the gallbladder and often perforation and necrosis of its wall. The stone may erode into any hollow viscus and produce a spontaneous internal biliary fistula. It may erode into the gastrointestinal tract and pass distally until an intestinal obstruction is produced. The dangers of complications of a large solitary gallstone are sufficiently great, in my opinion, to justify the recommendation that cholecystectomy be performed even though the patient is asymptomatic.

Treatment of Cholecystic Disease

Conservative or nonsurgical treatment of symptomatic gallbladder disease has little to offer the patient. Restrictive diets may lessen the frequency of colics and minimize dyspepsia. Medication can diminish or relieve the pain of acute attacks and conservative therapy can aid in the recovery from such episodes. However, no known medical treatment can dissolve gallstones in the gallbladder or return a diseased gallbladder to a normal anatomic and physiologic state. Procrastination and delay of surgical therapy frequently permits a disease which has been confined to the gallbladder and which could have been completely cured to involve other structures where the disease presents a greater hazard and where operative treatment cannot offer as high an incidence of good results. Yet statistics show that such delay in adequate treatment is the rule. The fault lies partly with the patient who usually is not urged to be operated upon during an acute attack and who feels so well between attacks that he hopes he will have no recurrences. The delay is often due to the family physician who does not urge the patient to be operated on and does not inform him of the hazards of delay. Both the patient and the physician may know of instances in which biliary tract surgery failed to relieve symptoms and thus are hesitant about employing operative therapy. An understanding by the profession of the causes of poor results of biliary tract surgery and diligence in avoiding them will allow proper surgical therapy of symptomatic cholelithiasis to assume its proper place.

Cholecystostomy.—Removal of stones from the gallbladder but failure to remove the gallbladder itself is rarely justifiable. Disease of the gallbladder wall almost invariably accompanies the presence of gallstones and is one of the greatest factors in their formation. If the gallbladder is merely evacuated, the incidence of re-formation of stones is very high and subsequent operation is often necessary to remove the organ and to attempt to correct complications of the disease. Cholecystostomy is more justifiable in the acutely inflamed or gangrenous gallbladder than in one which is chronically diseased.

The trauma and operative time are usually a little greater for removing than for draining a chronically diseased gallbladder. However, in a very poor risk patient or in an elderly and debilitated individual this little difference may be important and cholecystostomy may be justified.

Cholecystectomy.—Cholecystectomy is the operation of choice and when properly executed in an adequately prepared patient carries very little risk. The technic of these operations will be described in Chapter 11.

TUMORS OF THE GALLBLADDER

Benign tumors.—Papillomas of the gallbladder are relatively common lesions. They usually are small and may be multiple. The tumors themselves seldom produce symptoms. However, they are frequently associated with chronic cholecystitis and with cholelithiasis, both of which conditions may produce symptoms referable to the gallbladder. Often they are not diagnosed until the gallbladder has been examined at autopsy or after surgical removal. They can be detected by cholecystography if the gallbladder is able to concentrate dye (Plate 24, *F*). On roentgenograms they appear as filling defects which maintain their relative positions in the gallbladder despite changes of position of the patient. Roentgenograms taken from various positions will show the lesion arising from the wall of the gallbladder. Papillomas are always small, in contrast to adenomas which are rarely found but which may attain a fairly large size. Other benign tumors of the gallbladder are extremely rare.

Carcinoma.—Primary carcinoma of the gallbladder is a rare disease. Early medical literature reported an incidence as high as 5 per cent in all gallbladders treated surgically. More recent medical literature indicates its presence in from 0.5 to 2 per cent of patients with cholecystic disease. We have recently reviewed the records of 29 patients in whom the diagnosis of primary carcinoma of the gallbladder was established histologically. The incidence was slightly more than one of every 1,000 diagnoses of carcinoma. This low figure is partially accounted for by the fact that nearly all the patients were males, whereas carcinoma of the gallbladder is far more common in the female.

As the specific cause of carcinoma remains obscure, so also does the etiology of malignancy of the gallbladder. However, there seems to be a definite relation between gallstones and primary carcinoma of the gallbladder, and this relationship was found in a large series of medical reports summarized which showed that about 85 per cent of patients with carcinoma of the gallbladder also had gallstones.

Carcinoma of the gallbladder is a rapidly spreading disease with early extension into the liver, the bile ducts and their surrounding lymphatics and eventually to various organs of the body.

Symptomatology.—Because of the pre-existence of cholecystic disease with stones, there may be a history of gallbladder symptoms long before symptoms are produced by the malignancy. In our patients the symptoms most frequently encountered were pain, dyspepsia, weight loss and jaundice. The pain, an admitting symptom in over 90 per cent of patients, was usually located in the right upper quadrant or epigastrium, being intermittent or cramping in earlier stages but later becoming constant and progressive. Most patients complained of dyspepsia consisting of belching, nausea and vomiting. Over two thirds of the patients had noted a definite weight loss and more than half were jaundiced on hospitalization. A mass could be palpated in the right upper abdomen in about two thirds of the patients and there was often an associated tenderness. All patients on whom cholecystograms were made had nonfunctioning gallbladders. Barium studies of the gastrointestinal tract frequently revealed filling defects suggestive of an extrinsic mass in the right upper quadrant causing gastrointestinal deformities.

Treatment.—Because of the rapid spread of carcinoma of the gallbladder, the results of treatment are most discouraging. In all but three of the 29 patients an abdominal exploration was carried out and in nine a cholecystectomy was performed. In five of these the diagnosis was not suspected until pathologic studies of the gallbladder had been made. In two, a wedge resection of the liver at the site of the gallbladder bed was performed in an effort to remove any extension of the disease into the liver (Plate 7).

Results.—All 29 patients died of extension of the primary lesion. Death occurred in 20 patients in less than three months. The two longest survivors lived 18 months.

Prophylaxis.—It has been recommended that cholecystectomy be performed when gallstones are present to prevent the development of carcinoma of the gallbladder. Because malignancy of this organ is such a rare disease, this form of prophylaxis hardly seems justifiable. However, symptomatic cholelithiasis and large solitary gallstones, when neglected, produce other complications sufficiently often to make cholecystectomy advisable for relief of the disease and for prevention of such complications. In these patients the operation also serves as prophylaxis against carcinoma.

CHAPTER 8

Complications of Cholecystic Disease

DELAY IN THE surgical treatment of cholecystic disease, especially when stones are present, may lead to a number of complications. A gallstone may completely obstruct the neck of the gallbladder or the cystic duct. This will be followed by a gradual absorption of bile salts and pigment from the gallbladder and the secretion of mucus into the gallbladder, producing a hydrops. Such gallbladders may become greatly enlarged and may simulate other cystic conditions within the abdomen. Occlusion of the outlet of the gallbladder by stones may cause distention of the gallbladder and result in pressure of the neck of the gallbladder against the common duct, producing obstructive jaundice. This may occur even though no disease is present within the common bile duct. Occasionally pressure may be exerted against the portal vein and produce symptoms of portal hypertension. An adequate cholecystectomy will relieve these conditions.

Infections within the gallbladder, especially when associated with obstruction of the neck, may lead to varying degrees of suppuration, necrosis and peritonitis. These have been discussed under Acute Cholecystitis in Chapter 7.

BILIARY FISTULAS

Biliary fistulas are not uncommon complications of cholecystic disease. However, external fistulas are quite rare, and spontaneous external biliary fistulas are seldom encountered in modern day medicine. These usually result from an abscessed gallbladder pointing through the abdominal wall. Occasionally an abscess of the abdominal wall will form and, when incised, bile and gallstones may be extruded. Postoperative external biliary fistulas are more commonly seen and usually result from inadequate surgery upon the biliary tract. They not infrequently follow cholecystostomy or incomplete removal of the gallbladder. They indicate an inadequate drainage of bile into the duodenum and are associated with common duct stones, strictures and other obstructive lesions (Chapter 12).

SPONTANEOUS INTERNAL BILIARY FISTULAS.—These fistulas are not uncommon. I have encountered existing or healed fistulas in 3 per cent of patients operated on for biliary tract disease. They may exist between the gallbladder or common bile duct and any hollow viscus within the abdomen or between the intrahepatic bile ducts and a bronchus. Most internal biliary fistulas are formed by the erosion of gallstones through the wall of the gallbladder and into an adjacent viscus. It is usually a large gallstone which is likely to produce a fistula. The majority of fistulas exist between the gallbladder and duodenum. I have encountered them also between the gallbladder and colon, stomach and common bile duct. They have been reported extending into all parts of the gastrointestinal tract, the kidney pelvis, portal vein, ovarian cysts and bladder. Occasionally an inflammatory disease of an adjacent structure, such as a duodenal or gastric ulcer may perforate into the gallbladder or common duct or may render the sphincter action at the duodenal end of the common duct incontinent and produce a fistula in the reverse direction.

Symptomatology.—In our series of patients with spontaneous internal biliary fistulas, all have given a history of severe to intense attacks of colic for an average of eight years. Jaundice occurred in nearly all patients, being recurrent in a few and persistent in the majority. These patients were acutely ill, debilitated and gave a history of moderate to marked weight loss. The symptoms were more severe and the debility was greater than is usually seen in cholecystic disease. It has been stated that patients in whom spontaneous internal biliary fistulas develop have a history of long-standing gallbladder disease and then after a particularly severe attack are relieved of all symptoms. This was not true in any of our patients. Reflux of intestinal contents into the bile ducts produced an ascending cholangitis and hepatitis and, at operation, pronounced liver damage was noted in many of the patients. The result was the same whether the regurgitation was from the stomach, duodenum or colon. However, colon contents seemed to produce a more acute and virulent reaction. Large gallstones may erode into the intestinal tract and pass distally until they occlude the lumen of the small bowel, producing intestinal obstruction.

Diagnosis.—Cholecystograms are of little value in the diagnosis of internal biliary fistulas because of the severe dysfunction and disease of the gallbladder. Barium studies of the gastrointestinal tract often show a regurgitation of the opaque medium through the fistula, outlining the gallbladder and bile ducts and often demonstrating stones within them (Plate 26). Frequently air can be demonstrated in the gallbladder or bile ducts.

Treatment.—Treatment for spontaneous internal biliary fistulas consists of eradication of the fistulous tract, removal of the gallbladder, evacuation of all stones and debris from the common bile duct and drainage of the common bile duct. One must be certain that no obstruction to the flow of bile into the duodenum exists at the conclusion of the operation.

Results of treatment.—Because of the existence of a suppurative cholangitis and varying degrees of hepatitis the mortality in surgery for spontaneous internal biliary fistula is comparatively high and the end results are less satisfactory than those obtained in treatment of uncomplicated cholelithiasis. The dangers of this disease emphasize the importance of early surgical treatment of cholecystic disease before the development of such complications. When surgical therapy is instituted, intensive preoperative and postoperative management is essential for the protection of the diseased liver. If suppurative cholangitis exists at the time of operation, the patient should be carefully followed because of the danger of re-formation of stones within the bile ducts.

A. This patient had a cholecystogastric fistula. Barium outlines the stomach and is also seen in the intrahepatic ducts.

B.—This patient was given barium by mouth. A cholecystoduodenal fistula permitted entrance of the barium into the gallbladder where it is visualized radiographically.

C.—Following a barium enema, barium has entered the biliary tract through a cholecystocolic fistula and has disseminated gradually through the intrahepatic bile ducts.

D.—A choledochoduodenal fistula has permitted regurgitation of barium from the intestinal tract into the common bile duct and intrahepatic ducts.

E.—Barium was given by mouth to a patient with a cholecystoduodenal fistula. After barium had passed from the stomach and intestines, both barium and air remained to outline the gallbladder and bile ducts and to demonstrate an obstruction of the distal end of the common bile duct.

F.—When a fistula exists between the extrahepatic biliary tract and the gastrointestinal tract, air or gas frequently will pass into the bile ducts and will outline them radiographically.

Hepatobronchial fistulas frequently are preceded by the development of a subphrenic abscess and empyema, with eventual erosion into the bronchus (Plate 14). They may result from bile duct obstruction due to stones or from amebic abscesses in the liver. The presence of bile in the sputum is diagnostic of hematobronchial fistula.

PLATE 26

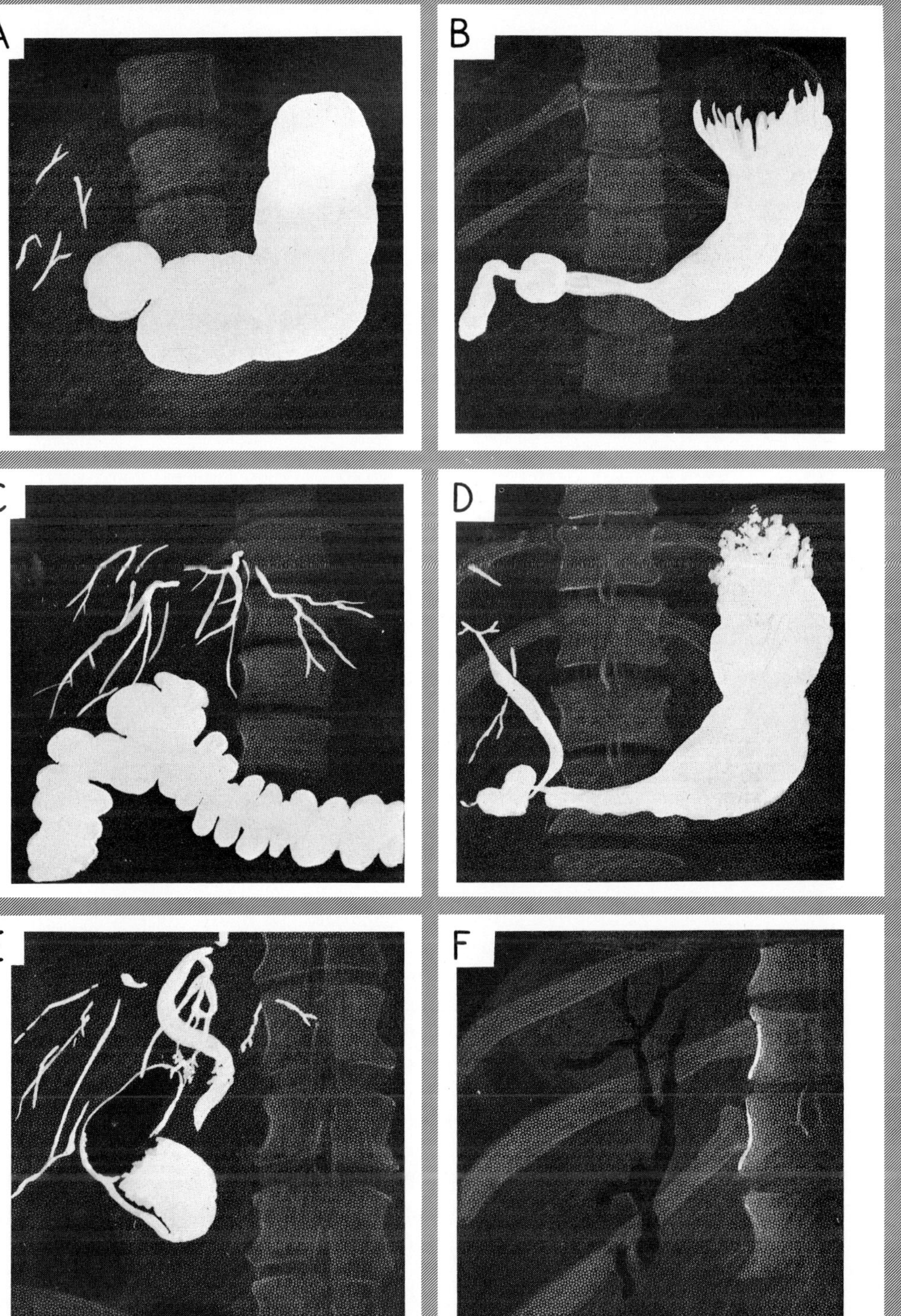

CHAPTER 9

Preoperative and Postoperative Management

PREOPERATIVE MANAGEMENT

THE LONG time interval between the onset of biliary tract symptoms and the institution of surgical therapy permits the development of many physiologic and pathologic changes which may add to the risk of operation. As in all fields of surgery, the dangers of the disease must be weighed against the hazards of its treatment. Elective operations are justifiable only after the completion of preoperative preparation which will minimize the incidence and severity of operative and postoperative dangers and complications. Acute diseases of the biliary tract which demand immediate surgical intervention fortunately constitute but a small percentage of surgical diseases of this system.

Much information can be learned from the history of the patient which will enable the surgeon to estimate the functional capacity of the liver and other involved organs as well as the extent of pathologic changes which have occurred in them. Patients with biliary tract disease are prone to limit their diet, either by their own volition or on advice of a physician, to a degree that nutritional deficiencies develop. One type of food after another is eliminated from the diet until an inadequate intake of many essential elements may increase the dangers of any surgical procedure. Laboratory studies may not reveal these changes. If a careful history of the patient's eating habits suggests the possibility of nutritional impairment, it may be necessary to delay operation for days or weeks to restore a safe nutritional state by proper dietary measures. Progressive weight loss may result in tissue impairment which will delay healing processes and functional activity. The surgeon must remember that an operation adds the insults produced by anesthesia and operative trauma to the already existing disease. The preoperative diet must contain an abundance of protein, calories, minerals and vitamins to restore nutrition to an optimal state. In debilitated patients this requires a longer time than is indicated by the return of functional tests to a normal level.

The results of laboratory studies should be carefully evaluated because many of the tests give abnormal findings only in the presence of pronounced physiologic or pathologic changes. Anemia should be corrected by medication or blood transfusion. In the presence of liver damage, careful selection of blood and meticulous cross-matching will minimize the danger of reaction and further liver damage. A prolonged prothrombin time may be corrected by the use of vitamin K. The levels of blood sugar, amylase and lipase and the estimation of digestion by stool studies will indicate the degree of pancreatic function and the possibility of coexisting pancreatic disease. Careful studies of the urine and of kidney function are of importance because of the frequency with which renal and hepatic damage coexist. It is a good rule to consider all patients with disease of the biliary tract to have functional impairment which must be corrected to as great a degree as possible by adequate preoperative preparation.

Psychologic factors are important in surgery of the biliary tract as in all types of surgery. The patient's apprehension must be allayed as much as possible. When disease is confined to the gallbladder, the patient must be assured that he can live comfortably and normally without this organ and with minimal restrictions after its removal. He may be consoled by the knowledge that the risk of operation is small, especially when compared to the dangers of complications of the disease. The surgeon must spend sufficient time with the patient to gain his confidence and allay his fears. The purposes of various preoperative and postoperative procedures should be explained, with emphasis on their importance in the prevention of complications, so that their institution will not cause undue alarm to the patient and his family.

The jaundiced patient requires intensive preoperative preparation. Diagnostic studies must establish, so far as possible, the etiology of the jaundice. Fortunately, the jaundiced patient seldom requires emergency surgery. Sufficient time usually can be taken both to establish the diagnosis and to prepare the patient adequately for operation. Surgical procedures upon patients with hepatocellular jaundice usually do not benefit the patient but add to the hazards of the disease. It is seldom necessary to operate at the time of an increasing jaundice. Patients with intermittent obstruction of the bile ducts due to stones usually have a fluctuating jaundice and may have less postoperative reaction if operated on when the jaundice is diminishing or has subsided. In patients with complete obstruction of the bile ducts there will be a gradually increasing jaundice which eventually levels off. The surgical risk is less at this stage than while the jaundice is increasing. Jaundiced patients require a maximal degree of liver protection. They should be placed on a high protein, high caloric diet containing adequate vitamins, especially vitamin K. It may be advisable to supplement oral feedings by the intravenous administration of glucose. Great caution should be exercised in the use of blood and plasma. When maximal improvement has been attained, the surgeon should select an operative procedure which will accomplish the desired purpose with the least amount of trauma and shock.

Hospitalization.—The crowded condition of many hospitals often necessitates a delay in the patient's admission. Many factors may develop during this period which will increase the hazards of operation.

Preoperative hours of hospitalization may considerably shorten the postoperative length of hospital stay. I believe all patients who are to undergo biliary tract surgery should be hospitalized for a minimum of 36 hours before operation. This permits time for careful re-evaluation of the patient and for essential laboratory studies. Febrile states can be detected, as can the presence of respiratory infection, suppurative skin disease and other conditions which might make it advisable to delay the operative procedure. Elderly and debilitated patients and those with considerable hepatic damage should be hospitalized for longer periods before operation.

Immediate preoperative care.—The patient should have a good night's sleep before operation to secure good mental and physical rest. Barbiturates usually are administered but should be given in small doses because impaired liver function may prolong their activity. Nembutal or Seconal, $\frac{3}{4}$ gr., usually gives good sedation in the absence of pain. Enemas usually are given before operation because of delayed bowel activity postoperatively. They have merit when needed but disturb some patients and I believe are unnecessary if the patient's bowels have been well evacuated the day before operation. It is our routine to administer 10 mg. of vitamin K intramuscularly twice daily before operation while the patient is in the hospital. Preoperative medication is discussed in Chapter 10. Doses of opiates should be minimal to lessen the immediate postoperative depression.

The intranasal insertion of gastric suction tubes before operation decompresses the stomach. This often facilitates the technic of the operative procedure by reducing gastric distention which may interfere with adequate exposure. If the operative procedure involves only the biliary tract, a single-lumen tube of Levin or Wangensteen type is very satisfactory. The tube should be of relatively small caliber to minimize discomfort in the nose and throat. It should be inserted on the morning of operation rather than the night before because irritation caused by the tube may keep the patient awake and prevent adequate preoperative rest. If the operation will include some form of gastrointestinal anastomosis, a double-lumen tube such as the Rawson-Abbott or Puestow-Olander tube should be inserted before operation. The feeding limb can be placed through the anastomosis and into the intestine at the time of operation to permit early intestinal feeding. In recent years, Foley catheter gastrostomies and polyethylene feeding tubes that extend into the distal jejunal limb and are brought out through the abdominal wall have been used extensively in place of nasogastric tubes.

The infusion of intravenous fluids (p. 147) should be started before the patient is anesthetized and should be continued throughout the operation and early postoperative period.

POSTOPERATIVE MANAGEMENT

PAIN.—The avoidance or relief of pain is one of the most important postoperative responsibilities. Morphine is probably the most satisfactory drug to accomplish this. Small doses usually are adequate and should be used to minimize respiratory depression. In most cases the dosage should not exceed 8.0 mg., especially in small or debilitated patients but 10.0 mg. may be given to large and robust patients. Demerol in doses of 50–100 mg. is effective in many patients. Much less medication is required to avoid the development of pain than to relieve it after it has become severe. It is well to administer the drug soon after the patient has recovered his reflexes and has emerged from the effects of the anesthetic agent but before pain has developed or become severe. If this is done, it is usually unnecessary to administer further sedation on the day of operation. Occasionally a second injection may be indicated on the evening of the operative day to encourage a good night's sleep. Repeated doses of opiates not only produce respiratory depression but interfere with intestinal motility and may be responsible for the development of nausea, vomiting, distention and gas pains. If pain relief is needed on subsequent days, Demerol or codeine usually will suffice.

INTRAVENOUS FLUIDS.—On the day of operation the patient should be given an average of 2,000 cc. of fluid by vein. In most patients, 1,000 cc. of 5 per cent dextrose in water and 1,000 cc. of 5 per cent dextrose in saline are adequate. Vitamins B, C and K may be added to these solutions. The solutions should be administered at a rate not greater than 60 drops per minute. If there is a large fluid loss from the body by gastric suction, bile drainage or from other sources, additional fluids should be administered to compensate for the loss. Intravenous fluids should be administered on subsequent postoperative days only as a substitute for or to supplement oral intake. If gastric suction is maintained, the patient should receive at least 2,000 cc. of fluid daily plus replacement for fluid loss. A sufficient amount of fluid should be administered to maintain a urinary output of approximately 1,000 cc. in each 24 hours. If there is evidence of potassium deficiency, Ringer's solution should be substituted for physiologic saline solution in addition to other potassium therapy. It is well to add vitamins to all fluids administered by vein.

GASTROINTESTINAL SUCTION.—The use of suction tubes in the stomach greatly aids in minimizing nausea and vomiting. These symptoms do not persist in a high percentage of patients beyond the first few postoperative hours. Suction tubes usually produce considerable discomfort to the patient and should be removed as early as possible. In most operations upon the biliary tract which do not include surgery of the gastrointestinal tract, the tubes can be removed at the end of operation or a few hours after operation. If vomiting subsequently occurs, the suction tubes may be reinserted.

When a gastrointestinal anastomosis is performed in conjunction with biliary tract surgery and a double-lumen tube is inserted to maintain gastric decompression and at the same time permit intestinal feeding, the tube must be left in place until the surgeon is convinced that the anastomosis is functioning and that oral intake will not be complicated by gastric distention and vomiting. This may not occur for from three to five days after operation. Gastric emptying through the anastomotic stoma may be verified by discontinuing suction upon the tube, administering liquids by mouth and in one to two hours re-establishing suction to determine if the stomach is empty. If there is no gastric retention, the tube may be removed. While the double-lumen tube is in place it permits intestinal feedings of an adequate diet during the early postoperative days. This is most important, especially to debilitated patients. Liquids may be administered which contain abundant amounts of all food elements. The feedings should not include food substances which may regurgitate around the tube and coagulate to obstruct the suction openings within the stomach. If Foley catheter and jejunal feeding tubes are used, they should be kept in place for at least 10 days after operation to prevent possible leakage of intestinal contents into the peritoneal cavity.

Oral feedings.—Gastric irritation resulting from operative trauma, medication and anesthetic agents makes it advisable to reduce oral feedings to a minimum on the day of operation. Intravenous infusion can satisfy the patient's requirements. Small sips of water may be given to relieve dryness of the mouth and throat. Large amounts of oral fluids should be avoided. On the day after operation liquids in the form of water, tea, coffee or broth should be given in amounts tolerated by the patient. If the oral intake does not approximate 2,000 cc., supplemental fluids should be administered intravenously. On subsequent postoperative days the diet should be increased as rapidly as can be tolerated by the patient. The diet should be high in protein to support the liver.

Dietary restrictions imposed by a long period of qualitative food distress produce a psychologic fear of certain foods which is difficult for the patient to overcome. It is well to administer such foods to patients during the postoperative hospital stay to assure them that with removal of the disease, they may lead a normal dietary life.

Care of the bowels.—The restriction of the oral intake of food on the day of operation and the early postoperative days leaves little residue to be evacuated from the bowel. One should not be concerned if the patient's bowels do not move during the first 48 or 72 postoperative hours. If the patient does not complain of abdominal discomfort, it is unnecessary to give enemas soon after operation. Early ambulation is conducive to the early return of normal bowel habits. Enemas should be given only when indicated.

Urination.—Many patients are unable to void while lying in bed. The loss of fluids by respiration and perspiration may delay bladder distention and a desire to void. Patients often will not void for 12–24 hours after operation. If there is bladder discomfort and percussion reveals a distended bladder, and if the patient is unable to void while lying in bed, he should be assisted to stand at the side of the bed to encourage spontaneous evacuation of the bladder. After the first voluntary urination, the patient seldom has difficulty. Catheterization should only be used as a last resort. When once performed, it is essential that it be repeated at sufficiently frequent intervals to avoid overdistention of the bladder, and urinary antiseptics must be administered to decrease the danger of a urinary tract infection.

Ambulation.—Early ambulation is of value to counteract the development of progressive weakness of the patient and may have some bearing on postoperative complications. Patients may be out of bed on the day after operation. Weak and debilitated patients should not be ambulated until they have recovered sufficient strength to avoid severe prostration from the effort of getting out of bed. The time at which patients are ambulated is an individual problem with each patient.

Antibiotics.—Because a large percentage of operations upon the biliary tract are performed for diseases which do not have an associated infection, antibiotics should not be used routinely. When infection exists, they are indicated. They also may be used when postoperative complications indicate the development of infection. However, these agents are not without danger and should be used judiciously.

Blood transfusions.—The administration of blood to patients with biliary tract disease should be carried out cautiously because of the possibility of liver damage. Cross-matching of blood must be accurate. Blood of the same type as that of the patient is preferable to blood from a universal donor. Blood transfusion is of value in the presence of progressive anemia or when there is persistent bleeding.

Care of the Wound

Penrose drain.—As mentioned under surgical technics, we believe it important to place a Penrose drain down to Morison's pouch or in the subhepatic space in all operations upon the biliary tract. Such drains are important to permit the escape of bile or intestinal contents if there should be any leakage of these fluids into the peritoneal cavity. We do not believe the drains prolong convalescence or weaken the abdominal wall. If no drainage occurs around the drains, they may be shortened on the third or fourth day and removed 24 hours later. When drainage occurs, the drains may be shortened but should be left in place until the drainage has become minimal or ceased.

T-tubes.—T-tubes should not be attached to any connecting tubing or receptacle because traction upon them might dislodge the cross-arm within the common duct and bile peritonitis may result. Spilling of bile upon dressings or bedding is inconsequential compared to the damage which can result from a displaced T-tube. Bile usually drains freely from T-tubes in the early postoperative days because edema of the distal end of the common duct resulting from the passage of instruments interferes with the free passage of bile into the duodenum. This temporary obstruction usually subsides in from four to eight days. If the patient is not jaundiced, the T-tube may be clamped on about the seventh postoperative day. The first clamping should remain for about one hour, with instructions that the clamp should be removed if right upper quadrant pain develops. If no distress occurs, the length of time the tube is clamped may be rapidly increased, until by the tenth day the tube may be clamped for 24 hours. If the patient has no distress and if, on removal of the clamp, bile does not flow from the T-tube until its end is lowered to the level of the anterior abdominal wall, the surgeon can feel assured that there is no increased pressure within the common duct and that bile is flowing freely into the duodenum. At this time, the tube may be removed by gentle traction. If there is evidence of increased intraductal pressure, the tube should remain in place until subsequent measurements establish that intraductal pressure is about equal to intra-abdominal pressure.

T-tubes inserted in the common ducts of jaundiced patients should be left in place without clamping until the level of serum bilirubin has subsided to near normal. Cholangiograms before removal of the T-tube are desirable if there is any question of the patency of the duct or the presence of calculi within it. If a fine polyethylene tube is passed well down into the lumen of the T-tube and the opaque medium injected through it, the danger of air bubbles being forced into the common duct where they may be mistaken for stones will be minimized. We do not secure cholangiograms routinely because of the occasional systemic reaction following the injection of dye into the common duct.

Removal of sutures.—The skin and retention sutures should not be removed until about the tenth postoperative day. In jaundiced or debilitated patients in whom tissue healing may be delayed, it is often advisable to permit these sutures to remain in place for a longer time. In such patients, or in those in whom the wound becomes infected, there may be a separation of the skin edges upon removal of the skin sutures. If this occurs, adhesive butterfly bridges should be used to approximate the edges of the wound and should extend around the abdomen for a considerable distance on each side of the wound. It is advisable to restrict any activity such as lifting or straining which might place undue tension upon the wound for a period of six weeks after operation.

CHAPTER 10

Anesthesia for Biliary Tract Surgery

BILIARY TRACT surgery presents to the anesthesiologist most problems common to all upper abdominal operations. Additional hazards are imposed by the nature of the contemplated operative procedure and by the physiologic and pathologic alterations of the diseased organ. Included in these changes are impaired function of the liver and other organs secondarily involved, the occurrences of reflexes such as the cholecystocardiac reflex and impaired nutrition. Preoperative diagnostic inaccuracies may increase the problem of the anesthesiologist.

Anesthetic agents should be employed which will produce adequate abdominal relaxation and yet possess a minimal degree of toxicity for the liver. There is no single anesthetic agent or method of administration which is universally safe. Certain drugs, including chloroform and trichloroethylene, are contraindicated because of their potential hepatotoxic properties. It must be remembered, however, that hypoxia or carbon dioxide excess and shock may produce much greater damage than any anesthetic agent.

The preoperative preparation of the patient is discussed in Chapter 9. A good night's rest before operation is important. It may be provided by small doses of barbiturates, such as ¾ gr. of Seconal or Nembutal. If the patient is unable to sleep because of pain, small doses of Demerol or morphine may be administered.

The immediate preoperative medication must be determined by the condition of the patient. Morphine sulfate, 1/12–1/6 gr., or Demerol, 50–75 mg., combined with atropine or scopolamine are satisfactory drugs for the good risk patient. They should be administered one hour before anesthesia if given hypodermically or 30 minutes before anesthesia if given intravenously. In emaciated or deeply jaundiced patients, small doses of short-acting barbiturates may be preferred to opiates. It should be remembered that most barbiturates are broken down in the liver and their effect will be prolonged in the presence of hepatic insufficiency.

Before the patient is taken to the operating room, the desired type of gastric suction tube should be inserted intranasally and should be tested to confirm its presence in the stomach. After positioning the patient upon the operating table, one or two 16 or 18 gauge needles should be inserted into accessible veins and intravenous infusion started. Properly typed and cross-matched blood should be available.

The type of anesthetic agent and the method of administration should be determined by the condition and age of the patient, the type and duration of the contemplated operative procedure and the skill of the anesthesiologist. Complicated anesthesia technics should be avoided by the administrator who has not had extensive training and experience.

Regional Anesthesia

Local anesthetic agents are less hepatotoxic than general anesthetic drugs but increase the difficulties of the operating team and may not permit an extensive operation. The duration of anesthesia, even with the use of long-acting drugs and with the addition of epinephrine, is limited, and supplementation by intravenous or inhalation agents may be required.

Infiltration.—Local infiltration in the immediate vicinity of the incision and down to the peritoneum is reserved for the very poor risk patient in whom a minor procedure such as incision and drainage of a subhepatic abscess or cholecystostomy is contemplated. Relaxation will be minimal. Visceral pain may be diminished by splanchnic block using 20–40 cc. of 0.5–1 per cent Xylocaine solution.

Field block.—In this type of regional anesthesia, the area of operation is surrounded by a barrier of anesthetic solution through all layers of the abdominal wall, thus interrupting the nerve supply to the region contained within the anesthetized area. This method affords better muscular relaxation than simple infiltration but requires a larger amount of the anesthetic solution and greater skill.

Nerve block.—Either intercostal or paravertebral block may be of value in biliary tract surgery. Unilateral block occasionally will be adequate but it is well to interrupt any overlap from the opposite side by a series of subcutaneous infiltrations or injections in the midline of the abdomen from the xiphoid process of the sternum to the umbilicus. The line of incision also should be infiltrated. A 0.5 per cent procaine solution is used for these infiltrations. Each of the intercostal nerves from the fifth to the eleventh thoracic should be blocked with 5 cc. of 1 per cent Xylocaine solution. These injections may be adequate to block visceral afferent sensation and reflexes, but a supplementary splanchnic block may be needed.

Spinal anesthesia.—In skilled hands, spinal anesthesia is quite satisfactory for biliary tract surgery. It offers good relaxation, is less toxic and will interrupt most reflexes from the operating field. To accomplish this, spinal anesthesia must extend to the fourth thoracic vertebral level. A decided fall in blood pressure may accompany spinal anesthesia at such levels and hypoxia may occur. Vasopressor drugs should be given prophylactically and repeated if a fall in blood pressure occurs. Oxygen should be administered throughout the operation to combat any tendency toward hypoxia. Shock is a contraindication to spinal anesthesia. Compensated shock must be recognized before operation since spinal anesthesia may break the compensation.

Continuous or fractional spinal anesthesia is less dangerous and less toxic than single dose methods because smaller amounts of the drug are used initially. This technic may maintain adequate anesthesia for any length of time and the administrator has greater flexibility in varying its level. Minimal doses may be administered to elderly and debilitated patients with excellent anesthetic and relaxant results.

Epidural or peridural anesthesia.—This form of anesthesia has increased in popularity among trained anesthesiologists with the advent of the more potent, better spreading agents such as Xylocaine (lidocaine) and Carbocaine (mepivacaine). This form of anesthesia may be of the single-shot variety or of the continuous or intermittent variety. It provides conditions similar to those of a spinal anesthetic with less hazards as to the complications of meningitis and postspinal headache, the difference being that the solution is injected around the dura rather than subdurally. It is a technique that is extremely useful for the management of pain as well as for the production of anesthesia.

General Anesthesia

Most agents used for general anesthesia have some hepatotoxic effects, the degree varying with the drug used and the condition of the patient. Most of these effects on the liver are reversible with the drugs in common use, but improper administration of a drug and the occurrence of hypoxia may be very harmful in the presence of liver damage.

Nitrous oxide.—This agent by itself is unsuited for any upper abdominal operation. It is a weak anesthetic and is incapable of affording a suitable degree of muscular relaxation. The narrow margin between anesthetic and hypoxic concentration renders it undesirable for a prolonged operation. However, nitrous oxide is valuable if combined with other anesthetic drugs, such as ether or Pentothal, which permit adequate oxygen to be given. This is true especially if curare is used to increase relaxation.

Ethylene.—Most comments regarding nitrous oxide also apply to ethylene. However, more oxygen may be given with this drug and the danger of hypoxia is thus reduced. The explosive quality of ethylene presents an added hazard.

Ether.—When correctly used, ether is one of the safest and most satisfactory anesthetic agents for biliary tract surgery. Deep ether anesthesia is toxic to a damaged liver and therefore should be used with caution. When administered in conjunction with intravenous or other inhalation agents, ether permits an adequate concentration of oxygen, a satisfactory degree of relaxation and relatively easy control of the patient. It is probably the anesthetic of choice if a highly skilled anesthesiologist is not available. It may produce vomiting, slight depression of liver function and slight hypotension, especially when a very deep level of anesthesia is maintained. Supplemented with curare, small doses of ether offer excellent anesthesia and relaxation with minimal toxic reaction if no hypoxia has existed. It is essential to supplement ether with adequate concentrations of oxygen when the open drop method is used.

Cyclopropane.—Cyclopropane is a controversial drug. Its action on parenchymal tissue is less than that of ether and its toxicity is somewhat lower. There is a moderate elevation of blood pressure and generalized oozing may be increased. When used with small amounts of ether, cyclopropane is an excellent agent for debilitated patients. The so-called "cyclopropane shock" which occurs when cyclopropane is withdrawn is probably the expression of carbon dioxide accumulation which has gone unrecognized during the operation and becomes manifest after the anesthesia has ended.

HALOTHANE (FLUOTHANE).—This agent has been growing rapidly in popularity and in the past seven years has been used in the administration of 15,000,000 anesthetics. It is not entirely without danger and 15 cases of liver damage have been reported as of late 1963. There have been implications that halothane has caused jaundice and liver death from acute yellow atrophy, but definite proof has not been established. Clinical studies suggest that it has produced no more deleterious effects on liver function than other commonly used drugs; however, until the safety of the drug has been established, it would be advisable to avoid its use in the presence of jaundice.

INTRAVENOUS ANESTHESIA.—Pentothal sodium is a useful drug for induction of anesthesia but should not be used to maintain anesthesia for biliary tract surgery. It does not give muscular relaxation unless combined with some other agent. It is a marked renal and respiratory depressant, does not block reflex activity and in the presence of liver damage its action may be strikingly prolonged. The administration of even moderate amounts of Pentothal sodium results in protracted postoperative sleep and increases the danger of pulmonary complications. This drug is useful as a supplemental agent. However, the greater the total dosage used, the more dangerous it becomes.

CURARES.—The muscle relaxants are of great value in all upper abdominal surgery. By their use it is possible to achieve profound relaxation with general anesthesia without the use of toxic doses. The muscular relaxation is comparable to that obtained with spinal anesthesia. However, the various curare drugs are not free from undesirable properties and disadvantages. They may contribute to hypotension and bronchospasm. Unless the dosage is correctly regulated, they may cause apnea from paralysis of the muscles of respiration. The tendency to administer too light a general anesthesia in conjunction with these drugs must be resisted because of unchecked and persistent reflex activity. When properly used, curare and its related relaxing agents are of great value to biliary tract surgery.

In the presence of severe liver damage, the pseudocholinesterase activity may be considerably diminished. This may result in marked prolongation of the effect of curare drugs. This implies that these drugs must be used with greater caution and minimal dosage, lest a residual paralysis develop. It has been recommended that, when this occurs, the administration of whole blood or plasma may help terminate the paralysis because of the pseudocholinesterase content. Of primary importance is maintenance of respiration by adequate use of pressure-breathing devices to assure adequacy of gas exchange.

Anesthetic Technic

The closed technic with carbon dioxide absorption is preferred for administration of most inhalation anesthetics. When nitrous oxide or ethylene is used, a semi-closed system is preferable. The use of a circle or to-and-fro system is a matter of individual preference. The use of endotracheal tubes assures a patent airway which is always important, especially in the presence of advanced disease. Such tubes permit a more controlled anesthesia in debilitated patients and in those with excessive secretions in the lungs. They should not be used by inexperienced personnel since they may cause varying degrees of local trauma and systemic reflex activities. Their use is seldom mandatory in biliary tract surgery.

Fluids should be administered intravenously as needed throughout the operation but excessive amounts should be avoided. Blood should be available but should be used sparingly, especially in jaundiced patients, because reactions may increase liver damage.

Summary

In general there are two types of anesthesia which are satisfactory for surgery upon the biliary tract. Spinal anesthesia administered in a single dose or by continuous flow has proved satisfactory when used by experienced personnel. If general anesthesia is preferred, nitrous oxide, ethylene, cyclopropane or Pentothal should be used for the induction, the choice depending upon the condition of the patient and the preference and experience of the administrator. Following induction, ether is given to maintain the patient in the upper second plane of the third stage of anesthesia, using the closed method. Curare is administered to obtain relaxation.

CHAPTER 11

Gallbladder Surgery

THE PATIENT should be placed squarely on his back on a flat operating table for all anterior abdominal approaches to the biliary tract. Breaking the table under the upper lumbar spine to hyperextend the spine and elevate the costal margin often results in unnecessary backache in the postoperative period. The use of sand bags or gallbladder lifts under the lower right thorax has a similar disadvantage, without increasing exposure to any appreciable degree. Retraction of the right costal margin by an assistant gives equally good exposure with far less postoperative distress. Hyperextension of the spine also increases the tension of the abdominal muscles by tilting the pelvis downward and thus increasing the distance between the costal margin and the symphysis. This diminishes the efficiency of retraction of the edges of the abdominal wound.

Before the operation is started, a 16 or 18 gauge needle is inserted into a vein for intravenous infusion of anesthetic agents and fluids containing nutritive materials, minerals and vitamins. If the patient is debilitated, deeply jaundiced or likely to require the administration of blood during the operation, it is well to start infusions in two separate veins. This will give added assurance of an available portal for intravenous therapy if it should suddenly be needed during operation. If the needle is inserted in a foot or ankle vein, both arms of the patient may be placed at his side on the operating table, giving more room for the operating team. The use of the lower extremities for infusions has the disadvantage of placing the fluids at a considerable distance from the anesthesiologist, making it more difficult for him to watch and control them. Thrombophlebitis following intravenous infusions is more common in the lower extremities than in the upper extremities. If an arm vein is to be used and the arm to be placed on an arm board at a right angle to the table, the left arm should be used as it is less in the way of the operating team. However, infusions can be given in either arm with the arm placed at the side of the patient. It is well to use an arm shield to protect the intravenous needle from being dislodged by pressure from the body of the surgeon or an assistant.

The placing of a gastric suction tube (p. 135) through the nose and into the patient's stomach before he is brought to the operating room will permit gastric decompression to be maintained throughout the operation and is often of great value. Its use is important in the obese patient and in the individual whose anatomic conformity or adhesions from previous surgery may make every aid to exposure and technic important. Intranasal gastric suction often is important both during the operation and in the early postoperative period. However, such tubes are one of the greatest causes of postoperative discomfort. If the operation is unlikely to interfere with gastrointestinal motility and there is a minimum of intra-abdominal trauma, the tube often can be removed at the end of operation or a few hours later with little danger of postoperative nausea and vomiting and with the advantage of eliminating irritation to the nasal passages and pharynx. The tube should always be removed as early as possible in accordance with the patient's postoperative response.

The skin of the operative field should be thoroughly and widely cleansed. The initial drapes should expose only enough skin to permit an adequate incision. Contamination from the skin edges should be minimized by the early placement of drapes to protect them. The availability of antibiotics is not an excuse to minimize aseptic technic.

Instruments

Simple instruments usually are satisfactory for gallbladder surgery. Fancy or complicated instruments may do more harm than good. A number of instruments I find most useful are shown in Plate 27. The C. W. Mayo retractor permits strong retraction of the right costal margin which facilitates rotation of the liver out of the abdominal cavity. It also is designed for the comfort of the assistant as it does not tire his hands and he is able to maintain better retraction. Aspirating and suction equipment should always be available to evacuate the gallbladder and bile ducts and to keep the operative field clean. An aspirating syringe and needle are essential since the surgeon should not incise what he thinks to be the common duct until he has aspirated it to be sure it contains bile and not blood. Anomalies or distortions due to previous surgery occasionally cause the portal vein to be mistaken for the common duct.

Various sizes of T-tubes are most satisfactory for draining the common duct. Some surgeons recommend the use of a T-tube with a long cross-arm, permitting it to extend through the ampulla of Vater and into the duodenum. I am opposed to the use of such T-tubes for several reasons. When the gallbladder is removed, the tonus of the sphincter of Oddi is relaxed and if its patency is determined to be adequate at the time of operation it is not necessary to have a tube passing through it. Temporary traumatic edema may occlude the distal common duct but this soon subsides to permit bile to flow freely into the duodenum; meanwhile the external limb of the T-tube furnishes an adequate escape for bile. The limb of a T-tube passing into the duodenum often permits regurgitation of intestinal contents into the bile ducts and out through the wound. This may complicate wound healing. There have been reports of compression of the opening of the pancreatic duct and the development of acute pancreatitis due to pressure of a long-limbed T-tube in the region of the ampulla of Vater. Medical literature records a number of deaths due to acute hemorrhagic pancreatitis associated with the use of a long-limbed T-tube.

The Judd-Allis forceps is an excellent instrument with which to grasp the bile ducts without causing damage. The curved Pean forceps is excellent for dissecting the bile ducts and vessels, clamping them and exploring the common bile duct. Malleable probes and scoops permit careful exploration of the ducts and of the patency of the ampulla without damage, when carefully handled. Their diameter should not exceed 5 mm., since larger instruments are likely to tear the distal common duct, with subsequent scarring and stenosis. Occasionally gallstone and kidney stone forceps are of value in removing impacted stones. Larger scoops are useful in evacuating stones from the gallbladder and from markedly dilated bile ducts.

Instruments for Biliary Tract Surgery

A number of instruments that are of particular usefulness in biliary tract surgery are illustrated.

1. C. W. Mayo retractor
2. Gallbladder trocar
3. Intestinal catgut on curved needles
4. Poole suction tube
5. Glass suction tube
6. T-tubes in various sizes
7. Syringe and needle
8. Judd-Allis forceps
9. Curved Pean forceps
10. Randall kidney stone forceps
11. Rochester gallstone forceps
12. Blake gallstone forceps
13. Mayo common duct probe
14. Mayo common duct scoop
15. Mayo cystic duct scoop
16. Mayo gallstone scoop
17. Russell gallstone scoop
18. Ferguson gallstone scoop

PLATE 27

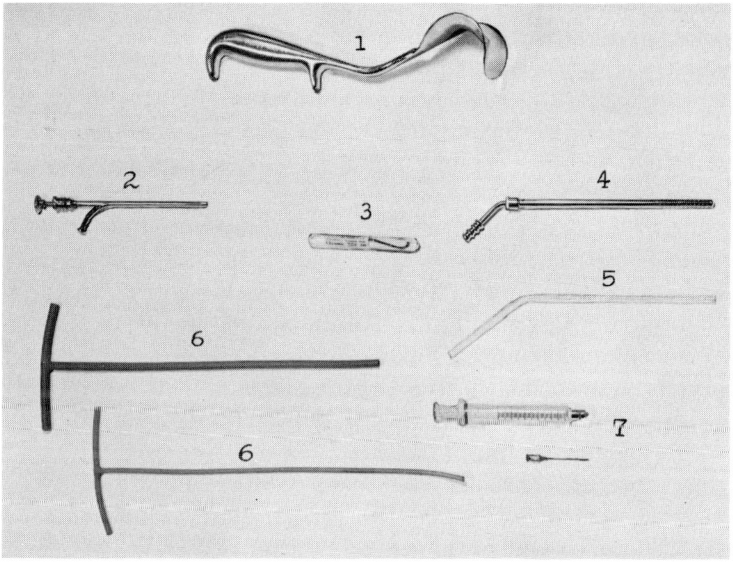

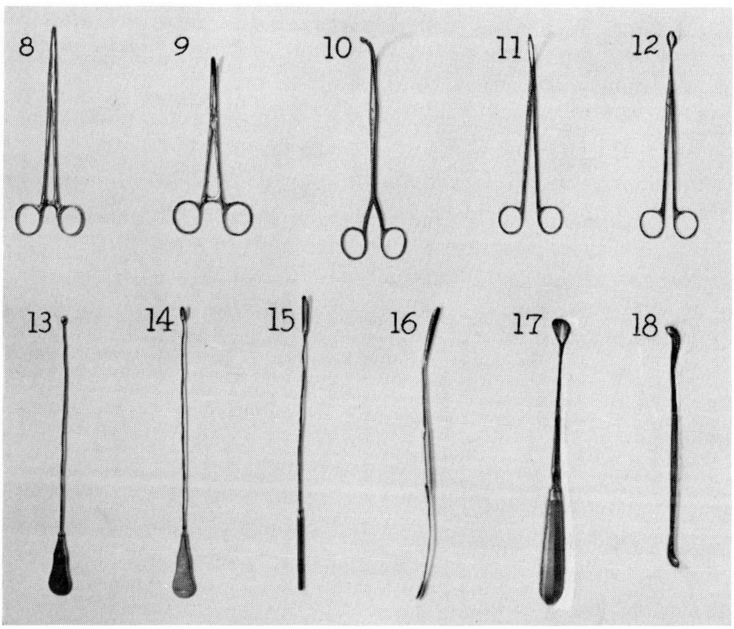

Careful dissection of the gallbladder, bile ducts and adjacent vessels is so important that an incision should be selected that will give a direct approach and ample exposure. The incision also should be adequate for exploration of the remaining abdominal viscera. This can be best accomplished by a vertical incision.

Vertical incision.—*A.*—The incision should begin as high as possible in the angle between the costal margin and the xiphoid cartilage. The skin and subcutaneous incision should be carried obliquely downward and slightly to the right, passing 1–2 in. to the right of the umbilicus. It should extend about 2 in. below the umbilicus. A vertical incision is then made through the anterior rectus sheath about 1 cm. to the right of the medial border of the rectus muscle.

B.—The rectus muscle may then be retracted slightly to the right for incision of the posterior sheath and peritoneum. I prefer to split the rectus muscle a few millimeters to the right of its medial border as I believe this facilitates closure and does not weaken the scar or the abdominal wall.

C.—The posterior sheath of the rectus and peritoneum are grasped with forceps in the upper portion of the incision where there is the least likelihood of injury to abdominal viscera. The peritoneum is incised under the full length of the skin incision. This gives excellent exposure of the biliary tract and permits complete abdominal exploration including delivery of the appendix into the wound when its removal is desired.

D.—Some surgeons prefer the shorter vertical incision to the right of the midline with a separate incision for access to the appendix. Occasionally when the diagnosis is in doubt and the surgeon does not know if surgery in the left upper abdomen may be indicated, an upper midline incision from the xiphoid cartilage nearly to the umbilicus may be made. After the abdomen has been explored, this incision may be elongated either to the right or to the left of the umbilicus.

[Subcostal and transverse incisions *on page 154.*]

PLATE 28

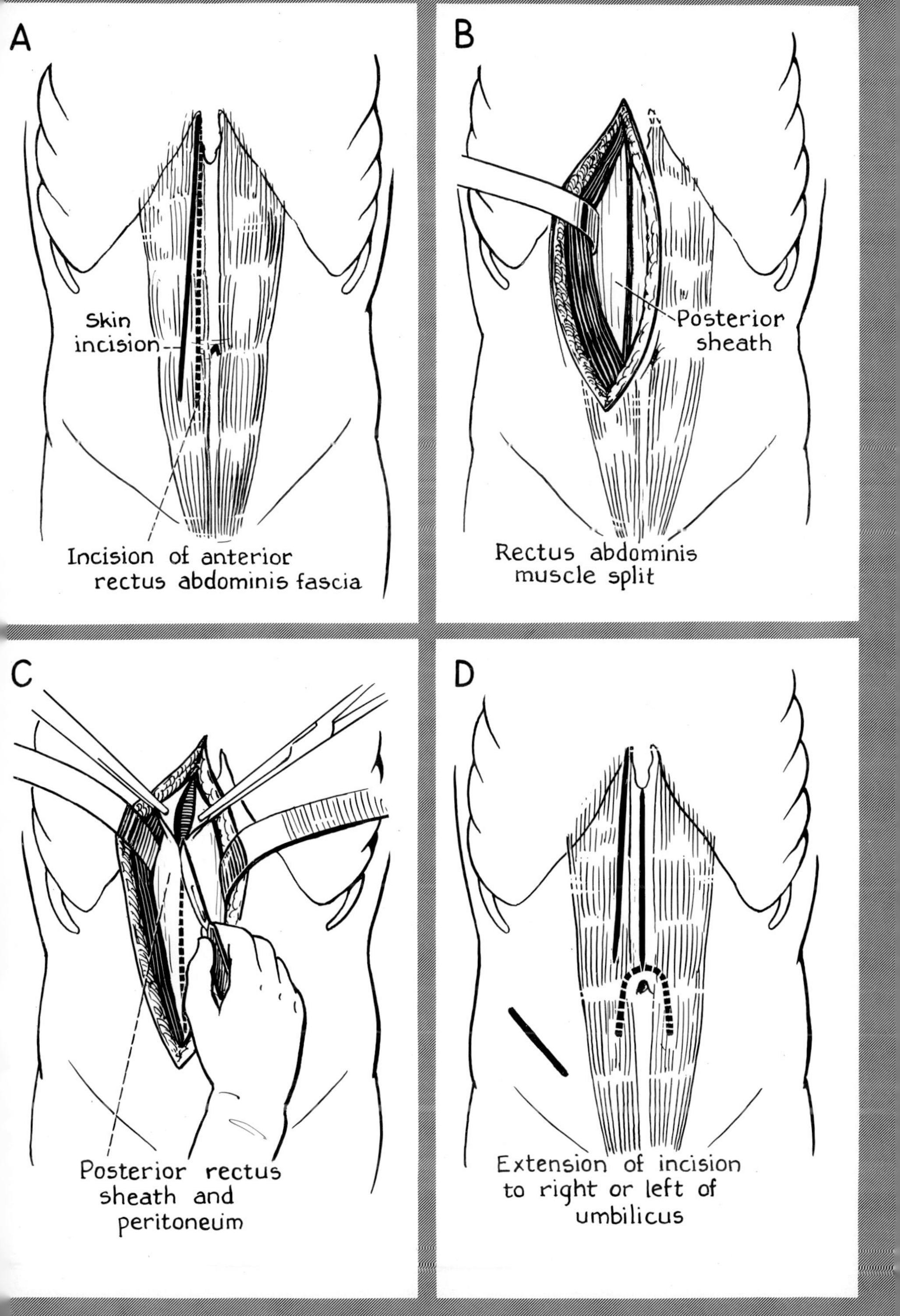
A
Skin incision
Incision of anterior rectus abdominis fascia
B
Posterior sheath
Rectus abdominis muscle split
C
Posterior rectus sheath and peritoneum
D
Extension of incision to right or left of umbilicus

SUBCOSTAL INCISION.—A right subcostal incision gives good exposure of the gallbladder and fairly good access to the bile ducts but does not permit a satisfactory examination of the other abdominal viscera. When an acutely inflamed suppurative or necrotic gallbladder is suspected, it may be approached through a subcostal incision with a minimum of danger of opening into the general peritoneal cavity and spreading infection.

E.—A small subcostal incision dividing the medial portion of the flat abdominal muscles and the lateral edge of the rectus sheath permits medial retraction of the right rectus muscle without necessitating its division. A gallbladder abscess can be drained through such an incision while maintaining maximal support of the abdominal wall.

F.—If cholecystectomy is to be performed, the incision may be carried across the right rectus muscle and midline and the medial portion of the left rectus sheath below the ensiform process. This approach gives satisfactory exposure but is more likely to leave a weakened scar in the presence of infection.

TRANSVERSE INCISION.—*G.*—The true transverse incision on the right divides the broad muscles of the abdominal wall and the right rectus muscle. It may be extended as far as desired to the left, dividing the left rectus sheath but retracting the left rectus muscle. This incision is considerably below the gallbladder and bile ducts and hampers access to them. The liver cannot be rolled out of the abdomen and it is often difficult to reach the cystic duct, particularly in patients with a narrow costal angle. A little better exposure can be obtained if the incision is arched upward as it approaches the midline.

[Closure of abdominal incision *on page 156.*]

E

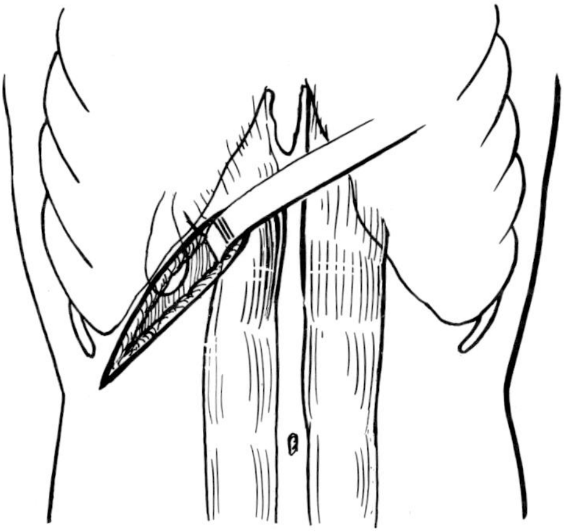

Retraction of right rectus abdominis muscle without its division

F

Right rectus abdominis muscle and medial portion of left rectus sheath incised

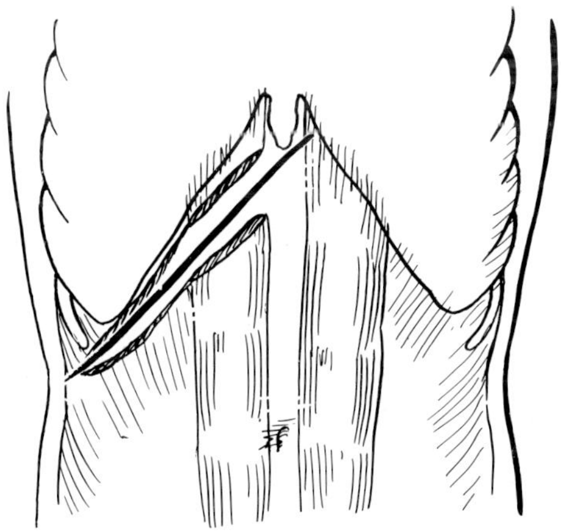

G

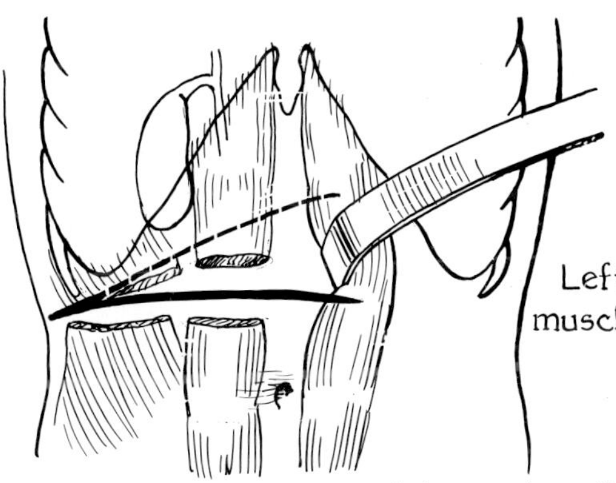

Left rectus muscle retracted

Right rectus and muscles of abdominal wall incised

The choice of suture material for closure of abdominal wounds is a matter of preference of the surgeon. Whether the material is absorbable or nonabsorbable plays but a small role in wound healing. The chief factors responsible for unsatisfactory healing of wounds are the impaired nutritional state of the patient and the development of wound infection, serum collections or other postoperative complications.

A.—For the closure of the peritoneal and fascial layers, I prefer to use a continuous suture of a double strand of 0 chromic catgut on a curved Mayo needle. The first layer includes the parietal peritoneum and posterior rectus fascia. These are approximated by a running stitch, except for the point of emergence of the drain where the suture is locked around the drain. So-called retention sutures then are passed through the skin and subcutaneous tissue and the external rectus fascia but not through the muscle as they would tend to cut the muscle when tied. They emerge from the skin about 1 in. to each side of the incision and are spaced 1½–2 in. apart. A nonabsorbable suture should be used, wire or silkworm tension sutures being very satisfactory. The cut edges of the anterior rectus fascia are next approximated by a continuous catgut suture.

B.—The transverse section through the wound illustrates the position of various suture rows.

C.—The skin is next closed with a continuous silk suture. Tension sutures should now be tied loosely, allowing enough space for the surgeon to be able to pass two fingers beneath them. Their main purpose is to obliterate dead space, and the swelling of the tissues will result in these sutures becoming snug but not so tight that they cut through the skin.

In all patients whose gallbladders are removed or whose bile ducts are explored a soft rubber drain should be placed in the right subhepatic space and brought out through the abdominal incision. I do not believe such drains interfere with wound healing or predispose to wound hernias. Drainage through separate stab wounds means additional unnecessary surgery.

D.—If an abdominal wound is closed without drainage, the tension sutures may be tied over a gauze roll. This aids in obliterating dead space and prevents the tension sutures from cutting into the skin.

PLATE 29

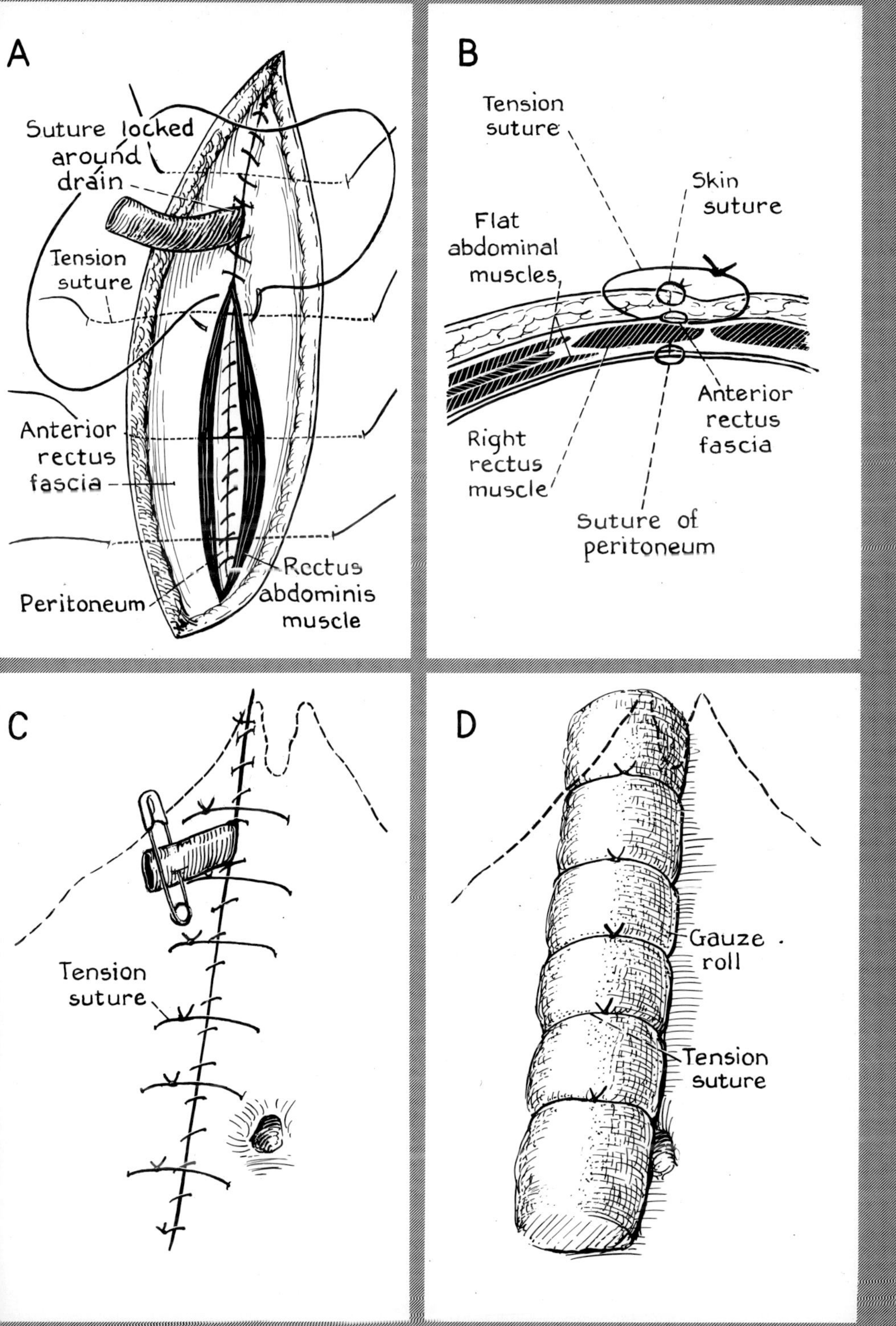
A
Suture locked around drain
Tension suture
Anterior rectus fascia
Peritoneum
Rectus abdominis muscle
B
Tension suture
Skin suture
Flat abdominal muscles
Anterior rectus fascia
Right rectus muscle
Suture of peritoneum
C
Tension suture
D
Gauze roll
Tension suture

Incision.—If the history and physical findings suggest a severe inflammatory process of the gallbladder, a subcostal incision gives adequate exposure and minimizes the danger of opening and contaminating the general peritoneal cavity. When evidences of a severe inflammatory process do not exist or when it is advisable to make a more extensive exploration of the upper abdomen, a vertical incision is preferable.

When the fundus of the gallbladder is exposed and adhesions are found which wall off that organ from the remainder of the peritoneal cavity, they should not be broken down.

A.—The fundus of the gallbladder is grasped with two Allis forceps a sufficient distance from the undersurface of the liver to allow an incision to be made and the edges to be inverted by pursestring sutures. If possible, the incision should be at least 2 cm. from the liver. A sharp trocar and cannula is forced into the gallbladder between the Allis forceps. The trocar is withdrawn beyond the side arm of the cannula to permit the liquid contents of the gallbladder to be aspirated by the attached suction apparatus.

B.—After evacuating as much of the contents as is possible, the trocar is withdrawn and the opening enlarged by sharp dissection.

C.—All calculi and foreign material should be evacuated by the use of forceps and scoops. If fine stones are present within the gallbladder, gauze should be introduced into it to help remove any stones that may have been overlooked.

D.—A finger is then inserted into the gallbladder and its lumen thoroughly explored well down to the neck and the beginning of the cystic duct to make sure that no stones which might interfere with free drainage of bile are lodged in this region.

[Cholecystostomy *continued on page 160.*]

PLATE 30

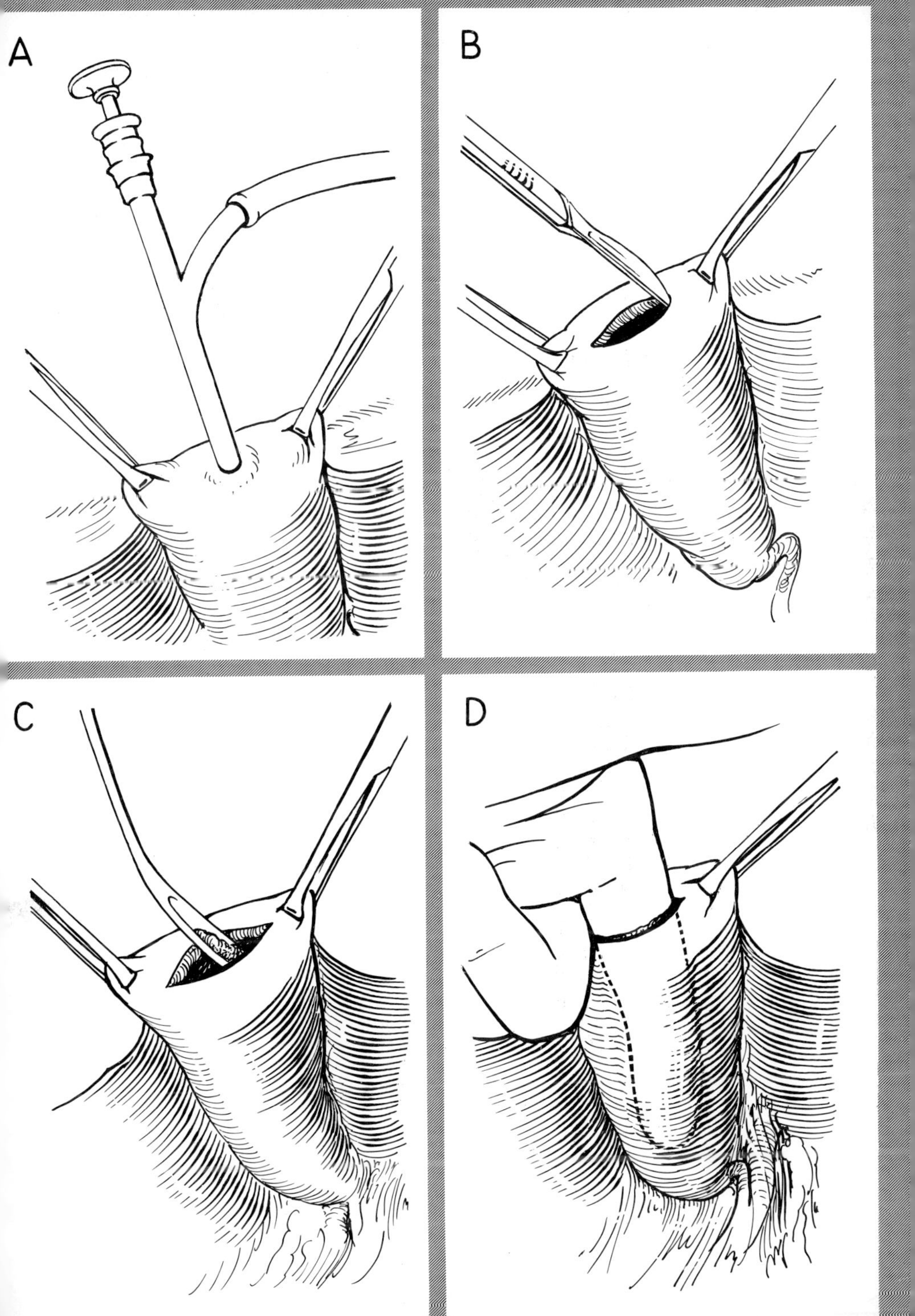

E.—When the free peritoneal cavity is entered and adhesions are not dense around the neck of the gallbladder and bile ducts, careful palpation should be made of these structures to make sure no removable stones are left behind. If any are encountered, an attempt should be made to milk them into the gallbladder and remove them with scoops or forceps. If possible a finger should be introduced into the foramen of Winslow beneath the ducts and vessels and the thumb approximated above them for accurate palpation.

F.—A pursestring suture of chromic catgut is placed around the opening in the fundus of the gallbladder. A large-sized Pezzer catheter with additional vents cut near the tip to minimize the danger of blockage is inserted into the gallbladder for a distance of about 2–3 in. The pursestring suture is then tied and the suture passed through the catheter where it enters the gallbladder to maintain the catheter at the desired level and to aid in inversion of the gallbladder wall when the next pursestring suture is applied.

G.—A second pursestring suture is placed around the first and is tied while pressure is being applied on the catheter to invert the serosa of the gallbladder.

H.—When the gallbladder wall is greatly thickened or partially necrotic, it may be impossible to invert the fundus with pursestring sutures. Under such circumstances the gallbladder should be closed around the tube with interrupted catgut sutures, anchoring the catheter in place by passing one or two sutures through its edges.

I.—If any omentum is available it should be brought up around the catheter and sutured to the fundus of the gallbladder.

J.—In closing the abdomen, the gallbladder should be sutured to the edges of the peritoneum to minimize the danger of leakage into the peritoneal cavity and to enhance the maintenance of an external biliary fistula after the catheter has been removed. It is well to anchor the catheter to the skin by one or two interrupted nonabsorbable sutures to prevent its displacement before removal is desirable. As a rule, the catheter should remain in the wound two to three weeks. If there is infection or contamination around the gallbladder, a Penrose drain should be placed in the subhepatic space.

PLATE 30

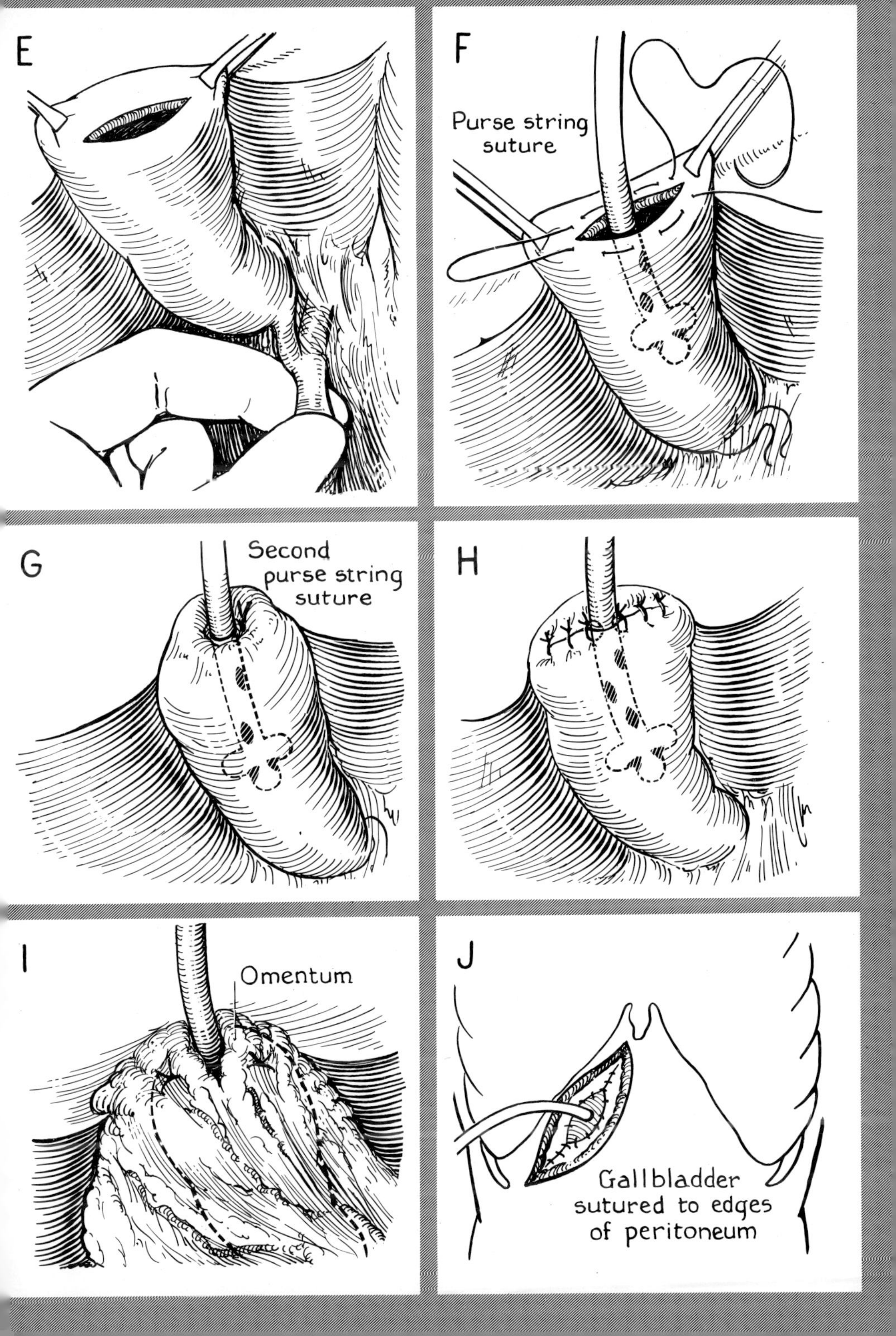
E
F
Purse string suture
G
Second purse string suture
H
I
Omentum
J
Gallbladder sutured to edges of peritoneum

Cholecystectomy is indicated for acute and chronic diseases of the gallbladder, especially when the gallbladder contains calculi and when contraindications do not exist. It is also indicated for benign and malignant tumors of the gallbladder if the operation is technically feasible.

Incision.—In chronic biliary tract disease an approach should be selected which not only gives good exposure of and access to the extrahepatic biliary tract but which permits a complete and careful examination of the rest of the abdominal viscera to rule out other disease which may be producing symptoms simulating those of biliary tract disease. I prefer a high and long, modified right rectus incision (Plate 28, *A*) because it meets these requirements, can be readily and satisfactorily closed and permits surgery to be carried out upon most of the gastrointestinal tract including the appendix. I have been able to remove the spleen and gallbladder at one operation through this incision.

A.—The round ligament and its surrounding falciform ligament which extend from the umbilicus to the interlobar notch are divided between clamps to the edge of the liver.

B.—The gallbladder is carefully palpated to determine the presence of stones.

C.—The abdominal contents are carefully explored. This should be done in a systematic manner to avoid overlooking existing disease. One method is to have an assistant grasp the anterior wall of the stomach at its greater and lesser curvatures and retract it to the left. This elevates the pylorus and duodenum and permits a careful examination of these structures for the possible presence of a peptic ulcer. The head and body of the pancreas should next be palpated.

D.—The surgeon should then palpate the entire stomach and carefully examine the esophageal hiatus to rule out the existence of a diaphragmatic hiatus hernia. He may continue to the left to examine the spleen and left kidney. The transverse colon may then be elevated and the entire large and small intestines examined. With an assistant retracting at the lower end of the wound, the cecum and appendix may be brought into the wound and an appendectomy performed. If the cecum is bound down, making delivery of the appendix difficult, the abdominal incision may be lengthened. I prefer to remove the appendix before biliary tract surgery is done.

[Cholecystectomy *continued on page 164.*]

PLATE 31

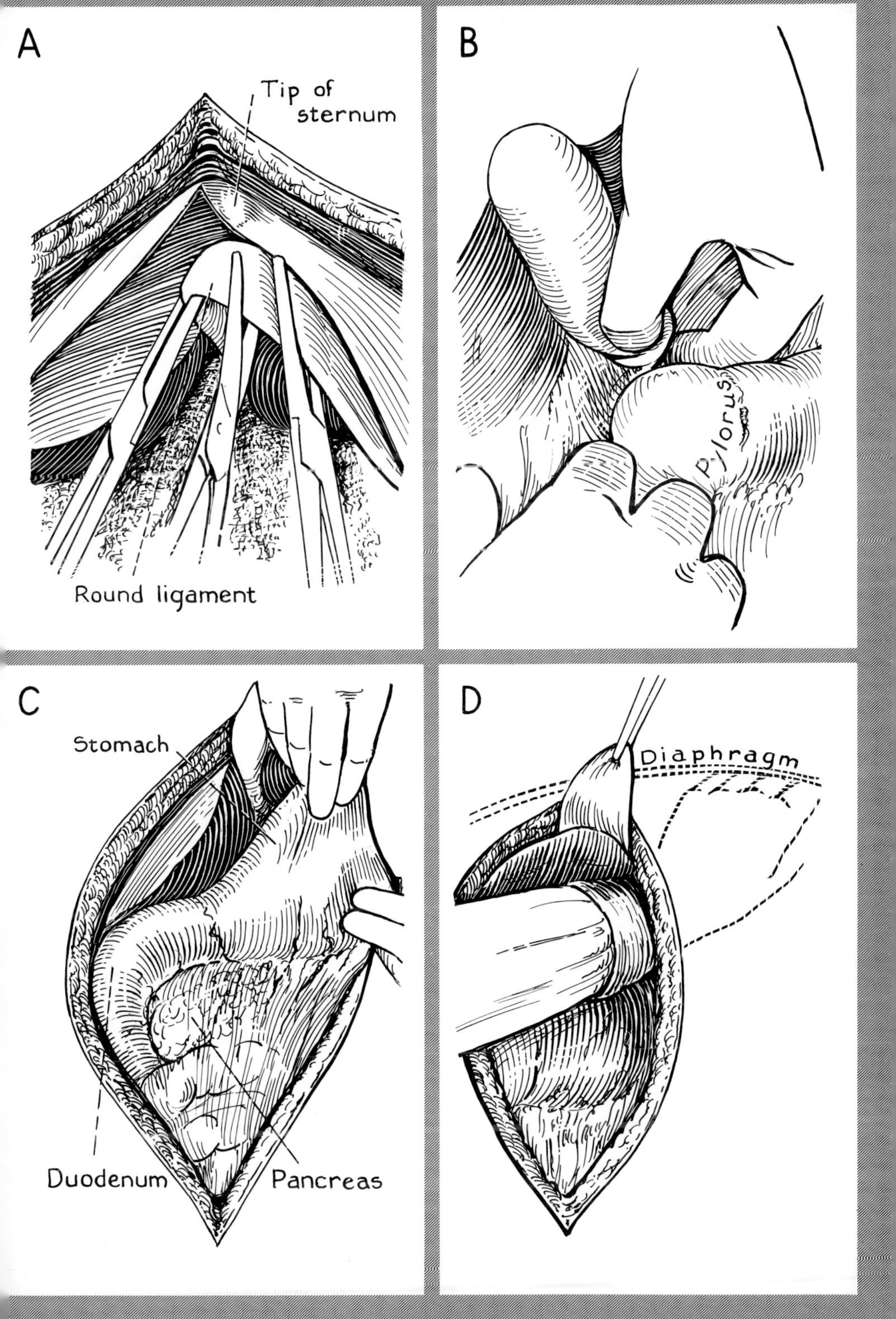
A
Tip of sternum
Round ligament
B
Pylorus
C
Stomach
Duodenum
Pancreas
D
Diaphragm

The extrahepatic biliary tract and its associated vessels can be elevated toward the anterior abdominal wall and made more accessible to careful dissection if as much of the liver as possible is rotated around the right costal margin. Good teamwork between the surgeon and his assistants is required.

E.—An assistant to the left of the operating surgeon on the patient's right side elevates the right costal margin with a retractor. The fundus of the gallbladder is grasped with a curved Pean forceps and the surgeon pulls downward. This retracts the liver downward and permits air to enter the subdiaphragmatic space. If adhesions exist between the liver and the undersurface of the diaphragm and prevent mobilization of the liver they should be separated by finger or scissor dissection.

F.—While traction is maintained on the gallbladder and round ligaments, the forceps are rotated anteriorly and then toward the head of the patient. This pulls the anterior edge of the liver forward and frequently will bring it around the costal margin. The posterior portion of the liver is pulled downward, giving better exposure of the hilar area. The inferior surface of the liver assumes a more anteroposterior direction.

G.—A large moist laparotomy pad is placed between the liver (above) and the hepatic flexure of the colon, duodenum and right kidney (below). A second laparotomy pad further separates the distal stomach and duodenum from the undersurface of the liver. An assistant standing at the left side of the patient and opposite the surgeon retracts downward with his left hand, placing the index finger to the left and the other three fingers to the right of the common duct. He should pull firmly toward the foot of the table and his hands should remain "frozen" and move only at the request of the surgeon.

[Cholecystectomy *continued on page 166.*]

E

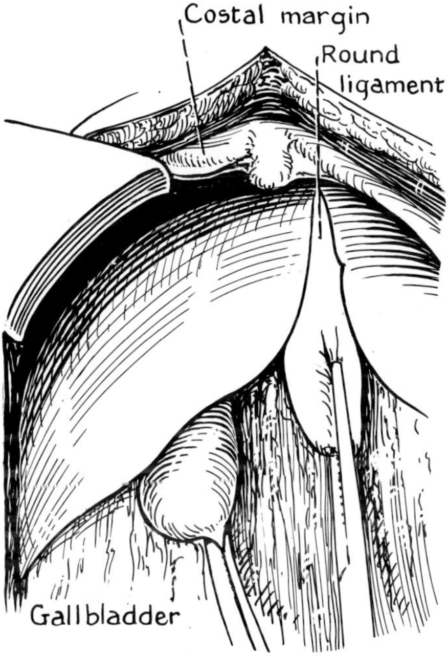

F

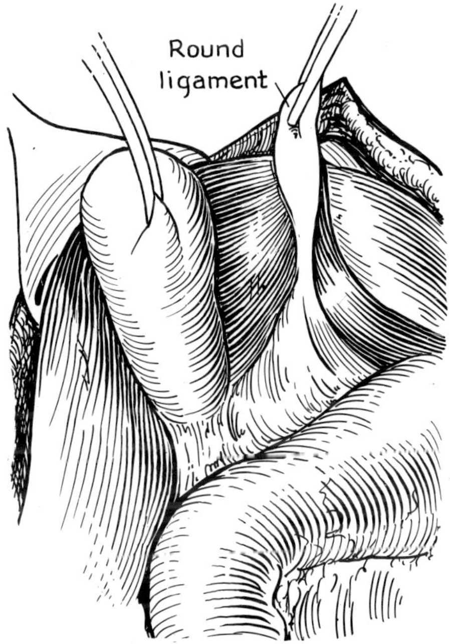

G

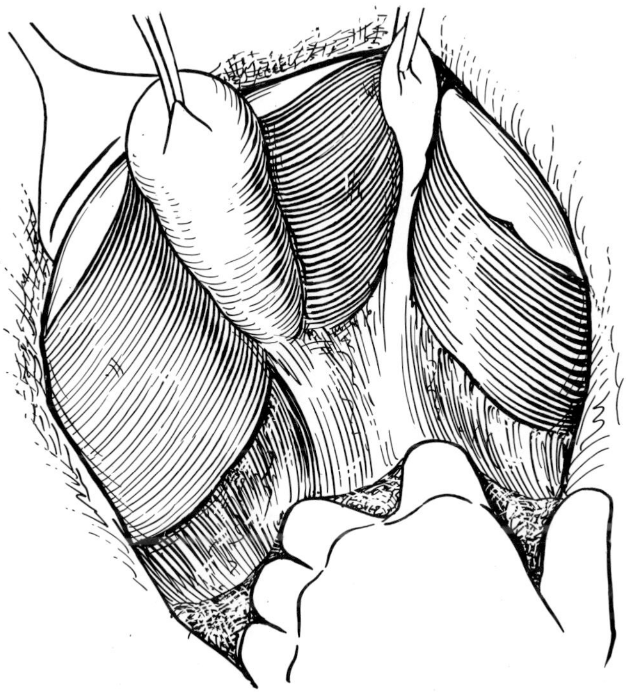

H.—The surgeon then grasps the neck of the gallbladder and, with gentle traction placed upon it, begins the dissection. This can be done safely by blunt dissection using a curved Pean forceps. The peritoneal fold which may be reflected from the neck of the gallbladder to the duodenum and often to the colon is gently pulled away from the gallbladder.

I.—Dissection is continued down the cystic duct to the common duct. The peritoneum overlying the common duct is divided by sliding the curved forceps under it and spreading the blades. The dissection should be continued until the cystic duct is completely isolated and its junction with the common duct accurately visualized.

J.—The index finger should be placed in the foramen of Winslow and the distal end of the cystic duct and the common duct should be palpated between it and the thumb. Careful search should be made for stones, especially any lodged in the distal portion of the cystic duct which might be left behind and produce subsequent symptoms. A curved clamp is then placed across the cystic duct about 5 mm. from its junction with the common duct. A second clamp is placed proximal to the first and the cystic duct divided between them. The stump is doubly ligated.

K.—The neck of the gallbladder is now elevated and the space behind it carefully dissected to isolate the cystic artery. This dissection should be carried well up toward the body of the gallbladder to identify the cystic artery accurately and to distinguish it from the right hepatic artery or any anomalous arteries. When the cystic artery has been carefully identified and freed, it is doubly clamped, divided and the stump ligated. Some surgeons prefer to isolate and clamp the cystic artery before dividing the cystic duct, others clamp the cystic artery and duct together. These practices may lead to surgical accidents to hepatic arteries or ducts.

[Cholecystectomy *continued on page 168.*]

PLATE 31

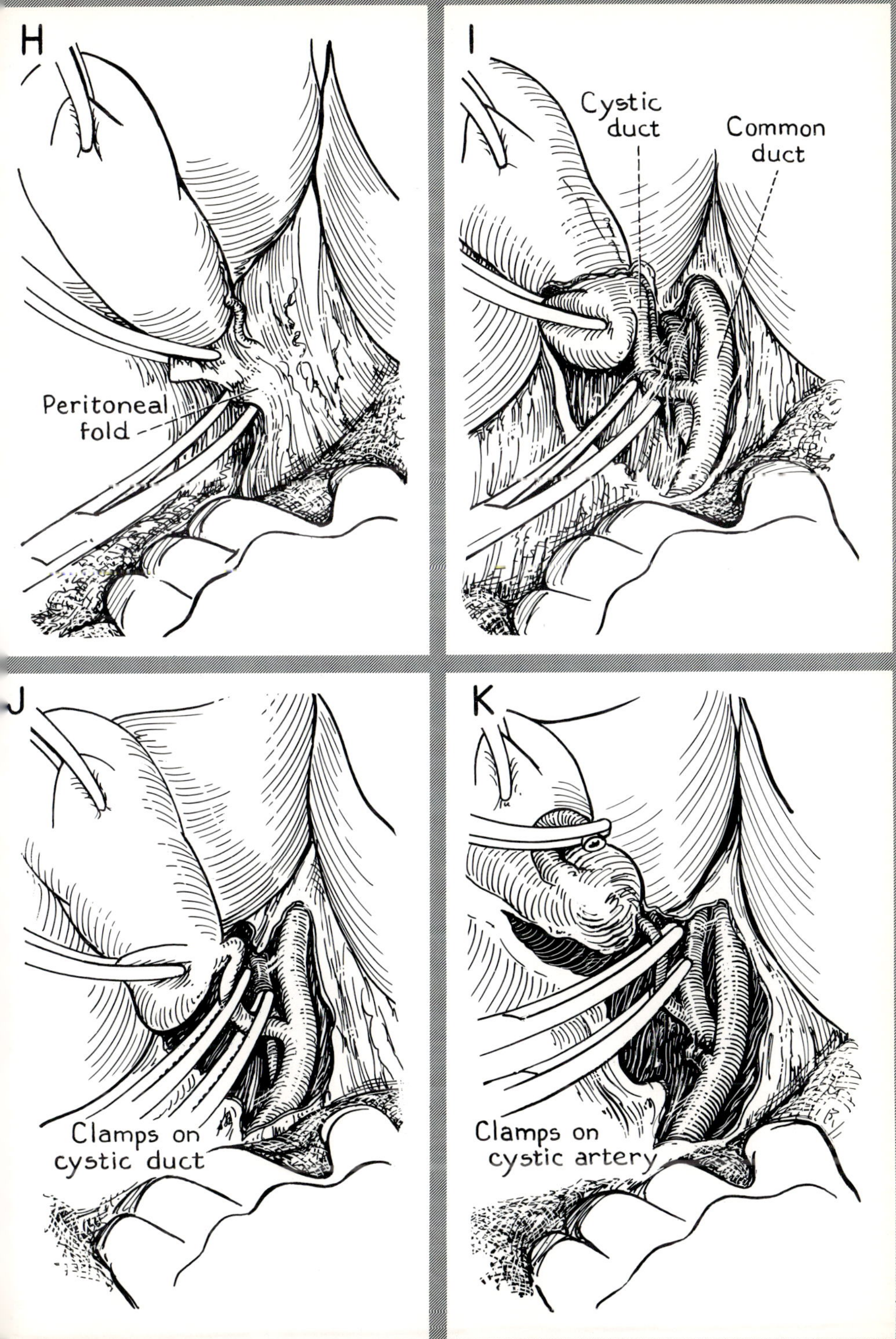
H
Peritoneal fold
I
Cystic duct
Common duct
J
Clamps on cystic duct
K
Clamps on cystic artery

L.—The gallbladder is dissected from its bed from below upward. The peritoneum which reflects from the liver onto the gallbladder should be incised as close to the gallbladder as possible. A fold of peritoneum should be left on each side of the gallbladder bed of sufficient length to permit their approximation to cover completely the denuded area of liver.

M.—Using chromic intestinal catgut on a curved needle, the bed is oversewn beginning at its distal portion. The surgeon should be sure that the first stitch is not placed too deeply because of the danger of including the right hepatic duct or artery in this suture.

N.—The gallbladder bed should be completely peritonealized if possible. The stumps of the cystic duct and cystic artery should be doubly ligated. No effort should be made to close the peritoneum over the common bile duct.

O.—A Penrose drain without a wick or a piece of soft rubber tubing should be placed down to the foramen of Winslow or to Morison's pouch and brought out through the abdominal incision. Before closing the wound it is well to place omentum between the undersurface of the liver and the duodenum.

PLATE 31

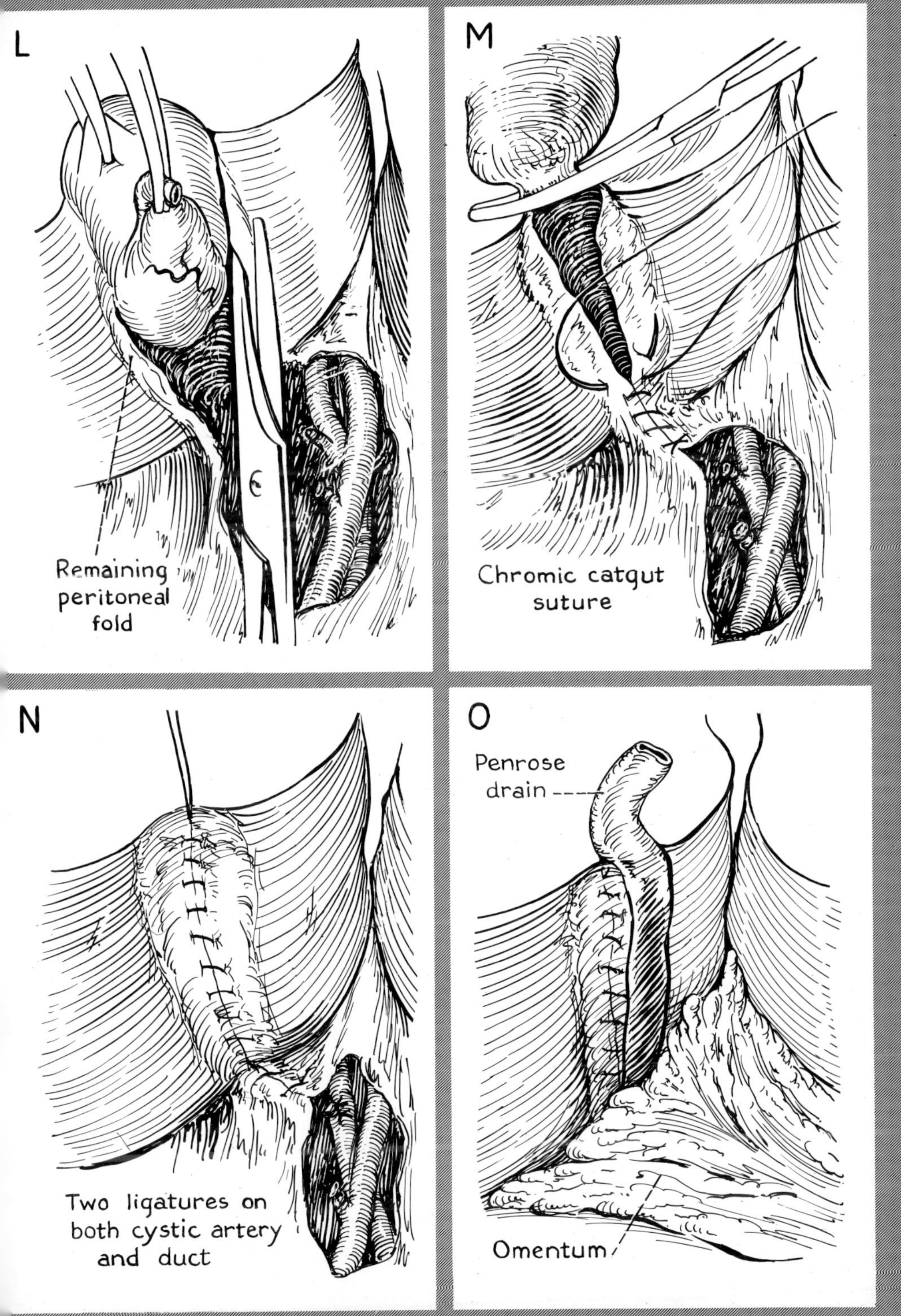
L
Remaining peritoneal fold
M
Chromic catgut suture
N
Two ligatures on both cystic artery and duct
O
Penrose drain
Omentum

A.—Occasionally the gallbladder is found to be so tense that it cannot be readily grasped with a forceps without danger of puncturing the wall. Under such circumstances, the surgeon may aspirate the gallbladder with a large syringe and large needle to lessen the tension and permit the gallbladder to be grasped with forceps. A Pean forceps should be placed around the needle before it is withdrawn so that the opening in the gallbladder can be closed with a minimum of leakage of its contents.

B.—In acute cholecystitis the gallbladder wall may be too thick or friable to permit it to be grasped with any instrument. Usually the gallbladder is sufficiently enlarged to permit a moist gauze sponge to be wrapped around the fundus. This sponge should be twisted snugly against the gallbladder and the ends grasped with a Pean forceps close to the gallbladder. Traction may then be placed on the forceps to elevate the gallbladder with little danger of rupture.

C.—In removing an acutely inflamed gallbladder it usually is impossible to preserve a peritoneal covering for the gallbladder bed. A raw and sometimes bleeding surface remains. By packing a hot wet laparotomy pad into the gallbladder bed and holding it in place for several minutes, bleeding usually is controlled.

D.—If definite bleeding areas persist, mattress sutures may be placed around them to include the capsule of the liver on each side of the bed if possible. These sutures cannot be tied too tightly or they will cut into the liver. Hemostasis can always be secured, and one should never leave a gauze pack in the bed of the gallbladder. I do not believe it advisable to leave hemostatic agents sutured into the bed of the gallbladder. The accumulation of any irritating substances around the common duct may eventually lead to a progressive obliterative cholangitis.

PLATE 32

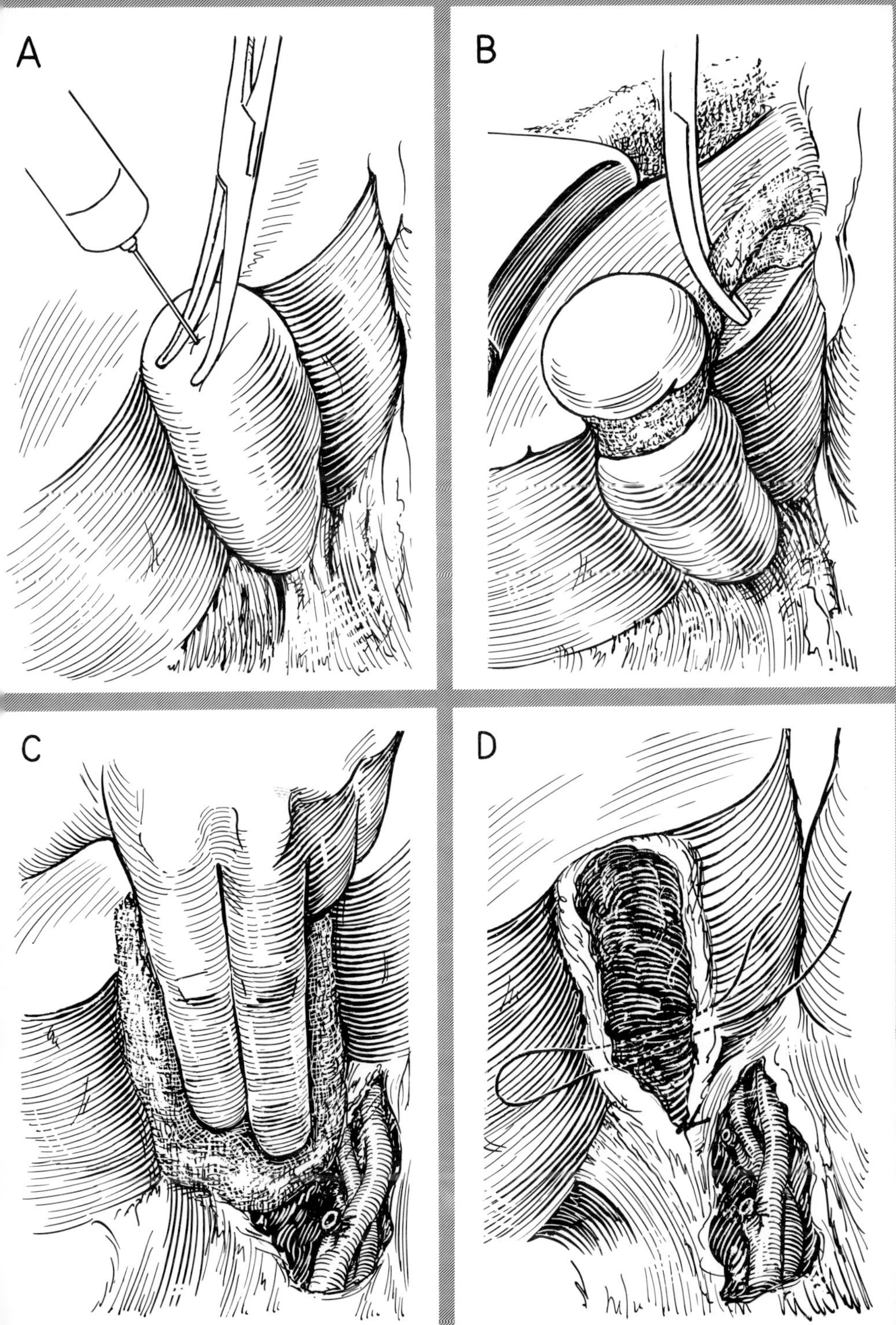

 Removal of Gallbladder from the Fundus Downward

There seldom is justification for removal of the gallbladder from the fundus downward. In so doing, considerable pooling of blood is encountered when the neck of the gallbladder and the cystic duct are reached. This may obscure the field and result in surgical accidents. It also complicates dissection and identification of the ducts and vessels.

A.—If the surgeon decides to remove the gallbladder from the fundus downward, the fundus is grasped with a curved Pean forceps. The peritoneal reflection from the liver onto the gallbladder is divided on each side. This division may be facilitated by injecting saline solution under the peritoneum, a procedure which elevates the peritoneum from the gallbladder and the liver.

B.—The peritoneum may then be divided by sharp dissection with less danger of cutting into either the gallbladder or the liver.

C.—When the gallbladder is completely freed, careful identification of the cystic artery and duct should be made before they are clamped, divided and ligated. It may be well to delay this procedure until oozing from the gallbladder bed is at a minimum. If the cystic artery can be identified and ligated first, a drier field may be obtained.

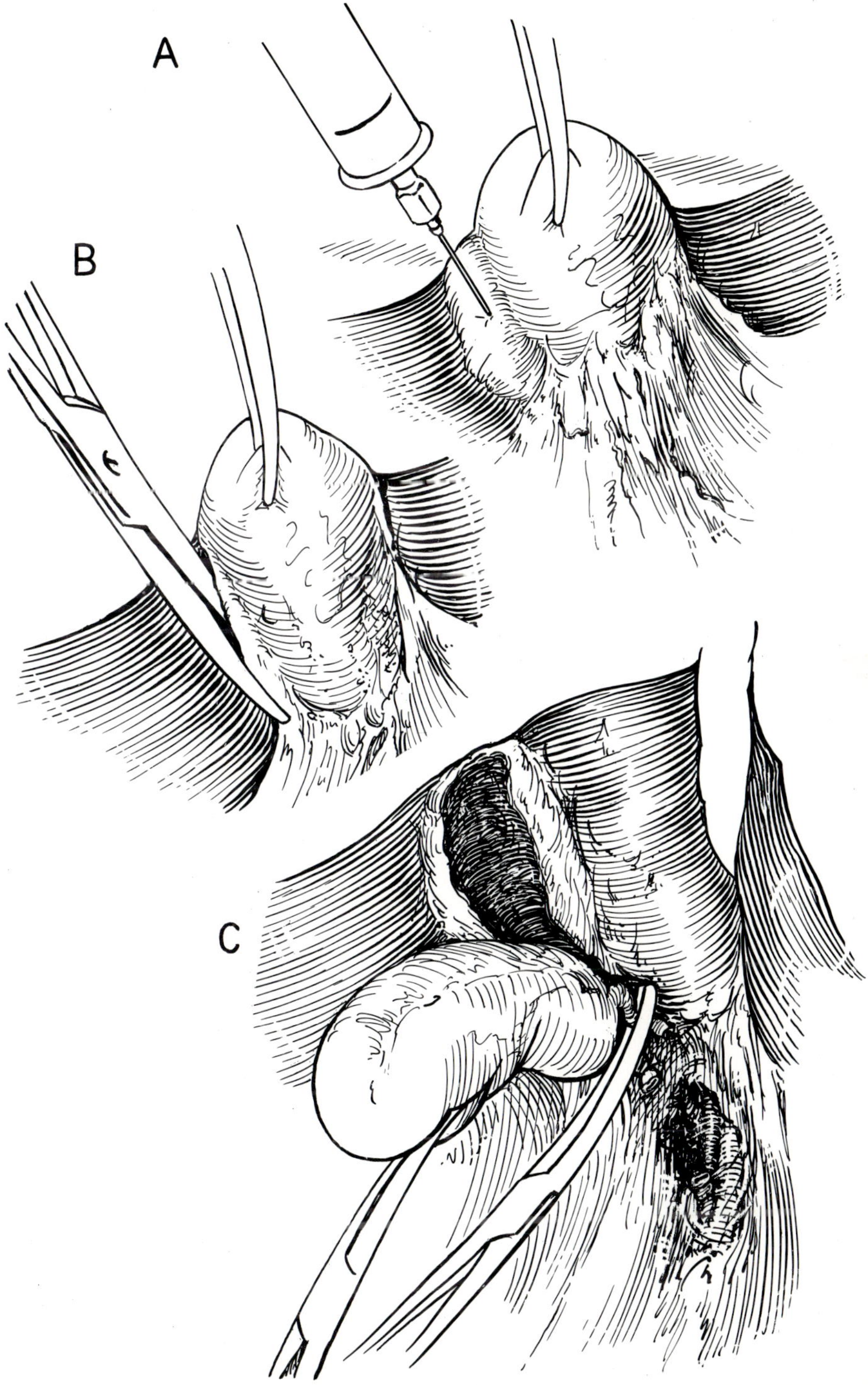
A
B
C

CHAPTER 12

Surgery of the Bile Ducts

SURGERY OF THE extrahepatic bile ducts may be indicated for the following lesions:

1. Lesions within the lumen of the duct
   - Parasites
   - Blood clots
   - Calculi
2. Lesions of the duct wall
   - Congenital anomalies
   - Inflammatory disease
   - Traumatic injury
   - Benign strictures
   - Tumors
3. Extraductal lesions involving the bile ducts
   - Inflammatory lesions
   - Lymphadenopathy
   - Malignant lesions

LESIONS WITHIN THE LUMEN OF THE DUCT

Surgical lesions within the lumen of the common bile duct other than calculi are extremely rare. Intestinal parasites occasionally invade the bile ducts. Ascaris lumbricoides is the parasite most commonly found in the bile ducts at operation or at autopsy. It usually is found in the intestinal tract and occasionally migrates through the ampulla of Vater into the bile ducts or gallbladder. Gallstones are often found in bile ducts invaded by parasites. Their prior existence may produce dilatation of the duct, resulting in easier access to it by the parasites.

Symptoms produced by the presence of Ascaris lumbricoides in the common bile duct simulate those of choledocholithiasis. Typical biliary colics are frequent and may or may not be associated with jaundice. Suppurative cholangitis may develop, with its characteristic symptoms of chills, fever and jaundice. The diagnosis usually is made at operation or at autopsy. Treatment consists of removal of the parasites through a choledochostomy incision and T-tube drainage of the common duct. The patient should also be treated medically for eradication of the parasites from the intestinal tract. Infiltration of the extrahepatic biliary tract by other parasites is seldom found in this country. Echinococcus cysts may compress the bile ducts by external pressure, or daughter cysts may form within them. Liver flukes are rare inhabitants of the bile ducts.

Traumatic injury to the liver may produce subcapsular tears of arteries and bile ducts within the liver substance. Bleeding may occur into the bile ducts and the blood may collect and clot within the common bile duct. The clots often produce temporary obstruction of the distal end of the duct with resultant colicky pains simulating those caused by calculi. Such clots usually will pass through the ampulla and surgical intervention is not necessary if other injuries do not demand an operation.

Choledocholithiasis

Many postmortem and operative studies have demonstrated that calculi are present in the choledochus in approximately 20 per cent of patients who have stones in the gallbladder. It is generally believed that most stones found in the common duct, and particularly cholesterol stones, originate in the gallbladder. Small cholesterol stones may pass from the gallbladder into the common duct where they may become enlarged by deposition of bile pigment. In the absence of infection of the bile ducts, stones found in the choledochus usually are firm, well formed and faceted and contain a large amount of cholesterol. Stones seldom re-form in the bile ducts after a cholecystectomy unless infection is present, and most stones subsequently found are those overlooked at the first operation. When suppurative cholangitis exists and cholecystectomy and choledochostomy are performed, bile pigment stones may re-form in the bile ducts. These usually are very soft and are associated with so-called "mud." Repeated explorations of the common duct may be necessary to remove the re-forming stones until the inflammatory process has subsided.

Symptomatology.—Although the symptoms presented by patients with stones in the common bile duct complicating cholecystic disease have many similarities to those of patients with residual stones after cholecystectomy, there are sufficient differences in the clinical pictures to warrant separate discussion.

When stones in the common duct complicate chronic cholecystic disease in the patient who has had no biliary tract surgery, there is usually a long history of biliary dyspepsia and colic. These symptoms are likely to be more definite and severe than those of disease confined to the gallbladder. In addition to the usual flatulence, belching and epigastric discomfort, the occurrence of nausea and vomiting soon after eating is more common. The colicky pain is apt to be more severe, of longer duration and more difficult to relieve but it differs little in location, being most commonly noted in the epigastrium or right upper quadrant and radiating through to the back or the right scapular region. Jaundice, although frequently noted, does not necessarily indicate the existence of stones within the common bile duct. Likewise, the absence of jaundice does not rule out choledocholithiasis, for many patients with the disease who have typical biliary dyspepsia and colic give no history of associated jaundice. When jaundice does occur, it usually appears soon after a severe colic, may increase to a moderate intensity and then diminish or entirely disappear. Similar episodes may recur at varying intervals. They are caused by the temporary obstruction of the distal end of the common bile duct, with the jaundice diminishing at the release of obstruction either by passage of the stone into the duodenum or by its dropping back into the common duct after dilatation of the duct releases it from its obstructing position.

Pain usually accompanies obstruction of the duct because the obstruction is relatively sudden, and rapid obstruction of any hollow viscus usually is accompanied by severe pain. Gallstones occasionally produce gradual obstruction of the duct unaccompanied by pain. Under such circumstances, the obstruction may be complete and the clinical picture may simulate that of obstruction due to malignant disease of the head of the pancreas or ampulla of Vater. Obstruction of the common bile duct by stones seldom is complete and some bile usually can be found in the duodenal contents and in the stools. This is particularly true when the obstruction is accompanied by pain. Chills and fever are associated with gallstone obstruction in less than one third of such attacks. Infection of the bile ducts does not usually accompany choledocholithiasis. When choledocholithiasis becomes symptomatic in association with gallbladder disease, the gallbladder often is functionless, sclerotic and small. It seldom can be palpated below the liver edge. Cholecystograms usually reveal a nonfunctioning gallbladder.

Residual stones in the common duct following cholecystectomy present a more difficult diagnostic problem. The realization that stones are present in the common duct in 20 per cent of patients with cholelithiasis and the statistical evidence that they are not completely removed in this high a percentage of cholecystectomies lead to the deduction that many patients are likely to have post-cholecystectomy symptoms due to stones. The symptomatology varies with the size, location and number of remaining stones. Very small stones may have been asymptomatic at the time of cholecystectomy and the patient may be symptom free for a considerable period after operation. As the stones gradually enlarge, the patient may develop a recurrence of biliary symptoms, consisting of dyspepsia and qualitative and quantitative food distress. Attacks of colic are frequent, may be severe and often are accompanied by nausea and vomiting. Jaundice may accompany the attack but frequently is absent, thus imposing a greater diagnostic problem. Only rarely are the stones opaque and visible on a plain roentgenogram of the abdomen. When noted, this is a great diagnostic aid, but unfortunately stones seldom are visualized. Roentgenographic studies have little value except in the elimination of other causes of the patient's symptoms. Chills and fever occasionally accompany the attack but are not common symptoms.

Large residual stones which are free in the common duct may produce symptoms soon after operation. There may be a repetition of the patient's preoperative history. If the common duct has been explored, large amounts of bile may drain through the T-tube for a longer period than that noted when the duct is completely evacuated and the ampulla is patent. If the T-tube is removed, severe colics with jaundice may occur in the early postoperative period. Stones impacted in the distal end of the common duct will manifest themselves in the immediate postoperative period if they have not been removed. If the common duct has not been explored or has been closed without drainage, bile will leak from the stump of the cystic duct or from the incision in the common duct, producing a bile peritonitis or profuse external drainage of bile. If a T-tube has been sutured into the common duct, bile will drain through it profusely and will not appreciably diminish in amount with the passage of time. Postoperative cholangiograms will demonstrate such stones.

Stones may be left in the common duct even though a careful exploration of the ducts has been made. Small stones may be overlooked in the common duct or may lodge in the intrahepatic duct and later migrate to the region of the ampulla and cause irritation or obstruction. Failure to explore the stump of the cystic duct carefully may cause the surgeon to overlook a stone in this region which can subsequently produce severe pain and biliary indigestion. Inadequate dissection of the cystic duct and failure to remove most of it may be followed by biliary distress. In a number of patients presenting postcholecystectomy symptoms, I have explored the common ducts and found no residual stones. However, in these patients a long cystic stump was found. After careful dissection of the common duct, removal of the cystic duct stump and drainage of the common duct, there was complete and permanent relief from symptoms. It is possible that the added dissection accomplished the release of the nervous control of the sphincter of Oddi which did not follow the first operation.

CHOLEDOCHOSTOMY

The indications for exploring the common bile duct in conjunction with cholecystectomy are: (1) a thickened and dilated common bile duct; (2) definite or questionable masses palpable within the bile duct; (3) a dilated cystic duct, especially if small stones are present in the gallbladder (a normal cystic duct has a diameter about equal to that of a kitchen match); (4) the presence or a history of jaundice, especially if it has been intermittent; (5) an inflamed common duct in conjunction with gallbladder disease.

Technic.—The following technic is recommended for patients who have had no previous surgery upon the biliary tract. The abdomen is opened preferably through a long, high, right rectus or right paramedian incision (Plate 28, *A*). The gallbladder, bile ducts and hepatic vessels are exposed by the method described under cholecystectomy (Plate 31). The peritoneum over these structures should be widely incised and the vessels and ducts positively identified.

It is my belief that choledochostomy should be performed before cholecystectomy. This is especially true if the patient is jaundiced. Choledochostomy may reveal certain abnormalities which may make it advisable to use the gallbladder as a route for internal or external biliary drainage. The presence of the gallbladder simplifies the exposure and exploration of the common bile ducts. If the gallbladder is removed first, oozing from the gallbladder bed may tend to obscure the field for choledochostomy.

Whenever the common duct is opened it should be drained. Adequate exploration of the duct is followed by temporary edema and partial occlusion of the distal end. This interferes with the free flow of bile and, if the duct is closed without drainage, may result in back pressure upon the liver and in leakage from the suture line. Bile peritonitis in the region of the common duct is one of the commonest causes for the subsequent development of obliterative cholangitis.

[Choledochostomy *continued on page 180.*]

A.—The common duct should be held taut and be exposed as widely as possible by upward retraction on the round ligament and gallbladder and downward retraction on the duodenum. The hand of the assistant retracting downward on the duodenum usually affords better exposure than retractors. The common duct is grasped with two Allis or Judd-Allis forceps placed opposite each other transversely on the anterior wall of the duct. Even though the surgeon is confident that he is dealing with the common duct, he should make doubly sure by aspirating its contents for bile with a syringe and needle.

B.—The anterior wall of the duct is incised between the Allis forceps by a knife incision longitudinal to the duct. The tip of an aspirator should be placed at the line of incision to minimize the spillage of bile. The incision may be enlarged longitudinally with either knife or scissors.

C.—The length of the incision in the common duct should be proportionate to the diameter of the duct and should not be curtailed if additional length would permit a more complete exploration of the duct. This diagram is made from a photograph of a common duct 2 cm. in diameter. The incision in the anterior wall was over 4 cm. long. It permits direct visual observation and careful probing and exploring of the right and left hepatic ducts. The distal common duct opening and the entrance of the cystic duct into the posterior wall of the common duct are visualized.

D.—It is well to begin the exploration with a curved Pean forceps. The forceps is inserted into the duct and the points are spread as widely as possible before the instrument is passed upward or downward in the duct. This facilitates the engagement of stones between the blades and reduces the probability of pushing calculi ahead of the instrument. The duct is carefully and repeatedly explored with the forceps, distally toward the ampulla and proximally toward the hepatic ducts as far as possible. Occasionally a stone will be encountered which cannot be grasped with the Pean forceps. Such a stone can sometimes be removed with one of the various types of kidney stone or gallstone forceps. A forceps should be selected which has a curve that will enable the grasping end to reach the stone.

[Choledochostomy *continued on page 182.*]

PLATE 34

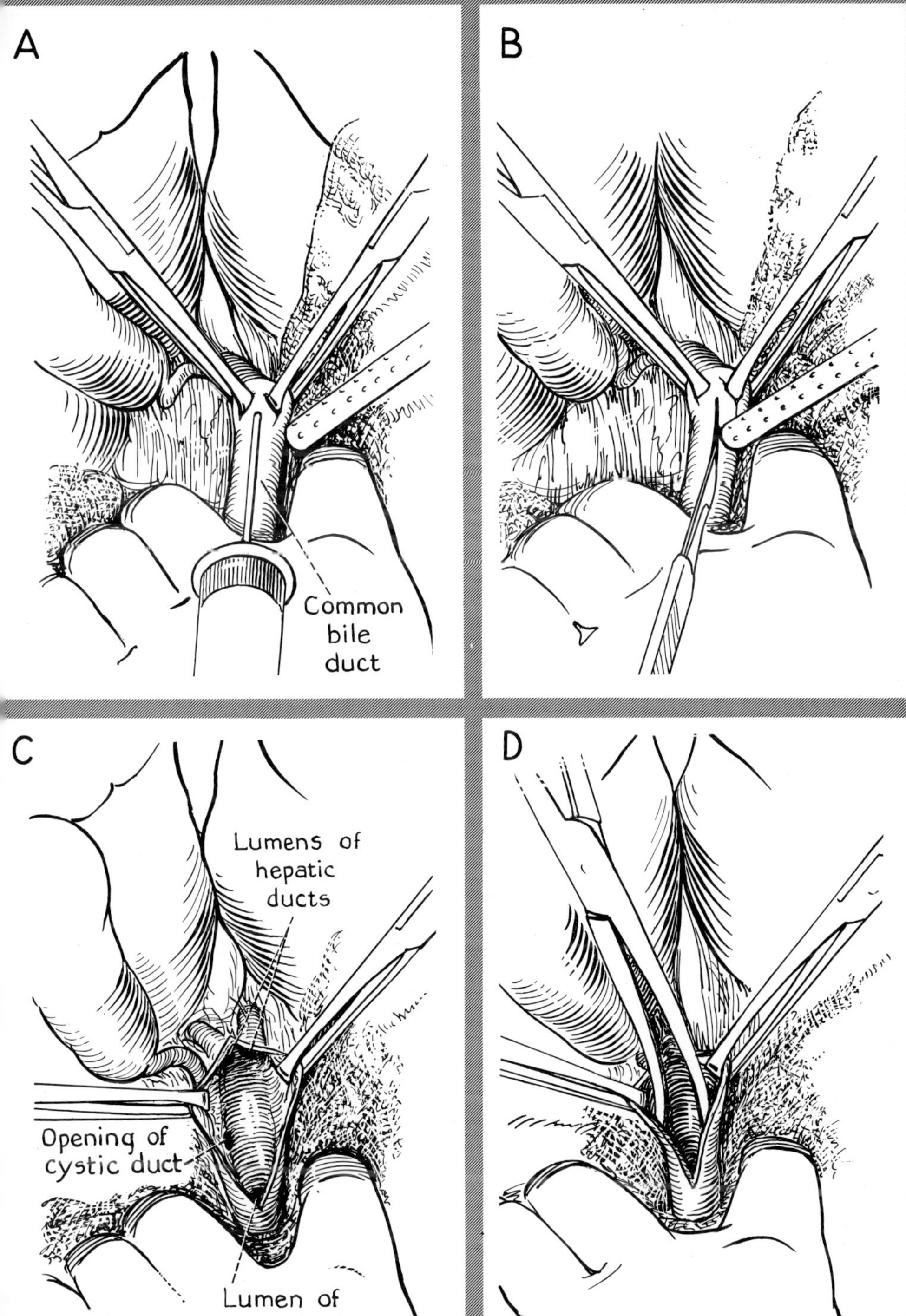
A
Common bile duct
B
C
Lumens of hepatic ducts
Opening of cystic duct
Lumen of distal common bile duct
D

E.—The duct is next explored with a scoop, such as the Mayo cystic duct or common duct scoop which has a malleable handle and a long narrow bowl. The handle should be bent so that the bowl will pass along the posterior wall of the duct to pick up stones within it rather than to force them ahead of it.

F.—After placing the scoop in the duct the surgeon palpates the duct over the scoop by placing the fingers posterior and the thumb anterior to the duct. In this manner, stones which were not previously detected can often be felt in contact with the scoop. By manipulation with the examining hand, the stones can sometimes be forced into the bowl of the scoop and removed.

G.—If possible, the scoop is passed through the ampulla of Vater and its tip identified under the anterior wall of the duodenum, thus assuring patency of the ampulla. If the scoop cannot be passed through the ampulla with gentle pressure, it should be removed and a malleable probe with a small bowl or tip inserted distally into the duct. The probe should be inserted carefully and the tip guided by the fingers of the surgeon to minimize the danger of producing a false passage.

H.—If the probe does not pass through, the ampulla should be approached transduodenally. Before incising the duodenum longitudinally, the scoop is passed into the common duct distally as far as possible to help identify the location of the ampulla of Vater. This is often well down on the second portion of the duodenum. The opening of the ampulla is enlarged sufficiently to permit the probe or scoop to pass readily through it. Closure of the duodenum should be in a transverse direction.

[Choledochostomy *continued on page 184.*]

PLATE 34

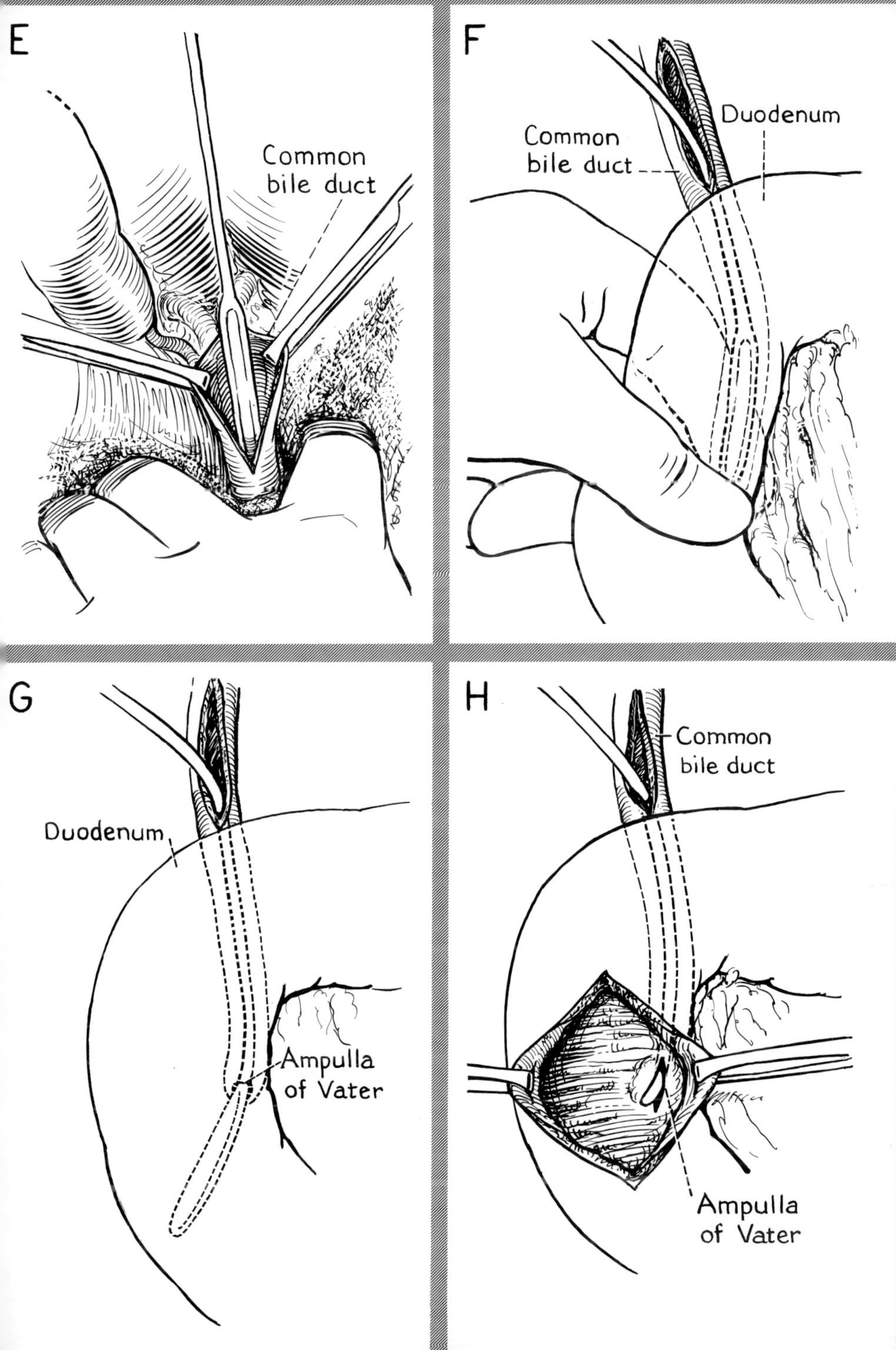
E
Common
bile duct
F
Common
bile duct
Duodenum
G
Duodenum
Ampulla
of Vater
H
Common
bile duct
Ampulla
of Vater

I.—When small stones are encountered in the common duct, aspiration and irrigation may remove overlooked calculi. A curved glass rod attached to suction is passed proximally and distally in the ducts in an effort to aspirate stones. A small catheter may then be passed into the ducts and saline solution forced through it with a syringe. This method is especially valuable in dislodging small stones from the intrahepatic duct.

J.—The cystic duct is now clamped about 0.5 cm. from its junction with the common duct, divided between clamps and ligated. When the cystic duct courses behind the common duct or alongside it for a considerable distance and one is not certain of the site of entrance into the common duct, it is well to open the distal end and probe it to be sure that no stones remain in the distal segment.

K.—Some surgeons prefer to explore the common duct through the cystic duct stump. Seldom is this of sufficient diameter to permit careful exploration. If the duct enters on the anterior wall of the common duct, it may be incised and the incision carried down the anterior common duct wall to permit adequate exploration. If the cystic duct enters on either side or the posterior wall of the common duct, it should not be used for exploration and for insertion of a T-tube because torsion of the common duct may result.

L.—After ligation of the cystic stump, the common duct is re-explored to make sure that no stones have passed into it during the manipulation following initial exploration. A T-tube is then sutured into the common duct, using a running intestinal catgut suture which should be locked around the vertical arm to hold it firmly in place. Before insertion, the tube is irrigated to assure the patency of its lumen. It is also carefully tested for any weakness at the junction of the vertical and cross-arms which could result in breaking of the tube during removal and require a duct exploration for removal of the cross-arm. The ends of the T are cut 1–2 cm. long. The size of the T-tube depends upon the diameter of the common duct. It should be of a size that will easily fit within the duct to permit adequate drainage and yet allow bile to flow around the intraductal portion of the tube should the lumen become occluded.

M.—The gallbladder may now be removed and its bed oversewn (Plate 31). A Penrose drain should be placed down to Morison's pouch and both T-tube and drain brought out through the abdominal incision.

[Choledochostomy *continued on page 186.*]

PLATE 34

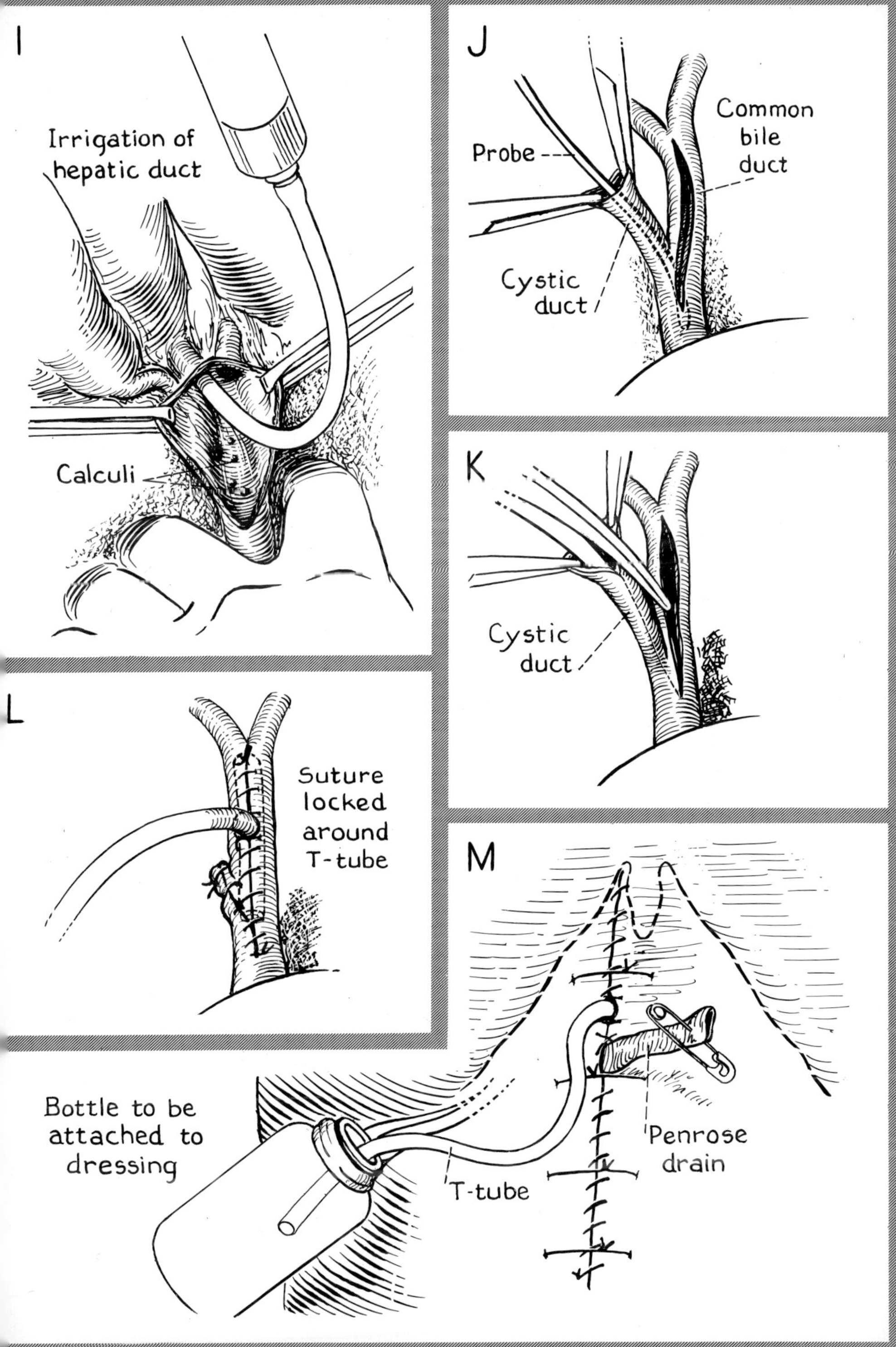
I
Irrigation of hepatic duct
Calculi
J
Probe
Common bile duct
Cystic duct
K
Cystic duct
L
Suture locked around T-tube
M
Bottle to be attached to dressing
T-tube
Penrose drain

The T-tube should not be sutured to the abdominal wall because movements of respiration or of the abdominal wall could dislodge the tube from the common duct or cause it to kink within the abdomen. It is most important that the end of the T-tube protruding from the abdominal wall is not attached in any manner that would permit traction on it and result in its dislodgment from the common duct. A bottle with a mouth of ample size to admit the T-tube may be attached to the patient's dressing. The spilling of bile upon the patient's dressings or bedclothes is of little consequence compared to the possible complication of early dislodgment of the T-tube and the development of bile peritonitis.

Dilatation of Ampulla of Vater

Some surgeons advocate dilatation of the ampulla of Vater with graded sounds to facilitate the subsequent passage of stones which may have been overlooked and also to overcome the tonus or spasm of the sphincter of Oddi. I personally am opposed to dilatation of the ampulla to any greater degree than that produced by small sounds or scoops. The passage of any instrument through the ampulla and the associated manipulation result in some edema which is apt to cause a temporary partial or complete obstruction to the passage of bile into the duodenum. This is not the result of spasm of the sphincter of Oddi which can be overcome by dilatation; our studies have shown that the sphincter loses its tone after an adequate cholecystectomy. The passing of large probes through the ampulla and sphincter may traumatize these structures and result in subsequent scarring and stenosis. However, as temporary edema and obstruction follow choledochostomy, it is imperative that the common duct always be drained after exploration to permit a free flow of bile and to prevent leakage into the peritoneal cavity. If the duct is closed primarily, the subsequent increased pressure within it may result in local bile leakage and peritonitis which may subsequently produce a progressive obliterative cholangitis.

Operative Cholangiography

In my opinion, no form of common duct exploration is more accurate than careful palpation of the duct (containing a scoop or probe) by the fingers and thumb of the surgeon. The accuracy of this method increases with the experience of the surgeon and the diligence with which the examination is conducted. A number of factors, however, increase the difficulty and affect the accuracy of such an examination. If the head of the pancreas is nodular and firm or if the duct passes through a groove within the head of the pancreas, detection of stones within the duct may be confusing. Dense adhesions from previous surgical procedures and inflammatory disease may make such an examination inaccurate. As it is most important to remove all stones in the bile duct at the first exploration, any aids to accomplish this are worthy of trial.

Many surgeons routinely take cholangiograms during the course of biliary tract surgery. Some claim this procedure has great diagnostic value in demonstrating a variety of conditions of the biliary system, including the number and position of stones, the anatomic configuration and variations of the extrahepatic biliary system, the patency of the ducts and sphincter of Oddi, any existing fistulous communications, displacements due to neoplasms or other tumors of the ducts and ampulla of Vater, the reflux of bile into the pancreatic ducts and the functional status of the sphincter of Oddi.

Technic.—A cassette tunnel is placed under the patient at the level of the upper abdomen and lower chest so that the entire biliary system will lie anterior to the film. Drapes should be applied in such a manner that the cassettes may be changed without contaminating the sterile operating field. Towels are sutured to the edges of the wound to avoid shadows made by towel clips. After the gallbladder and bile ducts have been exposed, a 35 per cent or 70 per cent aqueous solution of Diodrast (iodopyracet) is injected into the gallbladder or bile ducts by means of a syringe and fine needle. A scout film is taken to determine the accurate placement of the cassette. Bile is then aspirated from the gallbladder and replaced with 40–50 cc. of Diodrast. If the cystic duct is occluded, 15 cc. of Diodrast is injected into the common bile duct. It has been recommended that the common bile duct be transfixed with sutures to prevent the needle from passing through the posterior wall. After satisfactory cholangiograms have been obtained and studied the surgeon proceeds with the indicated operative procedure. If the common duct is explored and a T-tube inserted, Diodrast is again injected through the T-tube and a film taken to be sure all stones have been removed. Cholangiography has merit as an aid to biliary tract surgery but is not a substitute for careful exploration and is not without danger.

Gallstones may become firmly impacted in the distal end of the common duct so that removal through the ordinary choledochostomy incision is not possible. When this condition is encountered, one of two approaches may be used.

Retroduodenal Approach

A.—When the stone lies outside the duodenal wall a retroduodenal approach may be used. The peritoneal fold along the right border of the duodenum is incised. The posterior wall of the duodenum is mobilized and rotated to the left.

B.—The distal portion of the common duct is freed from surrounding structures until the stone can be palpated through it. A longitudinal incision is made in the duct over the stone and the stone removed with forceps.

C.—The opening in the duct wall is closed with continuous catgut sutures. The common duct is then re-explored through the original choledochostomy incision. After determining the patency of the ampulla, a T-tube is sutured into the common duct in the method previously described (Plate 34, *L*).

[Transduodenal approach *on page 190.*]

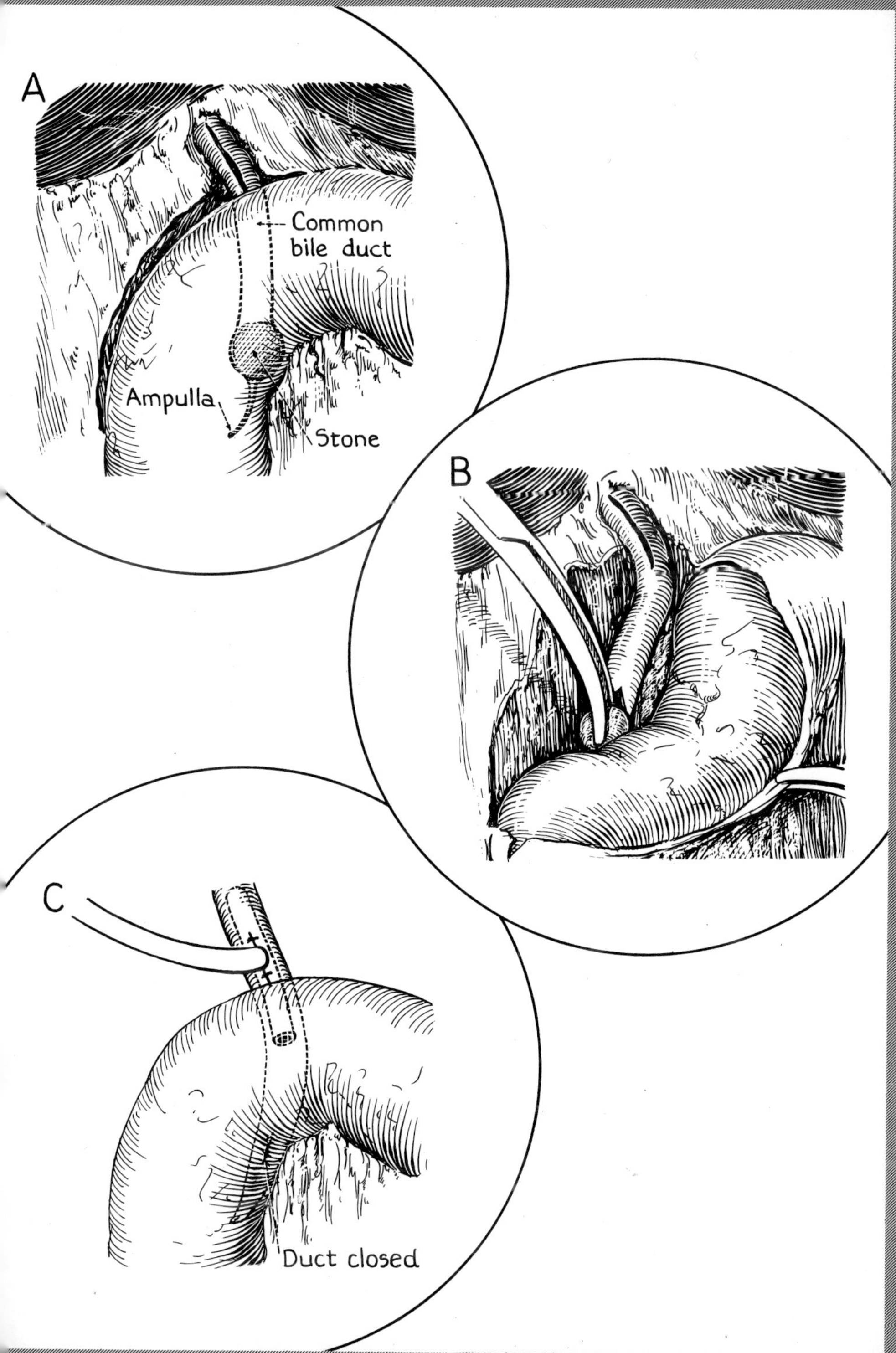
A
Common bile duct
Ampulla
Stone
B
C
Duct closed

Transduodenal Approach

A.—If the stone has passed through the duodenal wall and become lodged in the ampulla of Vater, it usually is necessary to remove it by a transduodenal approach. The common duct should first be explored and an attempt made to dislodge the stone. If this is unsuccessful, the stone is located by palpation and a longitudinal incision is made in the anterior wall of the duodenum directly over the stone.

B.—The opening of the ampulla is located and an incision is made through the posterior wall of the duodenum and the anterior wall of the ampulla directly over the stone. This is made only sufficiently large to permit removal of the stone.

C.—The duodenum is then closed transversely to minimize the danger of duodenal stenosis. The closure should be made with an inner continuous row of intestinal catgut and an outer row of interrupted cotton sutures. The suture line should be protected with omentum. A T-tube is sutured into the original choledochostomy incision.

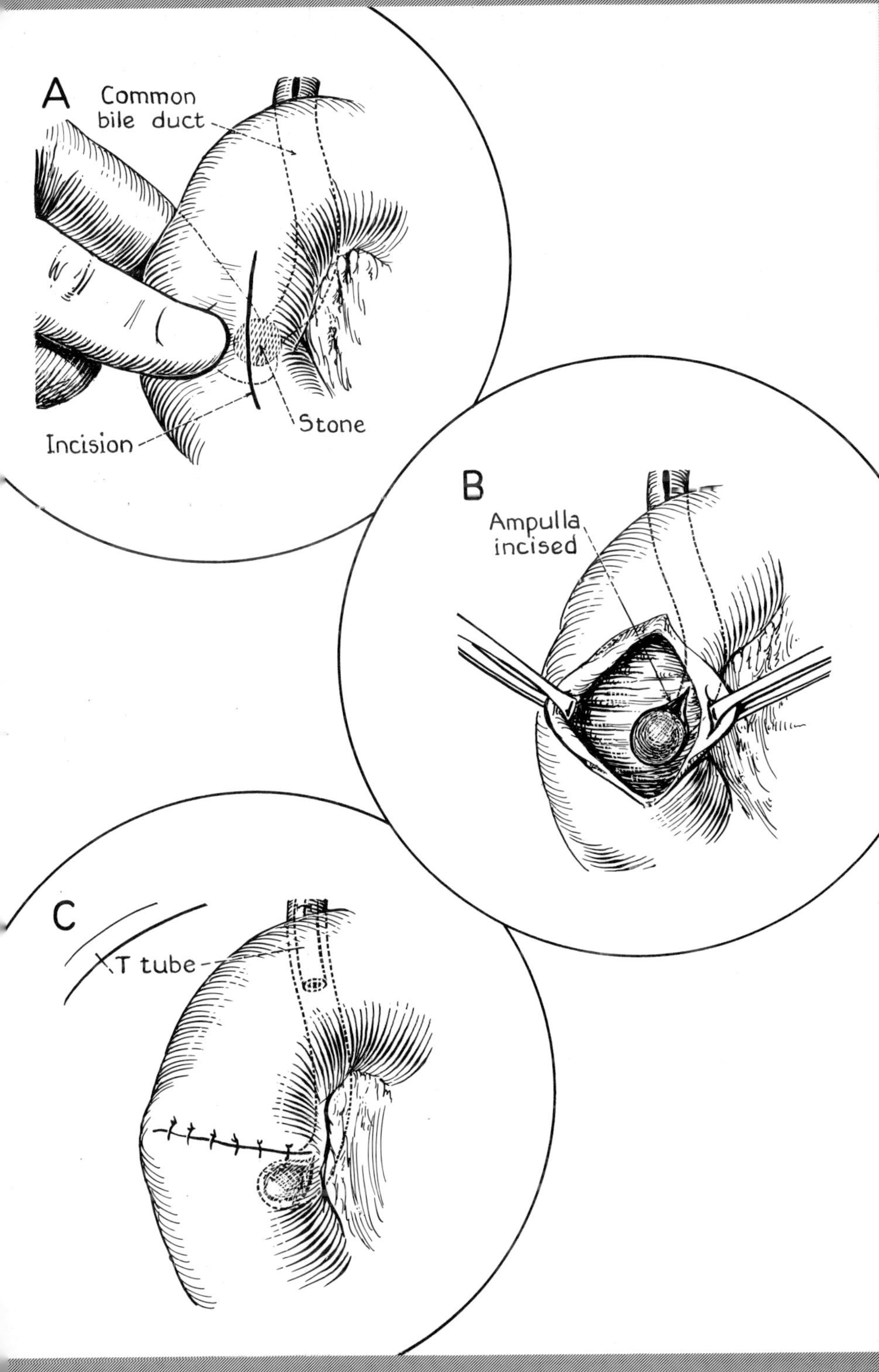
A
Common
bile duct
Incision
Stone
B
Ampulla
incised
C
T tube

LESIONS OF THE DUCT WALL

Congenital Anomalies

Any portion of the extraheptic biliary tract may be congenitally obliterated. Such occlusion of the common bile duct is rare and involvement of the hepatic ducts is even more infrequently encountered. These congenital lesions are thought to result from failure of proper canalization of the ducts. Though the lesions may completely occlude the bile ducts and prevent any bile from entering the intestinal tract, the diagnosis is not apparent immediately after birth and may be confused with icterus neonatorum. The latter condition, however, usually clears in a few days, whereas the jaundice due to congenital obstruction continues to increase. The liver and often the spleen may be greatly enlarged. The disease ends fatally in a very short time if some form of bile drainage either to the surface or into the intestinal tract is not established. Such operations are seldom successful.

Incomplete congenital obstruction of the distal portion of the common bile duct may permit the patient to live for a number of years, during which time a gradual dilatation of the common bile duct results in the formation of a choledochal cyst. The cyst may become very large and be palpable on abdominal examination. Intermittent attacks of jaundice, pain and fever often result. X-ray studies of the gastrointestinal tract may show a displacement of the stomach to the left and downward displacement of the duodenum and right portion of the transverse colon. Cholecystographic studies may demonstrate the cyst and show calcification in its wall. Treatment consists of the establishment of an adequate anastomosis between the cyst and an adjacent portion of the stomach or small intestine. The technic of these procedures is described under treatment of benign strictures of the common bile duct.

Inflammatory Disease of the Bile Ducts

Primary inflammatory disease of the bile ducts seldom is encountered. Cholangitis is usually associated with inflammatory diseases of the gallbladder, liver or pancreas or is produced by complications of these diseases, such as calculi, infected bile, suppurative drainage from the liver, spontaneous internal biliary fistulas or suppurative biliary tract surgery. It may follow failure to remove stones, inadequate cholecystectomy, the production of surgical strictures or the establishment of anastomoses which permit regurgitation of intestinal contents into the bile ducts. Progressive obliterative cholangitis occasionally may develop when there has been no surgical intervention but usually follows a surgical procedure although it may not develop for a number of years after operation. A gradually progressive periductal fibrosis as a result of inflammation around the duct is an etiologic factor.

Suppurative cholangitis presents a clinical picture of recurrent attacks of pain or discomfort, fluctuating jaundice, an intermittent septic type of fever, chills, leukocytosis and often a gradually enlarging liver. If the disease continues, the spleen may enlarge and the patient may become progressively emaciated. Treatment consists in the removal of the etiologic factor. If stones within the duct are the cause, their removal and prolonged drainage of the common duct may result in a cure. Treatment of other etiologic conditions is discussed under the respective headings.

Traumatic Injury of the Bile Ducts

The protected position of the bile ducts renders them less vulnerable to injury by external force than many other abdominal organs. However, they are occasionally traumatized and partially or completely severed by both penetrating and nonpenetrating injuries of the abdomen. During the course of exploration of penetrating wounds of the upper right abdomen, the bile ducts should be carefully examined. In non-penetrating wounds of the right upper abdomen there may be sufficient damage to the extrahepatic biliary system to cause leakage of bile. This will produce symptoms of local or generalized peritonitis. Such accidents demand early surgical exploration. If the common bile duct has been damaged or severed, it should be carefully exposed and a primary surgical repair completed whenever possible (Plate 38). If this is accomplished, the common duct should always be drained by the use of a T-tube. Similar repairs should be attempted on all penetrating wounds involving the bile ducts. If there is a considerable loss of substance, the duodenum and head of the pancreas can be mobilized to permit an end-to-end approximation of the severed ducts. The technics for these procedures are described in Plates 39 and 40.

Surgical accidents are the most common cause of benign strictures of the common bile ducts. The results of such accidents often are tragic and every possible precaution should be taken to avoid them. Some of the factors producing them are described here.

A.—Inadequate exposure to permit satisfactory visualization of the bile ducts is an important factor contributing to duct injury. Most patients upon whom I have operated for complications of surgical accidents have presented abdominal scars which indicated that previous incisions had not been carried high enough to permit good exposure of the ducts (see Plate 28).

B.—The common hepatic duct may be damaged by its inclusion in the clamp placed to occlude the cystic duct, cystic artery or both, which results from inadequate exposure and identification of the ducts and vessels. Even though the surgeon recognizes that he has included the common hepatic duct and releases the clamps, damage to the duct wall usually will result in a subsequent stricture if immediate repair is not performed.

C.—Hemorrhage from an accidentally torn or divided blood vessel sometimes induces the surgeon to stab blindly with hemostats to control the bleeding and in so doing the ducts may be injured. This is particularly true if a large hepatic artery is torn and bleeding is profuse. Sharp dissection behind the cystic duct or traction upon the neck of the gallbladder may result in a tear of the cystic artery or occasionally of the right hepatic artery.

D.—Such bleeding can be controlled by compression of the hepatic artery. This is accomplished by placing the index finger in the foramen of Winslow beneath the hepatic artery and the thumb anterior to it and compressing the artery between them. The blood should then be removed by suction and sponging. The end of the bleeding vessel should be carefully isolated and after identity of the vessel is definitely established, it should be clamped and ligated. Hemorrhage may also result from the tearing of anomalous vessels, particularly when the surgeon is not familiar with the numerous types of anomalies which may be encountered or when he does not make a careful dissection to identify the relationship of ducts and arteries (see Plate 23).

[Bile duct injuries *continued on page 196.*]

PLATE 37

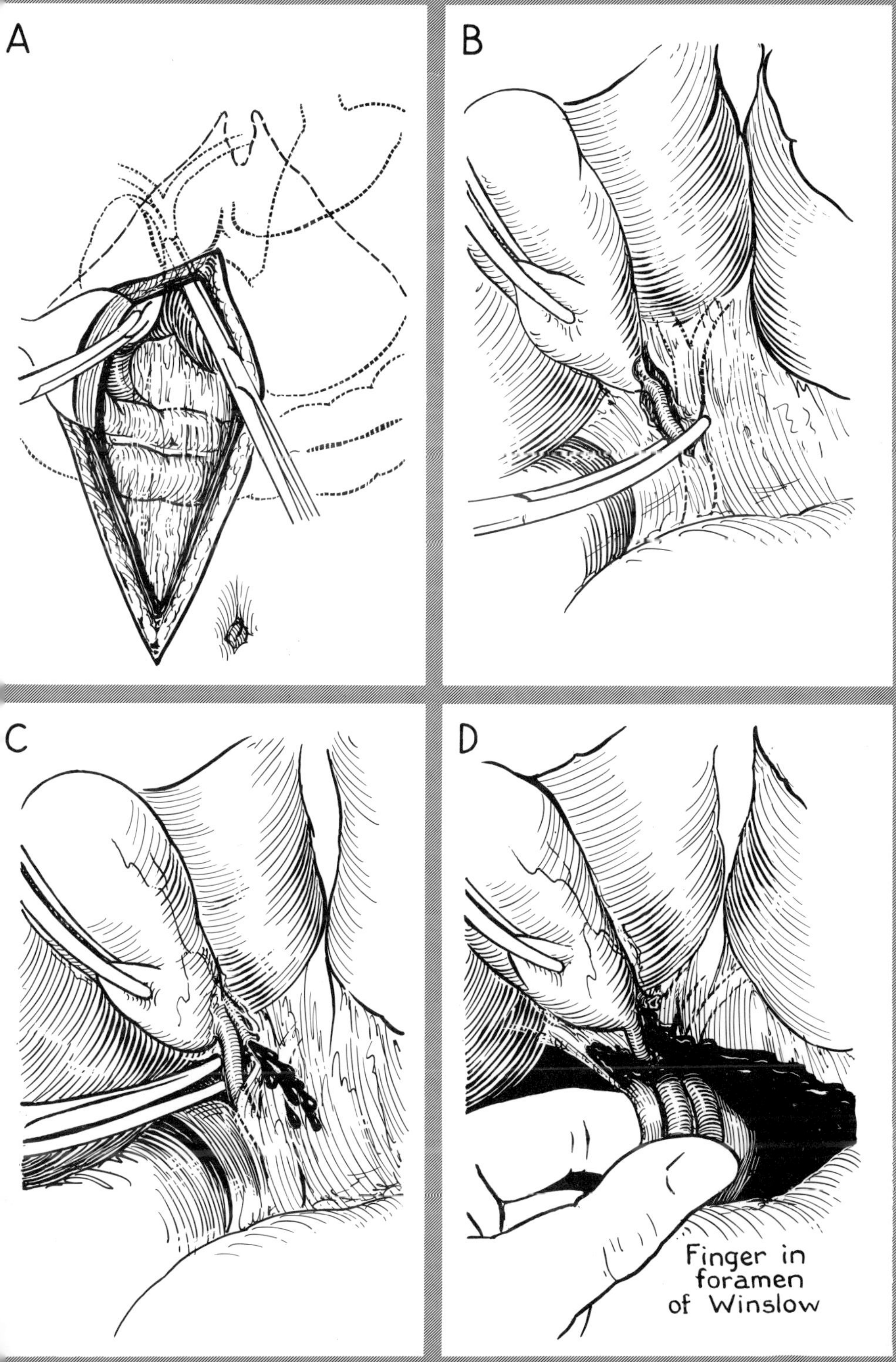

E.—One of the most common factors leading to common duct injury is angulation of the common duct by too much traction on the gallbladder and inadequate traction on the distal common duct by the assistant. Under such circumstances the angulated common duct may be mistaken for the distal end of the cystic duct and a ligature may be placed around the entire common duct. If this type of accident is not recognized and corrected at the time of operation, it usually produces immediate postoperative symptoms of obstructive jaundice, bile peritonitis or external biliary drainage. If the clamp and ligature only partially occlude the common duct, symptoms may not appear for weeks or months after operation when stenosis develops at the site of partial ligation.

F.—The packing of gauze in the bed of the gallbladder to be left in place and removed later through the wound may be the cause of a subsequent obliterative cholangitis and stricture formation. This procedure is particularly dangerous if the gauze is in contact with the common bile duct.

G.—Failure to identify and to ligate an aberrant hepatic duct can result in the pooling of bile around the common duct or in a generalized bile peritonitis, either of which can be followed by cholangitis with subsequent stricture formation. Bile leakage from a cystic duct stump from which the ligature has slipped can produce the same results. These dangers make it imperative to place a drain in Morison's pouch whenever cholecystectomy is performed.

H.—The common duct may be damaged during gastric resection. The danger is increased when there is extensive inflammation around the first portion of the duodenum and it is difficult to locate the pylorus. The common duct may be divided during the dissection or may be partially or completely occluded by suture in oversewing the duodenal stump.

[Repair of common duct injuries *on page 198.*]

PLATE 37

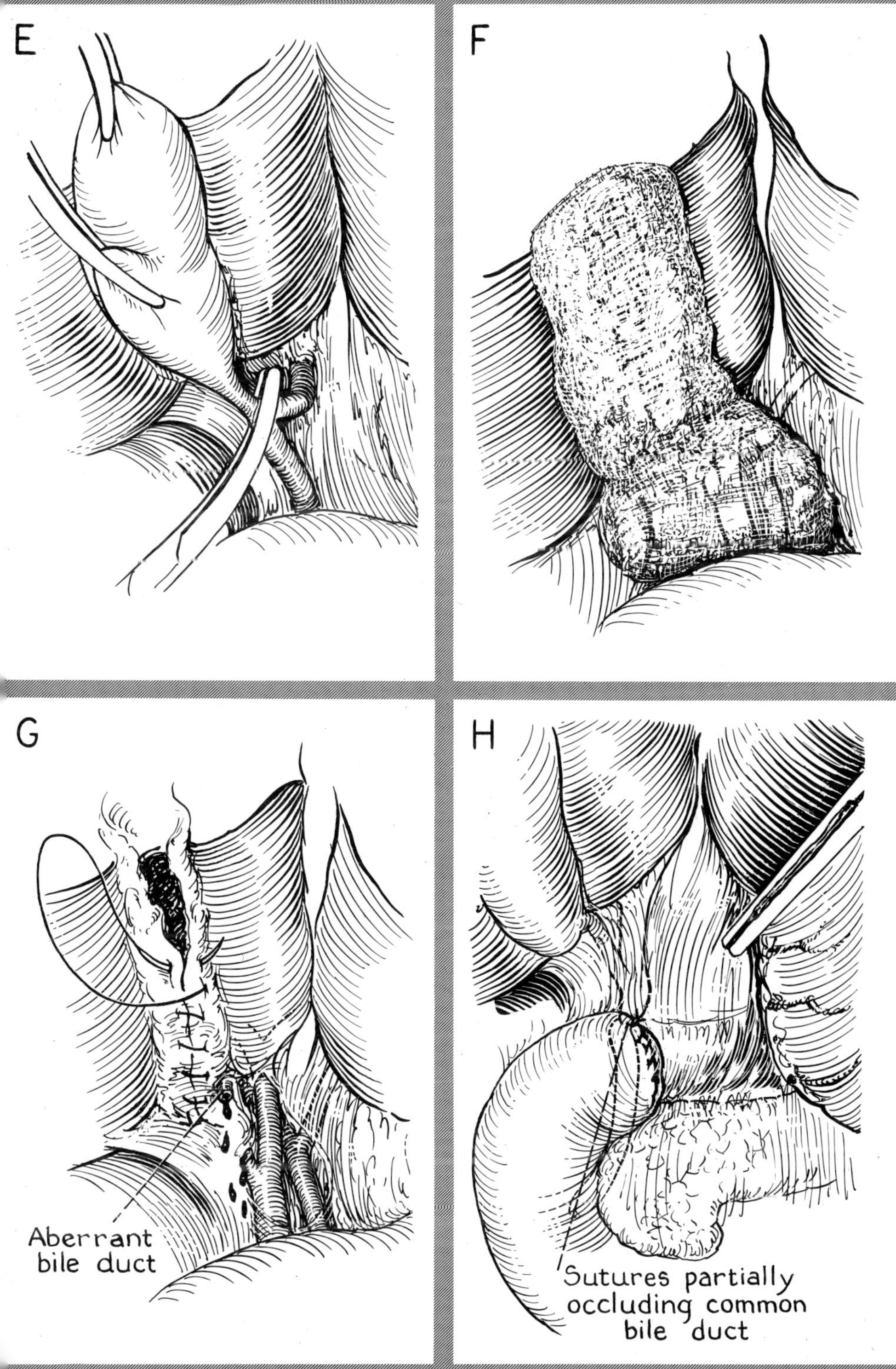
E
F
G
Aberrant bile duct
H
Sutures partially occluding common bile duct

If the surgeon recognizes or suspects that he has damaged the common bile duct during the course of an operation, he should make every attempt at an immediate repair. The common duct should be freed to give adequate exposure of the injured portion and of adjacent normal duct. If feasible, damaged portions of the duct should be excised so that normal duct wall can be approximated. Injuries to the common duct which are recognized shortly after operation should be repaired as soon as the condition of the patient permits.

A.—A longitudinal incision produced in the common bile duct by a sharp instrument may have a T-tube placed through the incision and the duct closed around it.

B.—Transection of the duct without crushing may be repaired by end-to-end anastomosis. The posterior row of fine interrupted cotton sutures is placed first. A longitudinal incision should be made in the anterior wall of the duct to admit the cross-limb of a T-tube but should not join the line of transection. It may be placed either above or below the site of injury, depending upon the amount of available duct in either location. A limb of the T-tube should extend through the site of anastomosis. The T-tube is sutured in place with continuous catgut sutures. An anterior row of fine cotton sutures completes the anastomosis.

C.—When the common duct has been angulated and clamped and both proximal and distal ends completely ligated, it is well to resect the duct beyond the area crushed by clamp or ligature. An end-to-end anastomosis is then accomplished as described in *B.*

D.—If a portion of the duct wall has been clamped and ligated, thus narrowing the lumen but not completely occluding it, it is not necessary to resect an entire segment of the duct. The ligature should be removed and the crushed portions of the duct wall debrided. After inserting a T-tube through a separate longitudinal incision, the opening in the duct should be closed transversely.

E.—When the common duct is divided close to the superior portion of the duodenum it may be possible to mobilize the duodenum and the head of the pancreas to permit an end-to-end anastomosis of the duct.

F.—If the distal portion of the common duct is damaged by division or occlusion during a gastric resection, a choledochoduodenostomy may be performed. Details of this procedure are described in Plate 44.

PLATE 38

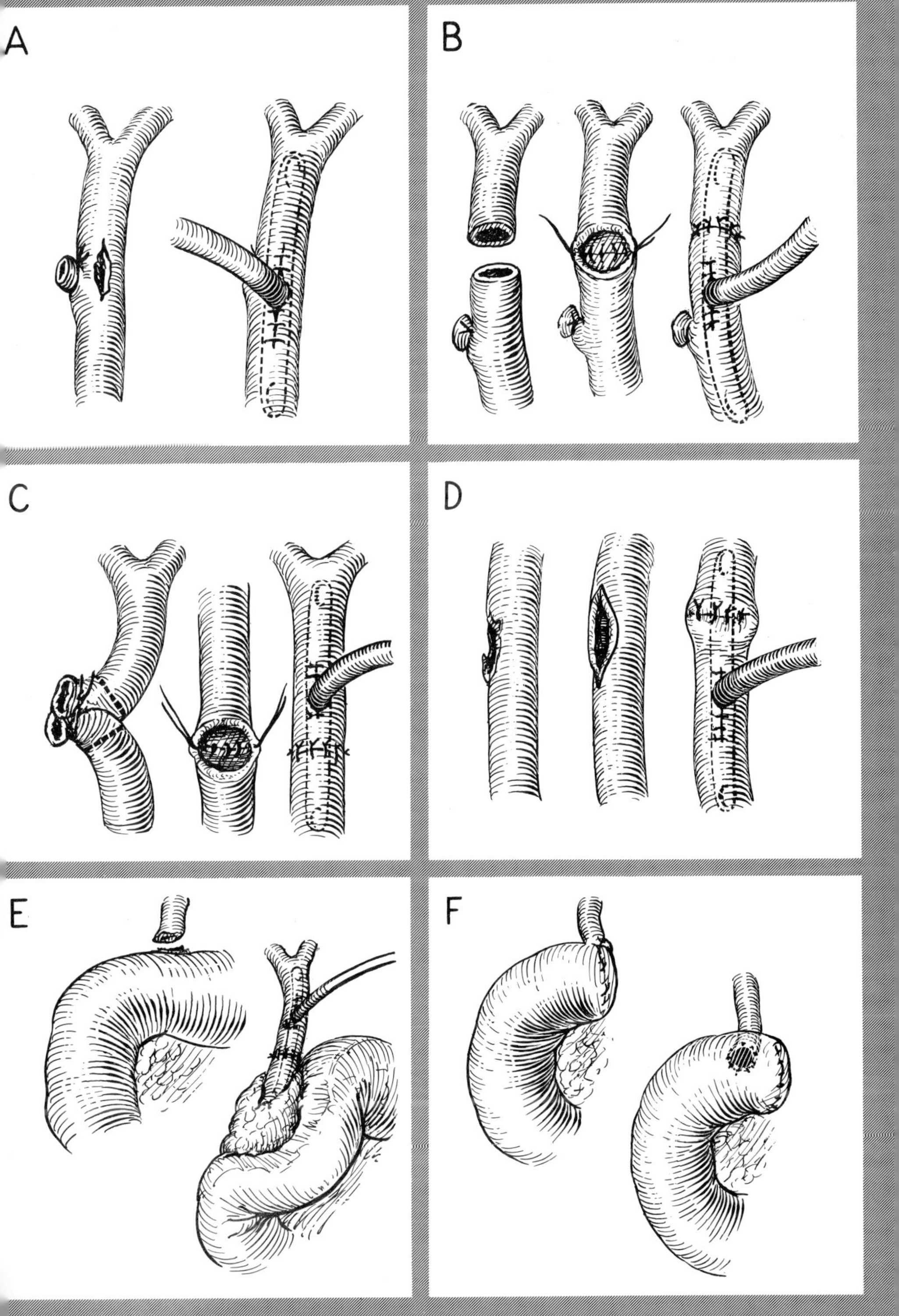

Exposure of the Common Bile Duct

The approach to a common duct stricture should be made through the scar of the previous operation if such an incision will give adequate exposure or can be extended to do so.

A.—Care must be taken in making this incision to avoid damage to any portion of the bowel or other viscera which might be adherent to the parietal peritoneum. The omentum and abdominal viscera must be carefully and widely dissected from the abdominal wall. This should include the anterior surface of the liver to permit better exposure. By grasping the parietal peritoneum and posterior rectus fascia with Kocher or similar forceps and elevating the abdominal wall, the plane of adhesions between the abdominal viscera and the peritoneum usually can be seen and separation accomplished by sharp dissection.

B.—The hepatic flexure of the colon, the duodenum, stomach and omentum usually are densely adherent to the undersurface of the liver. These structures should be freed from the liver by careful sharp dissection. It is well to begin dissection along the anterior margin of the liver on the right side. In the presence of jaundice, the capsule of the liver tears readily. Such tears should be avoided as they result in troublesome bleeding.

C.—By working from the right the hepatic flexure and omentum can be freed from the liver and the gallbladder bed with little danger of inadvertently damaging the bile ducts or vessels.

D.—The dissection should be carried posteriorly in an effort to locate and expose the foramen of Winslow.

E.—Frequently the duodenum will be densely adherent to the hilus of the liver and upon careful separation a hepaticoduodenal fistula will be found. This should be taken down and the duodenum closed by interrupted inverting sutures placed transversely in the duodenum.

[Exposure of the common duct *continued on page 202.*]

PLATE 39

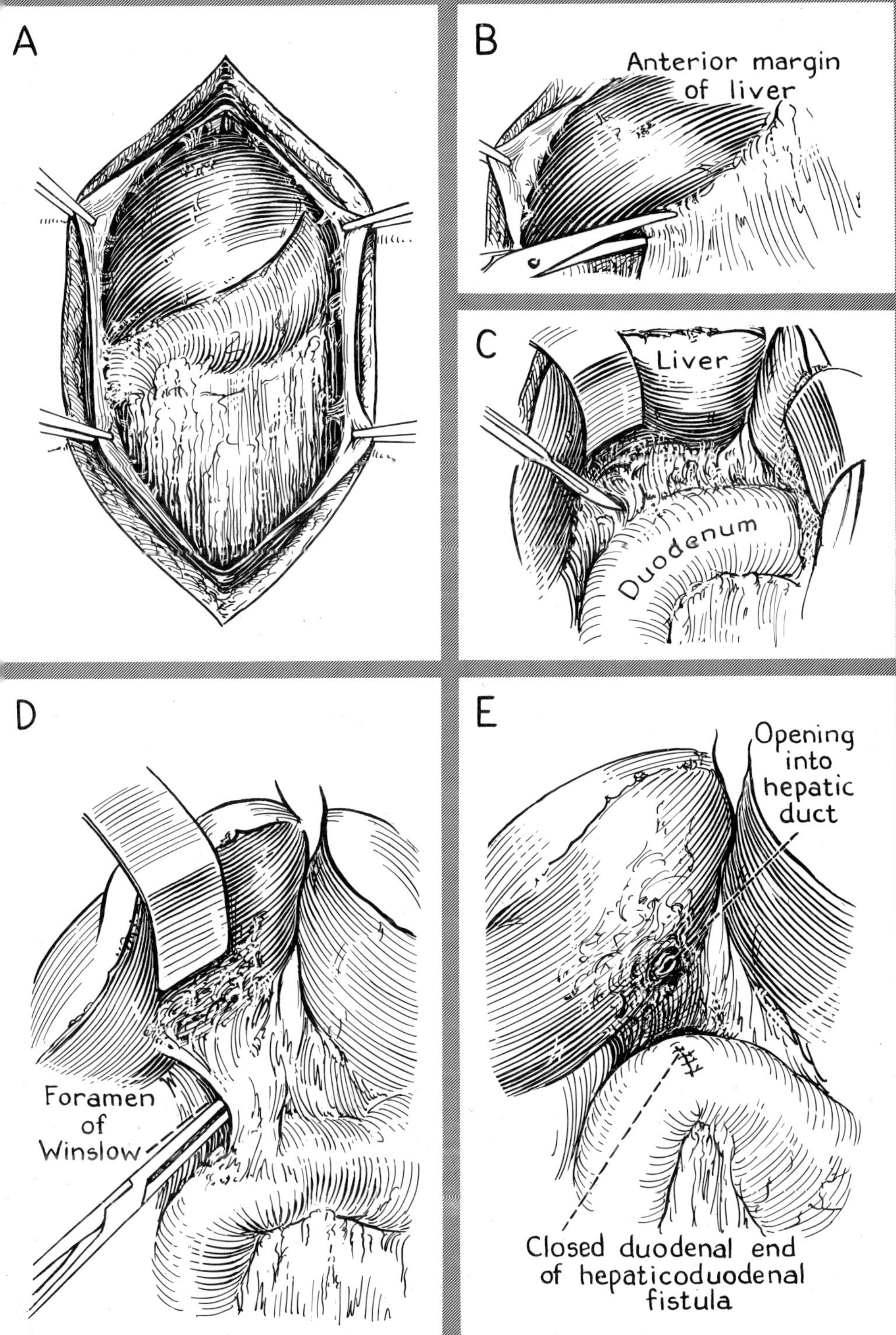
A
B
Anterior margin of liver
C
Liver
Duodenum
D
Foramen of Winslow
E
Opening into hepatic duct
Closed duodenal end of hepaticoduodenal fistula

F.—When the hilus of the liver is reached and the proximal end of the strictured bile duct is apparently located, the duct should be aspirated before being opened. If the duct is obliterated in the hilus of the liver, the portal vein may be mistaken for the common hepatic duct and an incision into it is time-consuming to repair.

G.—Upon identification, the proximal end of the duct is opened by a small longitudinal incision and the duct explored proximally and distally. With a probe extending distally to the point of stricture the surrounding duct can be more easily isolated. Every effort should be made to locate the duct distal to the stricture.

H.—If careful dissection above the duodenum fails to reveal the distal segment of common duct, it should be searched for retroduodenally. The intraduodenal, pancreatic and retroduodenal portions of the common duct seldom are damaged by trauma. It is most important to isolate them so as to repair the duct by an end-to-end anastomosis if possible. These portions of the duct seldom are strictured unless a cholangitis or sclerosing pancreatitis has been present. After careful exposure of the duodenum, the peritoneum is divided along its superior and right borders. The posterior surface of the duodenum is freed and rotated to the left. The head of the pancreas is mobilized on its posterior surface and likewise rotated to the left. This dissection should be carried out meticulously to minimize troublesome bleeding and avoid damage to the posterior wall of the duodenum. The common duct should be searched for proximal to the head of the pancreas. If it cannot be located, the duodenum should be separated from the pancreas or, if the pancreas extends posterior to the duodenum, an incision should be made through the pancreatic substance parallel to and a short distance from the medial posterior border of the duodenum. When the distal end of the duct has been located, it should be isolated from the pancreas and from surrounding scar tissue proximal to the pancreas until the point of stricture is reached.

I.—A considerable length of patent and comparatively normal duct frequently can be found and because of mobilization of the duodenum and pancreas can be elevated to meet the proximal end where an end-to-end anastomosis over a T-tube can be accomplished.

[End-to-end anastomosis *on page 204.*]

PLATE 39

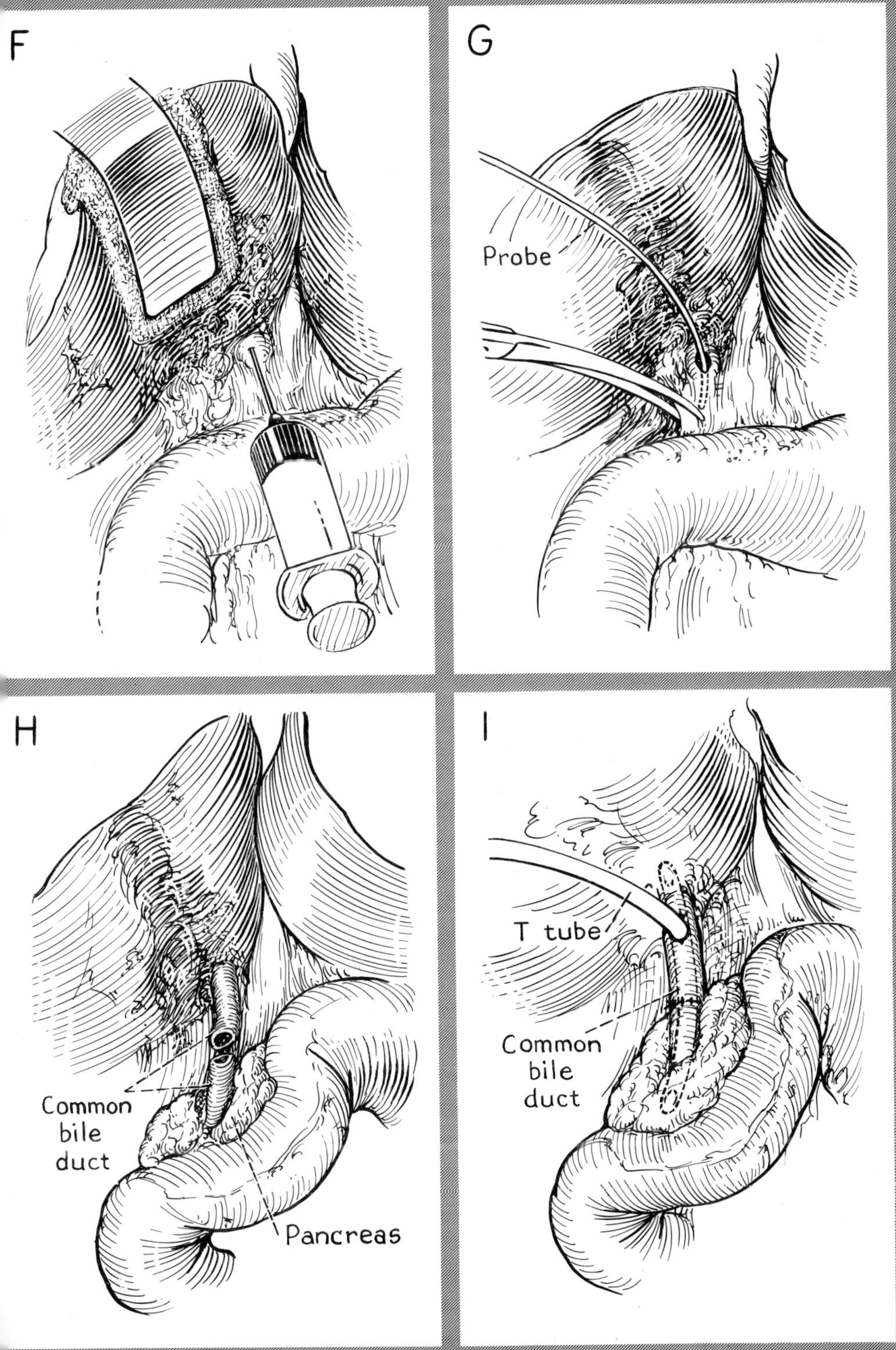
F
G
Probe
H
Common
bile
duct
Pancreas
I
T tube
Common
bile
duct

End-to-End Anastomosis

Narrow strictures of the duct lend themselves best to repair by end-to-end anastomosis and this type of repair gives the most satisfactory permanent results.

A.—Upon isolating such a stricture a longitudinal incision is made through it, extending into the proximal and distal patent segments.

B.—The scar tissue is cut away by sharp dissection. If the stricture has a lumen and the posterior wall does not appear to be too scarred, it is well to leave a small bridge of tissue in this region. However, most of the scar tissue must be cut away in order to approximate comparatively normal duct wall.

C.—An end-to-end anastomosis is then accomplished. The longitudinal incisions in both segments should be sufficiently long so that the diameter of the duct at the site of anastomosis will be larger than the smaller of the two segments of duct. Interrupted sutures of a very fine nonabsorbable material, preferably cotton, make a satisfactory anastomosis. The sutures should be placed about 2 mm. apart, and a single row of sutures is adequate. The posterior row is placed first.

D.—A longitudinal incision is made in either the proximal or distal segment but not to the line of anastomosis. A T-tube is placed in this incision with one limb extending through the anastomosis. The longitudinal incision may be closed around the T-tube with a continuous catgut suture. Following this, the anterior row of interrupted sutures is placed to complete the end-to-end anastomosis.

E.—Frequently a stricture will be found at the hilus of the liver with little or no normal duct extending beyond the liver capsule.

F.—Often by careful dissection through the liver capsule a sufficient amount of hepatic duct may be freed to permit an end-to-end anastomosis. If the stricture is short, the distal end can be brought to the proximal end without mobilization of the duodenum and pancreas. After removal of the scar tissue, the distal limb should be split anteriorly until its lumen is equal to that of the proximal duct. An end-to-end anastomosis is then accomplished with interrupted sutures.

G.—A T-tube is placed through a separate incision in the distal limb with a cross-arm extending into the liver beyond the suture line.

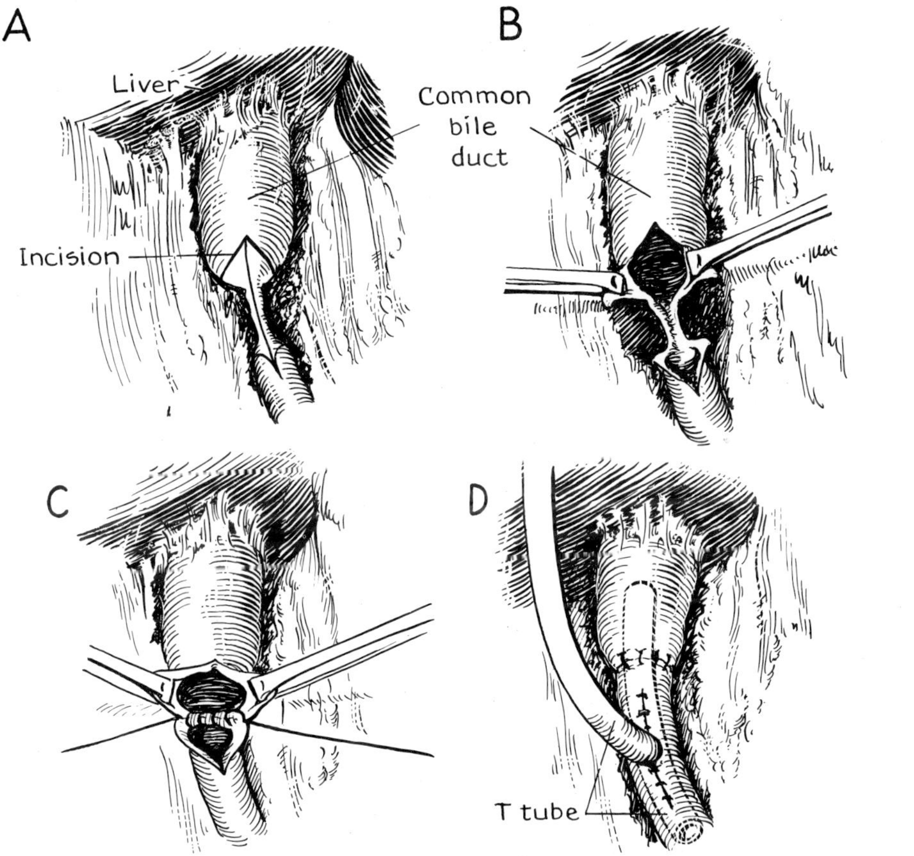
A
B
Liver
Common
bile
duct
Incision
C
D
T tube

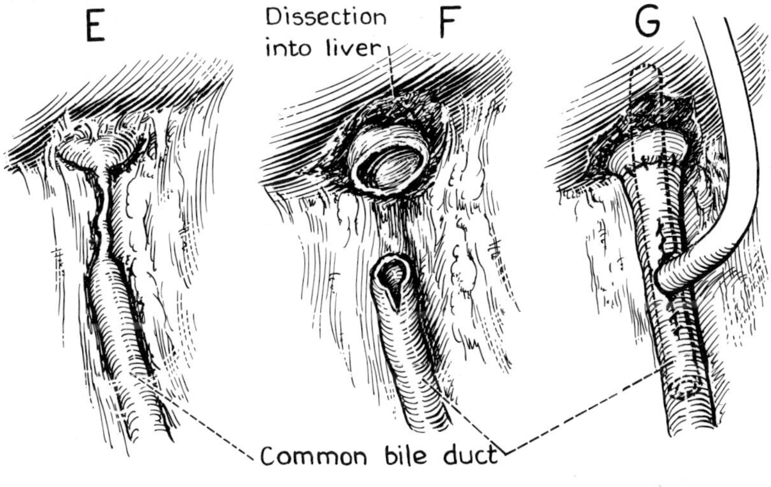
E
Dissection
into liver
F
G
Common bile duct

It is generally agreed that operations for stricture of the common bile duct which utilize the remaining patent portions of the duct with preservation of the functions of the intraduodenal portion and ampulla give more satisfactory results than direct anastomoses between the proximal end of the hepatic duct and the stomach or intestine. Dragstedt has described an operation which accomplishes the former in certain difficult cases. The distal end of the common duct often is difficult to locate, particularly if the stricture has extended down to the intrapancreatic portion of the duct. Although this portion of the duct usually escapes obliteration, it often is difficult to locate by retroduodenal dissection. Dragstedt's operation simplifies the identification of this portion of the duct.

A.—The inferior surface of the liver should be carefully freed from all adhesions (Plate 39). The proximal end of the strictured common hepatic duct is located and freed as much as possible from surrounding structures. There may be very little duct extending beyond the hilus of the liver but an attempt should be made to secure a small section of comparatively normal duct wall. (The drawings *A-H* are modified from those by Gladys McHugh.)

B.—The entire descending portion of the duodenum should be exposed. It may be necessary to mobilize the hepatic flexure and right portion of the transverse colon to accomplish this. The peritoneum is divided along the right border of the duodenum and the duodenum and head of the pancreas are elevated.

C.—A longitudinal incision is made on the anterior surface of the duodenum in its descending portion over the ampulla of Vater. Dragstedt has emphasized that the ampulla may be more distally located than expected and the incision should be carried well down on the descending portion of the duodenum.

D.—After the ampulla of Vater is located, it should be dilated by a hemostatic forceps to a size sufficient to admit a rubber catheter.

E.—A catheter as large as can be passed into the proximal duct segment is inserted through the ampulla and passed upward through the intraduodenal and intrapancreatic portions of the common duct until it meets the point of obstruction.

[Transduodenal reconstruction of bile duct *continued on page 208.*]

PLATE 41

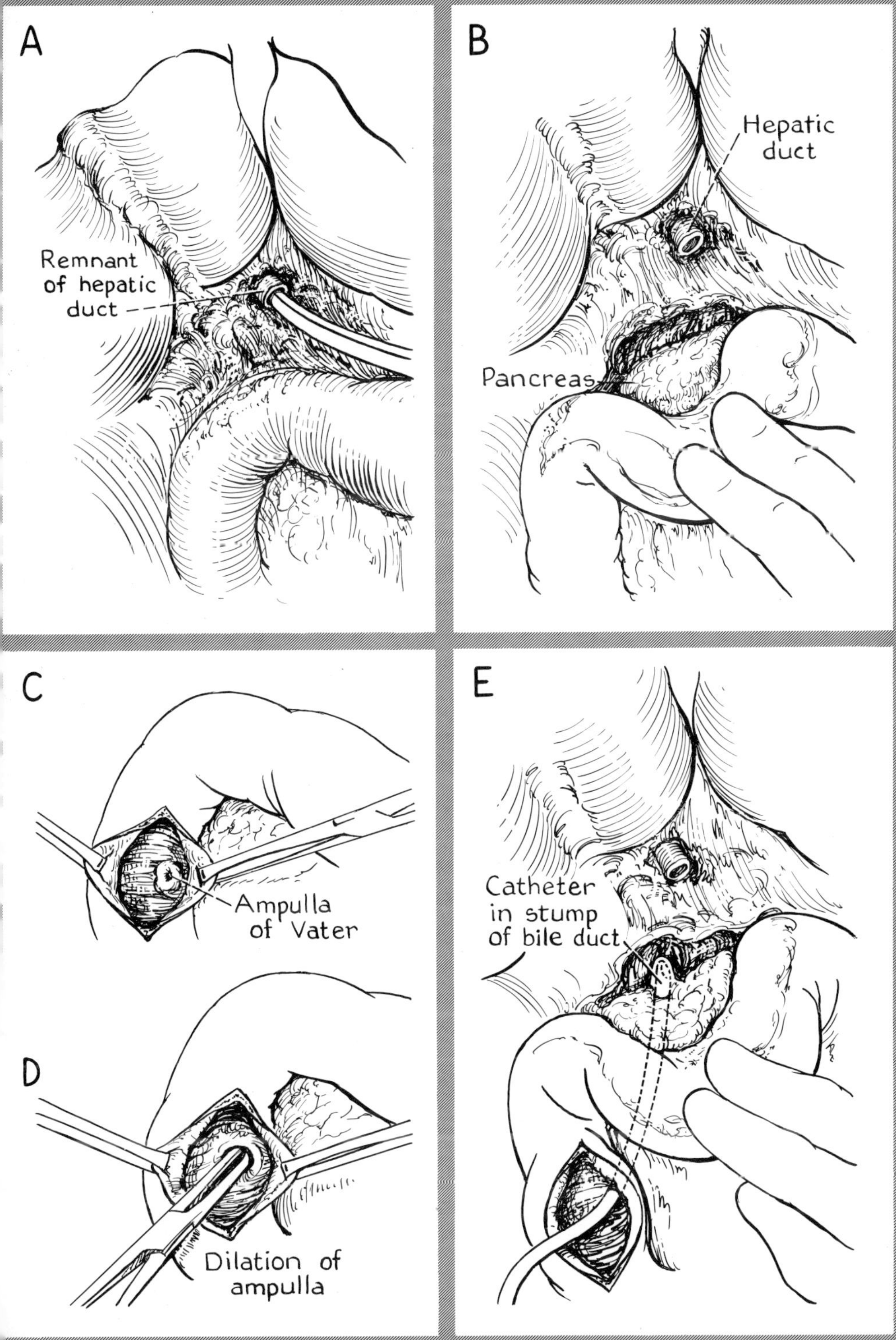

A
Remnant of hepatic duct
B
Hepatic duct
Pancreas
C
Ampulla of Vater
D
Dilation of ampulla
E
Catheter in stump of bile duct

F.—The point of obstruction of the distal end of the common duct can be located and carefully exposed. The scarred end of the distal segment of duct is resected to a point where comparatively normal duct wall is reached.

G.—The catheter is pushed upward into the proximal end of the common hepatic duct and well into the liver. The duodenum and pancreas are advanced toward the hilus of the liver to permit the ends of the duct to be approximated.

H.—An end-to-end anastomosis is made with interrupted, fine non-absorbable sutures. Care must be taken to have a minimal amount of traction upon the suture line. The duodenum is closed around the catheter which is fastened to the duodenum with chromic catgut at its point of emergence. Dragstedt wraps omentum around the catheter and sutures it to the duodenum to cover the incision. The catheter is brought to the exterior through a separate stab incision. A Penrose drain is placed under the liver and the wound closed.

I.—I have found this operation to be successful and a valuable aid in the performance of an end-to-end anastomosis of the common bile duct. My personal fear of the danger of leakage of duodenal contents around the catheter would make me reluctant to bring the catheter through the duodenal wall if this could be avoided. It is generally desirable to leave a rubber catheter through a point of stricture for about one year after operation, and a catheter placed by the Dragstedt method can be controlled as to its time of removal. If, after passing a catheter through the ampulla and locating the distal portion of the duct, it is possible to isolate sufficient duct to permit the placing of a T-tube into the common duct with one horizontal limb extending through the anastomosis, I would prefer this method.

J.—One could also place the distal end of the catheter in the duodenum, anchor it to the common duct by catgut sutures and completely close the duodenal wall in a transverse manner. Such a closure lessens the incidence of duodenal narrowing and minimizes the danger of a duodenal fistula but does not permit the surgeon to control the time of passage of the catheter.

PLATE 41

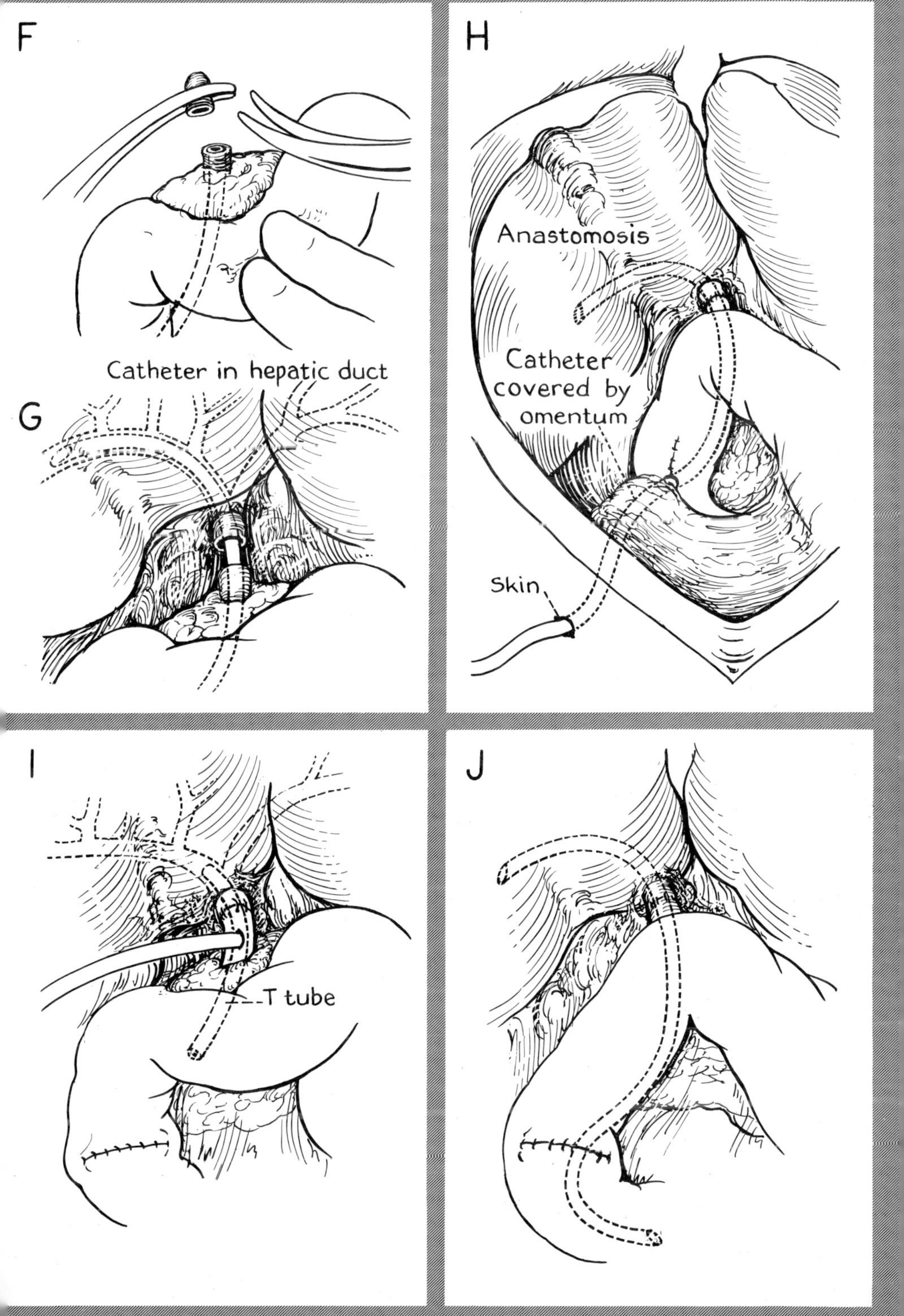
F
Catheter in hepatic duct
G
H
Anastomosis
Catheter covered by omentum
Skin
I
T tube
J

Strictures of the intraduodenal portion of the common duct or of the ampulla of Vater may result from large calculi impacted in this region for a considerable period of time. Pressure of the stone against the mucosa of the distal duct and ampulla may produce a necrosis which will be followed by fibrosis and stricture formation. This can occur whether the stone passes spontaneously or is removed surgically. It may take many weeks or months for the stricture to develop sufficiently to produce symptoms. The obstruction may be complete or a small amount of bile may pass into the intestine. Jaundice usually is progressive and quite constant. Frequently, infection of the bile ducts accompanies such a stricture and the patient will have chills and fever with some fluctuation in the degree of jaundice.

A.—This cholangiogram reveals the normal picture of the bile ducts, as outlined by the opaque medium, showing the patent distal end with its narrowed intraduodenal portion and with the medium passing freely into the duodenum.

B.—This patient had a stone impacted in the distal end of the common duct which subsequently passed into the duodenum. A stricture developed in the region of the ampulla, followed by the development of cholangitis. Her physician tapped the liver by an intercostal aspiration and entered a peripheral intrahepatic bile duct, establishing external biliary drainage through a fine catheter. Injection of opaque medium through this catheter visualized dilated bile ducts with a distal common duct stricture. This diagram is shown not as a recommendation for hepatic aspiration but to demonstrate the cholangiographic evidence of ampullary stricture.

[Repair of distal common duct strictures *on page 212.*]

PLATE 42

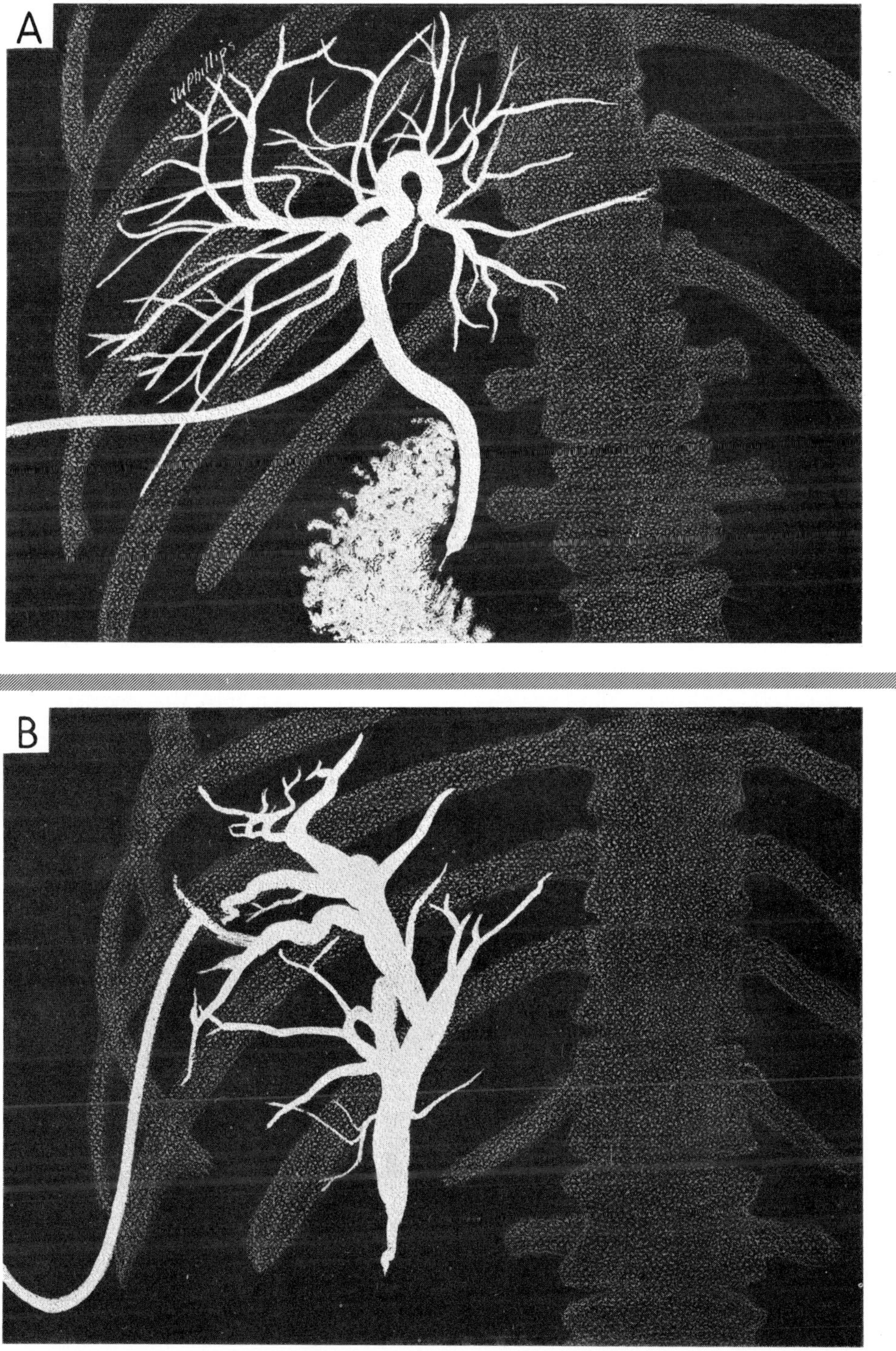

The abdomen should be opened and the common duct exposed as previously described (Plate 39). The duct, which usually is markedly dilated, should be opened through a longitudinal incision made above the duodenum. It should be carefully explored with forceps, probes and scoops. The point of stricture can be located with the end of the scoop.

A.—When the stricture is found to be at the terminal end of the common duct, it may be repaired by a transduodenal approach. The anterior wall of the duodenum is opened longitudinally opposite the tip of the scoop.

B.—A longitudinal incision is made through the posterior wall of the duodenum and the anterior wall of the common duct, using the bowl of the scoop as a guide and as protection against damage to underlying structures. The incision should be 1–2 cm. long.

C.—A continuous suture of intestinal catgut is used to approximate the cut edges of the posterior wall of the duodenum and the anterior wall of the common duct.

D.—This shows the anastomosis completed.

E.—A T-tube with a long limb should be placed in the original choledochostomy incision. The limb should be sufficiently long to pass through the anastomosis and well down into the duodenum. The opening in the duodenum is then closed transversely with an inner continuous row of intestinal catgut and an outer row of interrupted cotton sutures. The common duct incision is closed around the T-tube.

Results of this procedure are not always satisfactory. The absence of the valvelike action of the duodenal musculature and the mucosal folds in the ampulla of Vater allow regurgitation of intestinal contents into the bile duct and an ascending cholangitis may result. However, it is believed that this procedure should be tried first and more extensive procedures reserved for those patients in whom complications demand subsequent operative care. If the anastomosis becomes occluded, the Roux-Y procedure as shown in Plate 48 may be employed. If the anastomosis remains patent but an ascending cholangitis and hepatitis are sufficiently severe to demand surgical intervention, the pylorus may be resected, the duodenum closed and a gastrojejunostomy performed as shown in Plate 46.

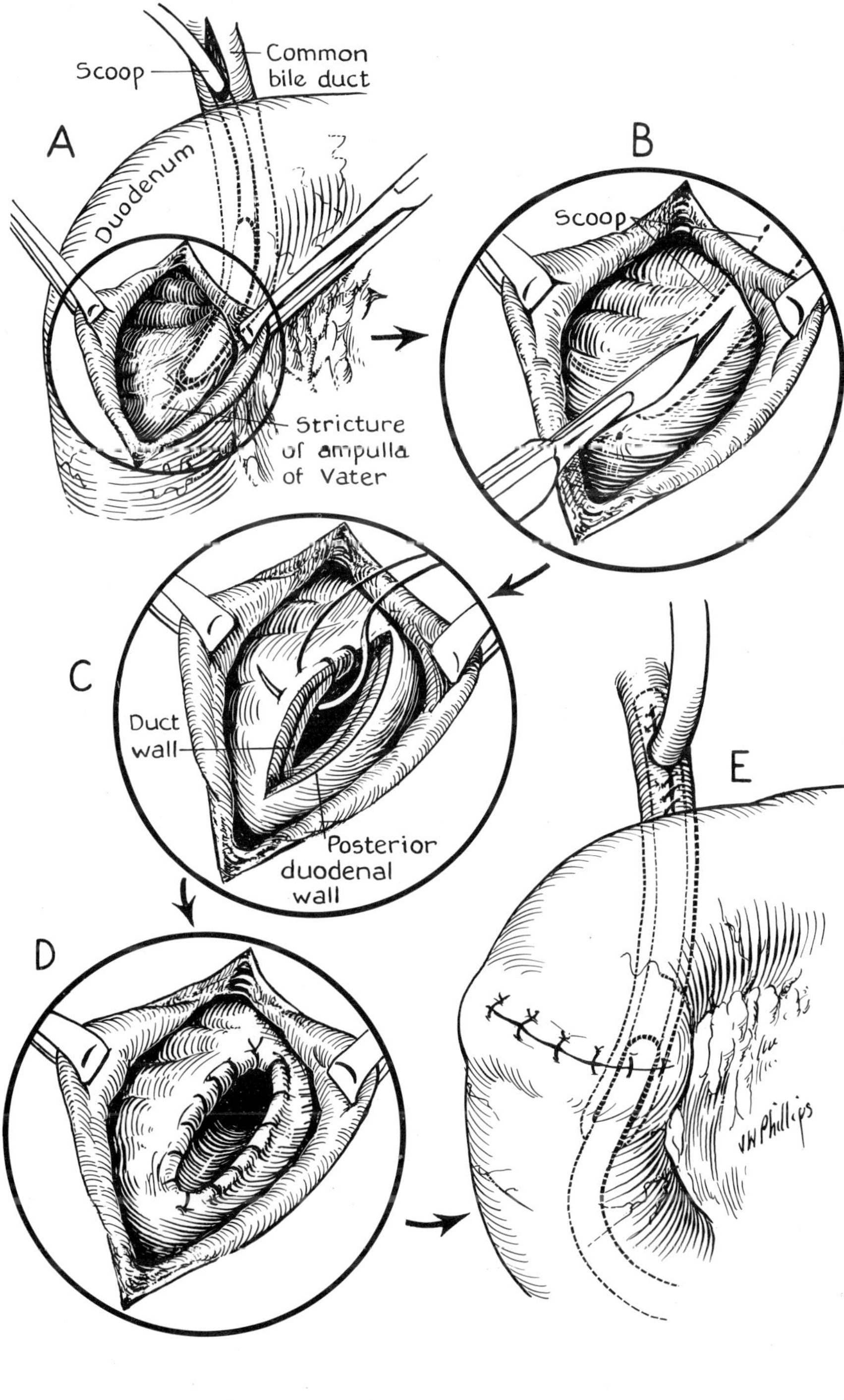
A
Scoop
Common
bile duct
Duodenum
Stricture
of ampulla
of Vater
B
Scoop
C
Duct
wall
Posterior
duodenal
wall
D
E
VW Phillips

More extensive strictures of the distal common duct may result from inflammatory disease of adjacent organs, such as sclerosing pancreatitis and peptic ulcer. Such strictures may be so extensive that a transduodenal anastomosis is technically not feasible. Under such circumstances a choledochoduodenostomy can relieve the obstruction.

A.—The common bile duct should be extensively exposed, opened by a longitudinal incision and carefully explored.

B.—After determining the level of the superior limit of the stricture, the posterior outer row of sutures for the establishment of a choledochoduodenostomy is placed. These sutures unite the anterior wall of the choledochus above the level of the stricture to the superior surface of the duodenum. The sutures are placed transversely on the common duct and longitudinally on the duodenum. A transverse incision then is made through the anterior wall of the common duct about 3 mm. proximal to the suture line and extending the entire diameter of the common duct. A longitudinal incision of equal length is made through the entire thickness of the duodenum an equal distance anterior to the suture line. The inner posterior row of sutures for the anastomosis consists of a continuous suture of fine intestinal catgut joining the distal cut edge of the common duct to the posterior cut edge of the duodenum.

C.—A long cross-limb of a T-tube is passed through the incision in the common duct and through the choledochoduodenostomy to extend well down into the duodenum.

D.—The choledochoduodenostomy is completed by an inner row of continuous catgut sutures joining the proximal edge of the transverse incision in the common duct to the anterior edge of the longitudinal incision in the duodenum. An anterior outer row of interrupted cotton sutures completes the anastomosis. The longitudinal incision in the common duct should be closed around the T-tube. It is well to reinforce the suture line with omentum. The T-tube may be left in place for several weeks or months.

The results of this operation frequently are unsatisfactory because of regurgitation of intestinal contents into the bile ducts and development of an ascending cholangitis. If this complication becomes severe, it may be advisable to resect the pylorus, close the distal end of the duodenum and perform a gastrojejunostomy.

PLATE 44

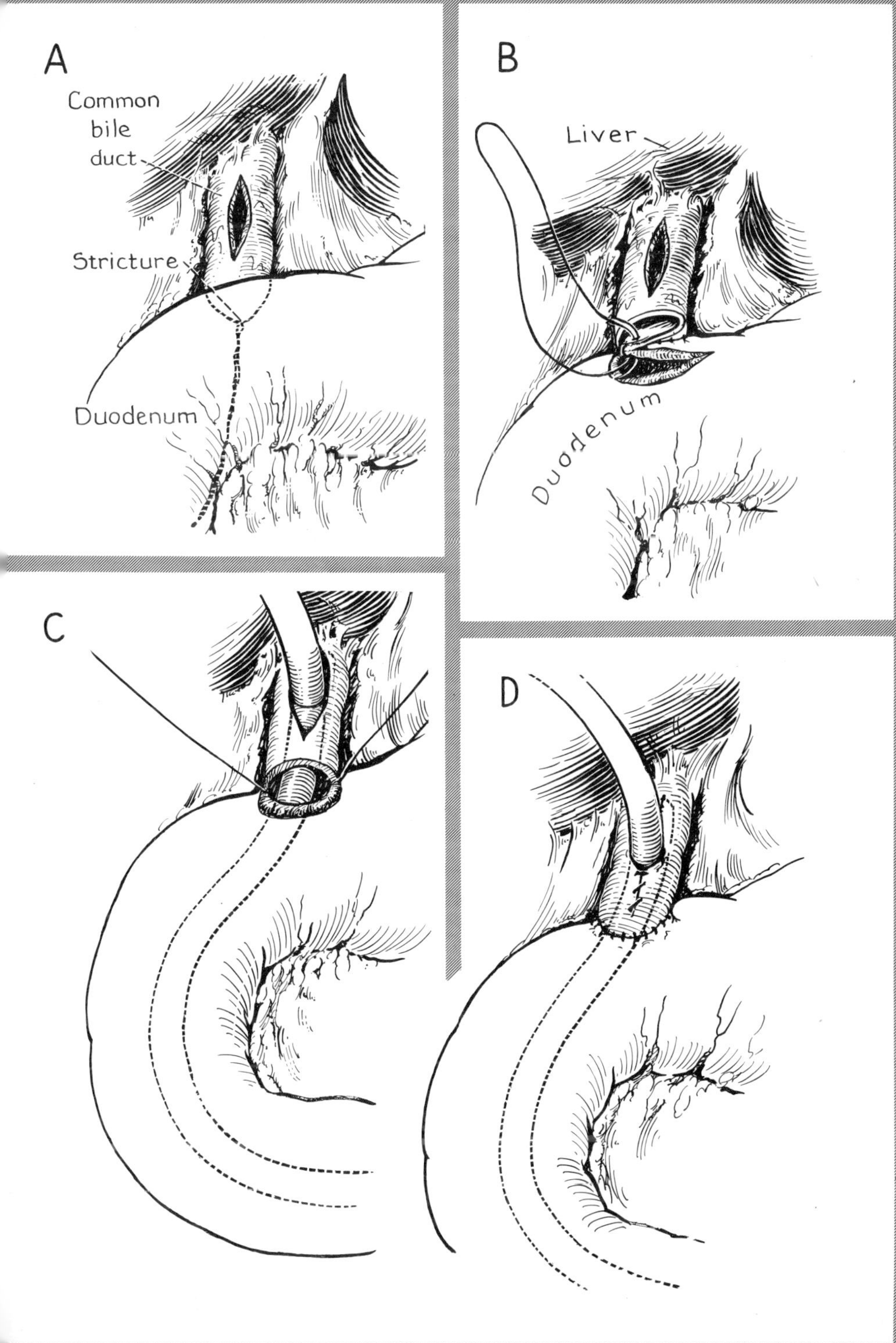

Hepaticoduodenostomy

Extensive strictures of the common duct which obliterate this structure from the hilus of the liver to the distal end of the duct or in which a distal portion of normal duct cannot be located present a difficult surgical problem. Hepaticoduodenostomy has for many years been used for the surgical treatment of such strictures, but the results are not permanently satisfactory in a high percentage of patients. As the operation gives good results in some patients and usually results in temporary improvement and relief from jaundice, it may be utilized in patients in whom more extensive procedures would be hazardous.

A.—The strictured common duct is located and the dilated proximal end is freed from adhesions and opened. As much normal duct as possible should be exposed beyond the liver capsule. A careful search should be made for a normal portion of the distal common duct. If this is unsuccessful, an anastomosis may be made between the proximal end of the duct and the duodenum.

B.—An outer row of interrupted cotton sutures should be placed between the superior surface of the duodenum and the capsule of the liver, posterior to the exposed proximal end of the hepatic duct. A longitudinal incision is made in the duodenum equal in length to the diameter of the exposed hepatic duct and a 3–5 mm. anterior to the previously placed suture line.

C.—The posterior inner row of sutures consists of a continuous suture of fine intestinal catgut, joining the posterior edges of the cut hepatic duct and duodenum. Some surgeons prefer to insert a catheter or rubber tubing, with one end extending into the liver and the other into the duodenum. This is held in place by a catgut suture at the line of anastomosis. The posterior inner row of sutures is continued around as the anterior inner row, joining the anterior edge of the hepatic duct to the anterior edge of the incision in the duodenum.

D.—An anterior outer row of fine interrupted cotton sutures is placed between the serosa of the duodenum and the capsule of the liver. These sutures should be extended well beyond the area of anastomosis to anchor the duodenum firmly to the undersurface of the liver. This completes the anastomosis. The suture line may be further protected by attaching omentum over it. A Penrose drain should be placed in the region of the anastomosis and brought out through the abdominal wound to permit escape of any leakage of bile or intestinal content.

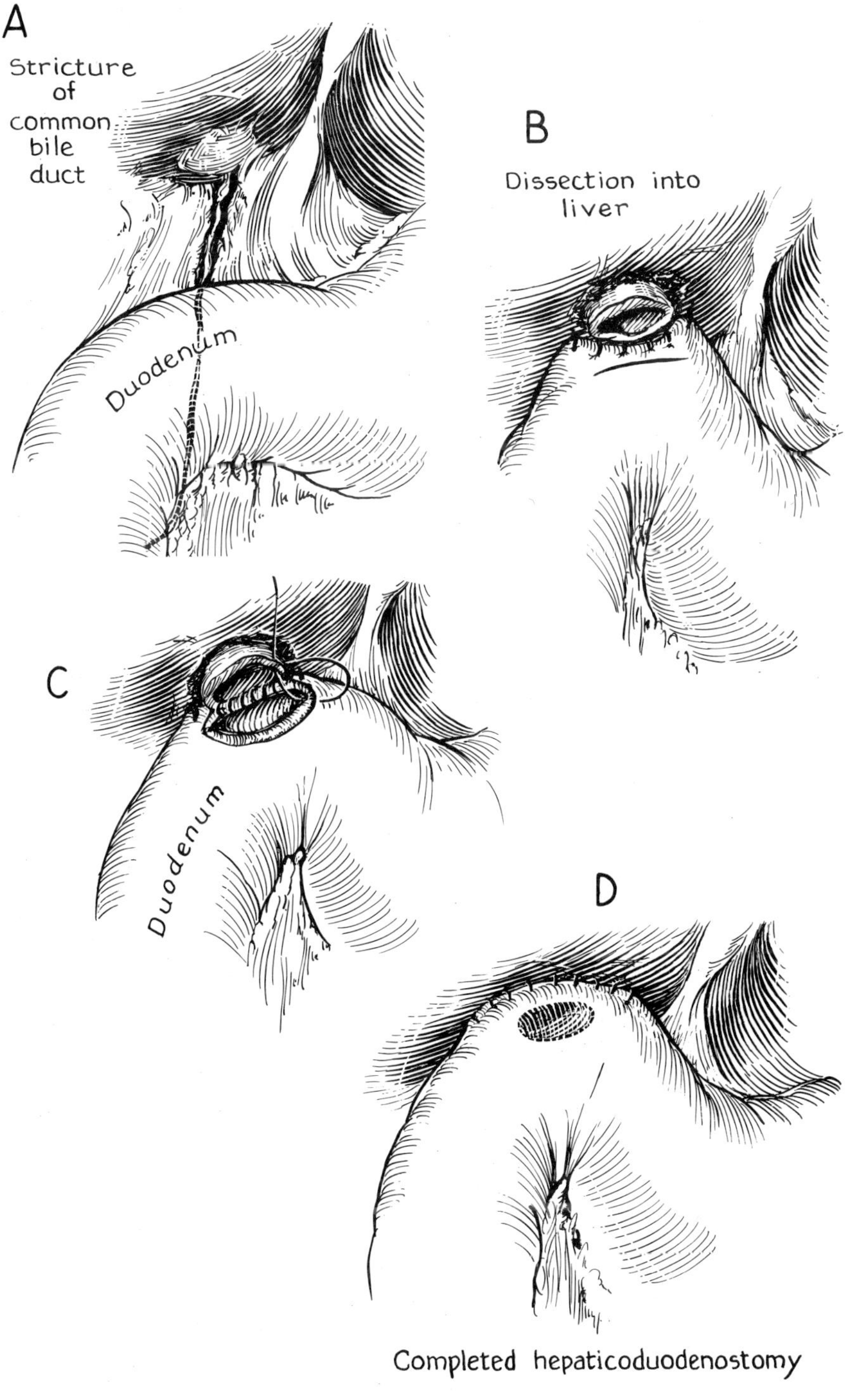
A
Stricture
of
common
bile
duct
Duodenum
B
Dissection into
liver
C
Duodenum
D
Completed hepaticoduodenostomy

Gastric Resection Subsequent to Hepaticoduodenostomy

After a hepaticoduodenostomy has been performed, many patients will manifest symptoms of an ascending cholangitis as a result of regurgitation of intestinal contents into the bile ducts or stenosis at the line of anastomosis. It has been contended that cholangitis will not occur if the anastomosis is adequate in size to permit a free flow of bile into the duodenum. This has not been true in all the patients we have seen. Some have had chills, fever and jaundice even though the anastomosis was large. We have relieved such patients of their symptoms by resecting the pyloric end of the stomach, closing the distal end of the duodenum and performing a gastrojejunostomy.

A.—The pyloric end of the stomach is mobilized and a clamp is placed on the duodenum just distal to the pyloric muscle. The duodenum is divided distal to the clamp and the hepaticoduodenal anastomosis is inspected from within the duodenum to determine its patency. If the opening is adequate to permit a free flow of bile into the duodenum, the open end of the duodenum is closed by an inner row of continuous catgut and an outer row of continuous cotton sutures. If the anastomosis has become stenosed and will not permit free flow of bile into the duodenum, it should be enlarged to correct the stenosis. It may be possible to perform a plastic procedure from within the duodenum to excise the scarred and narrowed area at the point of anastomosis and re-establish an adequate lumen. If this cannot be satisfactorily accomplished, it is advisable to take down the original anastomosis and create a new hepaticoduodenostomy.

B.—A second clamp is placed above the pyloric antrum and the distal stomach removed. Some form of gastrojejunostomy should be performed. This diagram shows a posterior Polya type of anastomosis. The proximal jejunum is brought through an opening in the transverse mesocolon and the divided end of the stomach is anastomosed to the jejunum, using two rows of continuous intestinal catgut. The edges of the opening of the transverse mesocolon should be sutured to the stomach proximal to the line of anastomosis.

PLATE 46

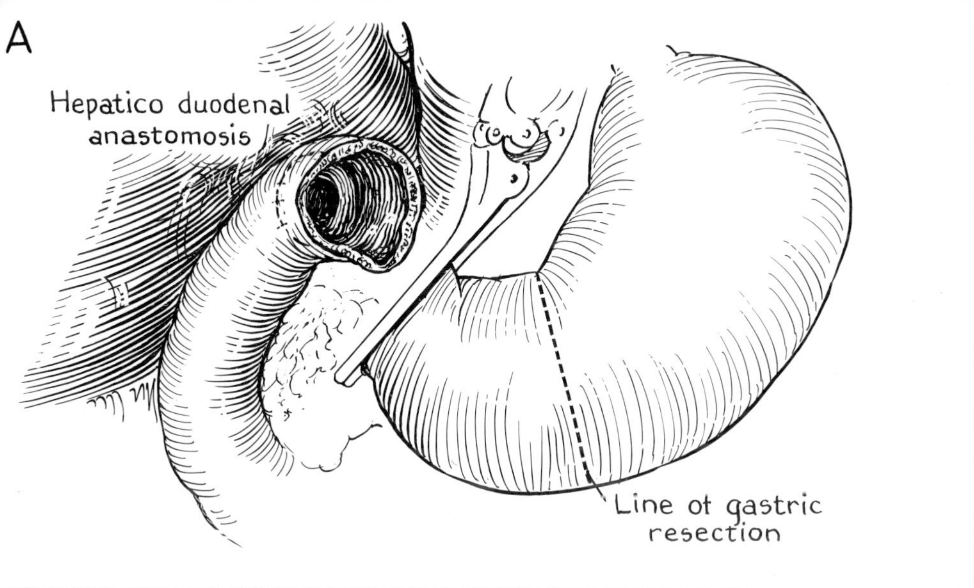
A
Hepatico duodenal anastomosis
Line of gastric resection

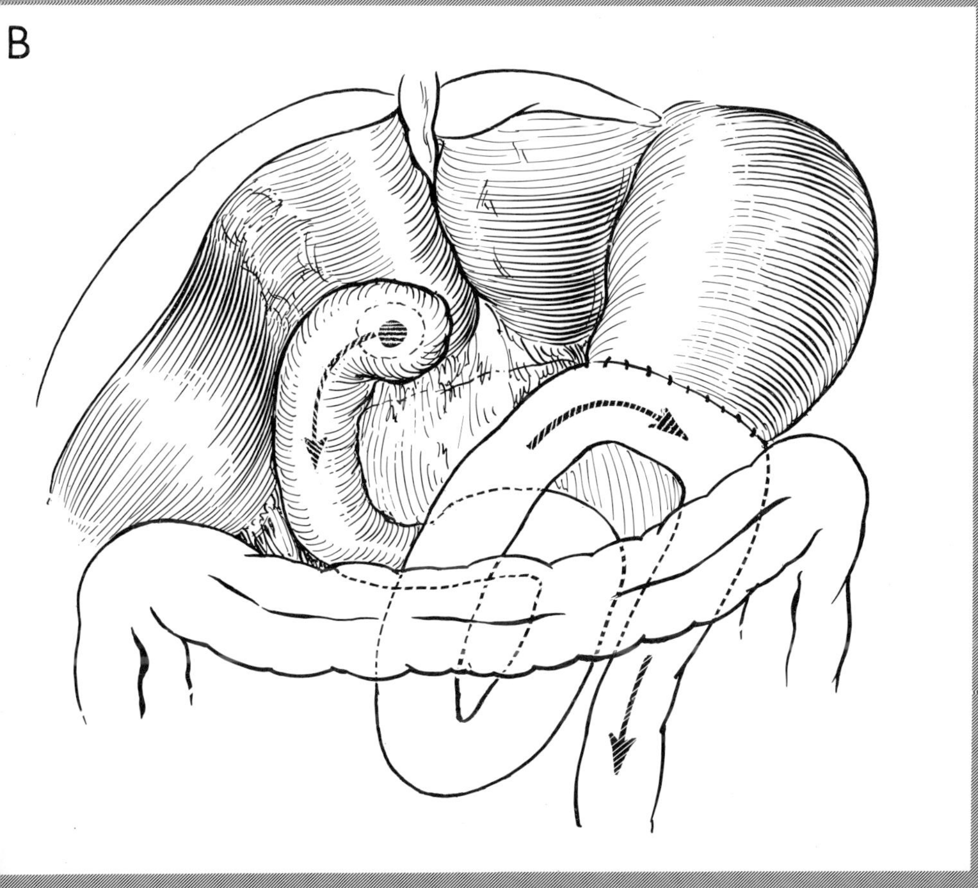
B

In our experience, the Roux-Y procedure for stricture of the common duct occasionally has been followed by the development of duodenal ulcer. I believe this is due to the shunting of bile away from the duodenum and into the jejunum a considerable distance below the duodenum. It would be preferable to have bile enter the duodenum and at the same time prevent regurgitation of intestinal contents into the hepatic ducts. The combination of hepaticoduodenostomy and subtotal gastric resection with gastrojejunostomy can accomplish this.

A.—Where it is impossible to perform an end-to-end anastomosis of the common bile duct and a moderate amount of common hepatic duct extends beyond the liver, this portion may be anastomosed to the end of the duodenum. The duodenum is divided below the pyloric muscle and its distal end anastomosed to the end of the common bile duct. This is accomplished by a mucosa-to-mucosa anastomosis, using an inner row of continuous catgut and an outer row of interrupted cotton.

B.—If there is an inadequate amount of duct extending beyond the hilus of the liver to perform a satisfactory end-to-end anastomosis, the open distal end of the duodenum may be sutured to the capsule of the liver around the opening into the hepatic duct. The technic is similar to that employed in the Roux-Y anastomosis (Plate 48). It is usually simpler to close the distal end of the duodenum and to use the side of the proximal duodenum for the hepaticoduodenostomy. Before starting the anastomosis, the edges of the duct at the hilus of the liver should be sutured to the liver capsule to maintain the lumen of the duct. The superior surface of the duodenum is sutured to the capsule of the liver posterior to the hepatic duct orifice. A longitudinal incision is made in the duodenum anterior to the previously placed row of sutures and opposite the opening in the liver. It is well to place a piece of rubber tubing into the intrahepatic ducts with the distal end extending into the duodenum and fastened with a single catgut suture. The anterior edge of the incised duodenum is sutured to the capsule of the liver anterior to the hepatic orifice. An outer row of interrupted cotton sutures is placed between the serosa of the duodenum and the liver capsule.

C.—The pyloric antrum is removed and the proximal jejunum is then anastomosed to the stomach. Because of adhesions from previous operations and debility of the patient an antecolic anastomosis may be simplest and will give very satisfactory results.

PLATE 47

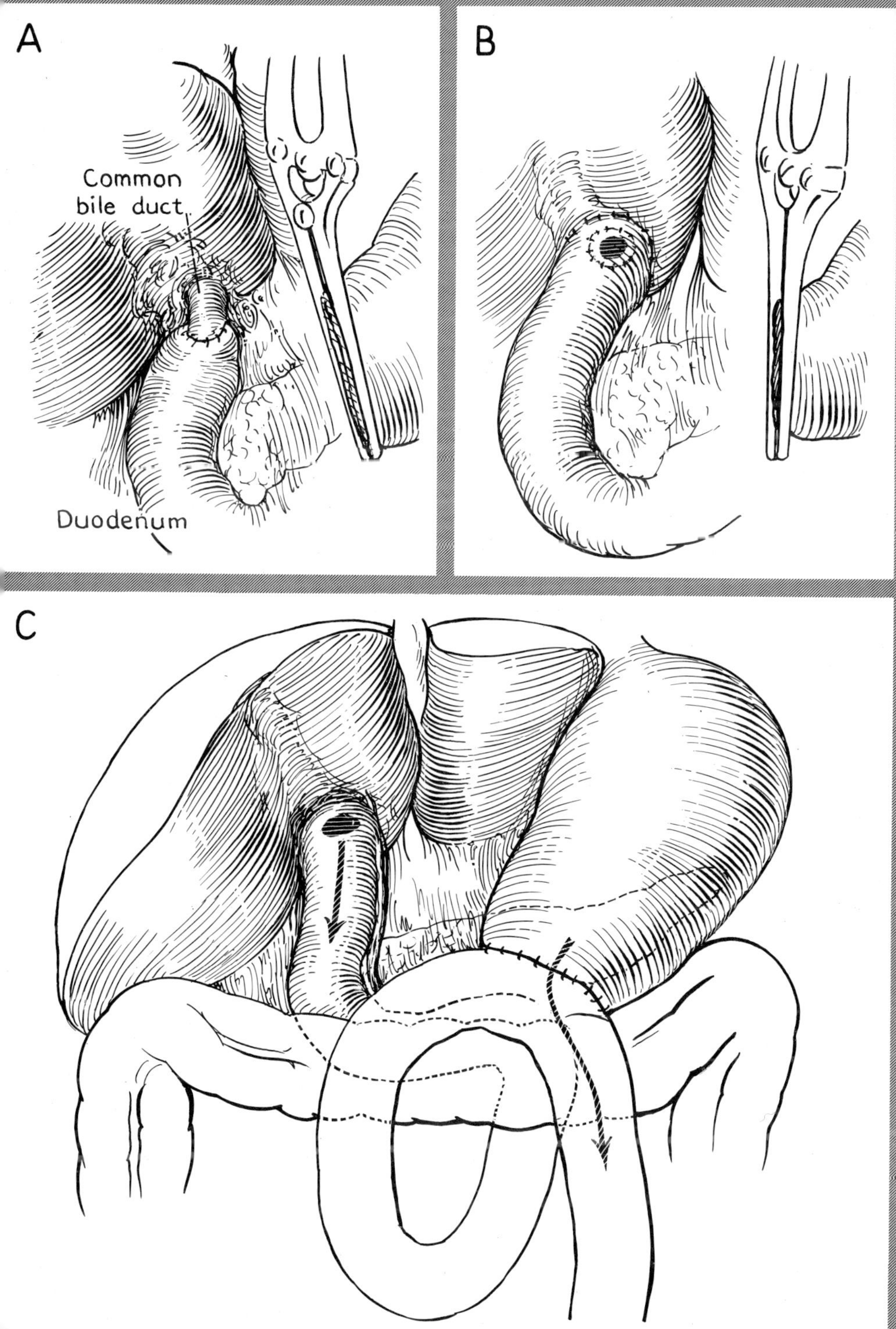

The high incidence of unsatisfactory results of anastomoses between the hepatic ducts and the duodenum where end-to-end anastomoses of strictures of the common duct have been technically impossible has led to a search for a more satisfactory method of repair. Experimental and clinical studies have shown that intestinal contents normally will not travel against the normal direction of peristalsis. When the intact duodenum is anastomosed to the hepatic duct or when a loop of bowel is brought up to it, intestinal contents can regurgitate into the biliary system and produce an ascending cholangitis. To avoid this the Roux-Y procedure was devised. In principle, it is an anastomosis of the hilus of the liver to a segment of bowel in which peristalsis runs from the liver distally and which is of sufficient length to prevent regurgitation of intestinal contents into the liver. This procedure does not supplant an end-to-end anastomosis. It has been argued that a mucosa-to-mucosa anastomosis minimizes the danger of a recurrent stricture. I am not in accord with this belief with regard to high strictures of the common bile duct. Mucosa-to-mucosa anastomoses between the bile duct and the bowel are frequently followed by a stricture at the suture line. In the technic of Roux-Y procedure described here there is no attempt to make a mucosa-to-mucosa anastomosis.

A.—The proximal end of the stricture of the common duct is dissected free and all possible scar tissue is removed.

B.—The proximal hepatic duct is opened as widely as possible and its edges are sutured to the surrounding capsule of the liver. The dissection of the hilus must be complete and be carefully accomplished to avoid damage to the portal vein and hepatic artery. The adjacent liver capsule should be exposed for a distance sufficient to permit anastomosis of the bowel to its surface around the opening of the hepatic duct.

C.—The transverse colon is now elevated and the jejunum located at the ligament of Treitz. It should be followed distally for a distance of about 15 in. and a point located where the mesentery can be divided between the arcades of blood vessels without interference with the blood supply to either end. The jejunum is clamped with two Kocher forceps and the bowel divided between them. The mesentery is divided to its root, carefully ligating the vessels during the course of the dissection. An opening is made through the transverse mesocolon between its vessels and slightly to the right of the midline.

[Roux-Y anastomosis *continued on page 224.*]

PLATE 48

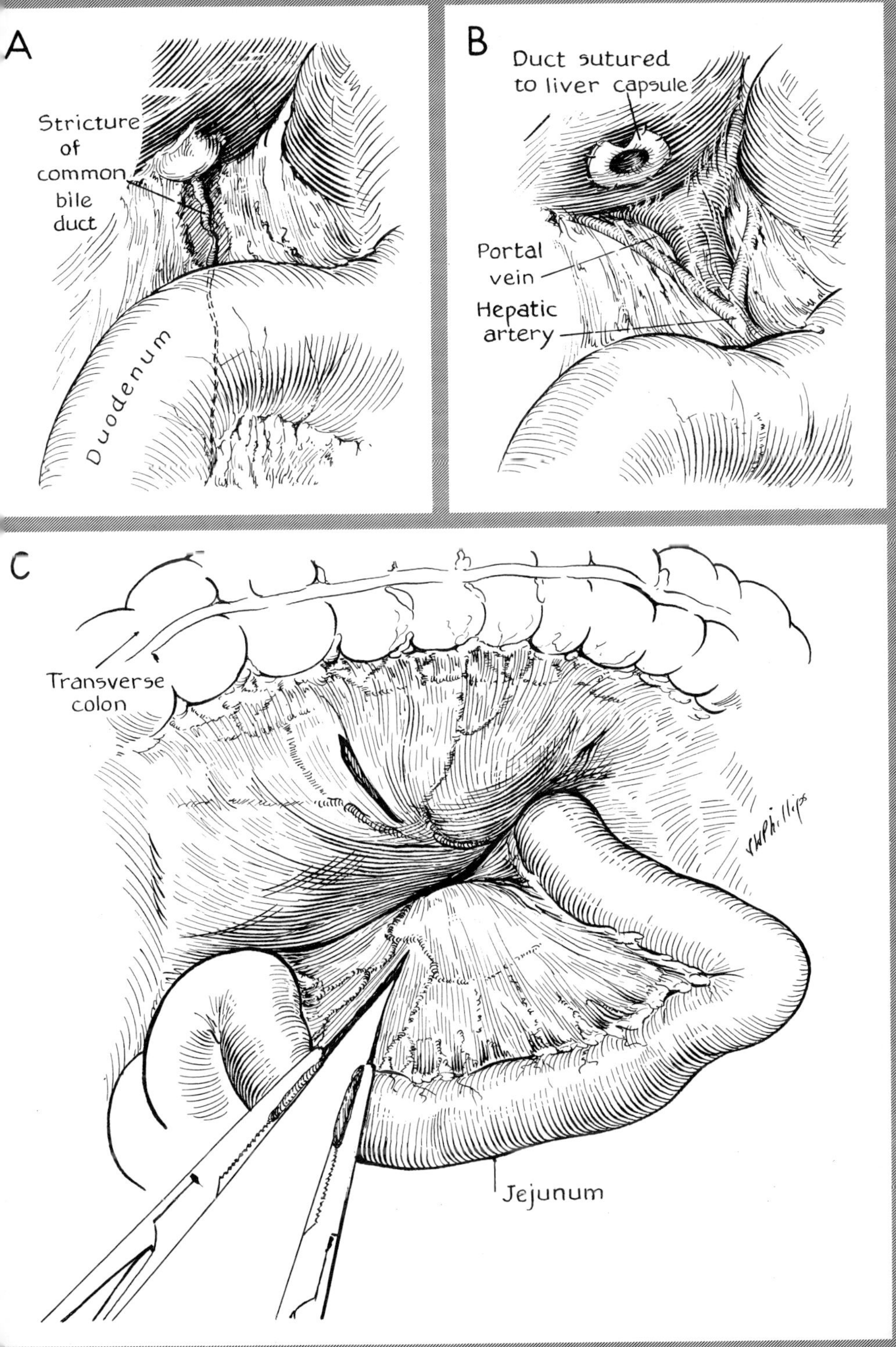
A
Stricture of common bile duct
Duodenum
B
Duct sutured to liver capsule
Portal vein
Hepatic artery
C
Transverse colon
Jejunum

D.—The distal segment of divided jejunum must be brought to the hilus of the liver without tension. For this reason it is important to select a point for the division where the mesentery is sufficiently long to permit the distal end of jejunum to be brought through the transverse mesocolon and to the hilus of the liver. Transillumination of the mesentery of the jejunum will greatly facilitate the location of its arcades of arteries and help determine the most feasible point of division. A Kocher forceps is passed through the opening in the transverse mesocolon from above downward to grasp the distal jejunal segment just below the previously applied clamp. The point of this forceps should be on the antimesenteric side of the bowel. This permits the bowel to be approximated to the hilus of the liver with the mesentery toward the medial portion of the body, which is the shortest distance between its origin and the liver. The small segment of jejunum held in the first applied distal clamp is cut off by sharp dissection between the two Kocher hemostats and the distal end of the jejunum is brought up through the opening in the transverse mesocolon.

E.—After bringing the distal end of jejunum through the transverse mesocolon it is held near the undersurface of the liver with its mesentery placed medially. Interrupted cotton sutures are inserted to approximate the serosa of jejunum to the capsule of the liver around the opening of the hepatic duct. These sutures should be so placed that the anastomosis between the hilus of the liver and the jejunum will equal the diameter of the jejunum. Great care must be taken in inserting the sutures posterior to the hepatic duct so that the portal vein or hepatic artery will not be included in them. The sutures should be spaced at intervals of about 3 mm. around the anastomosis. The jejunum is approximated to the hilus of the liver and all posterior sutures are tied. The hemostat then should be removed. A section of rubber catheter about 4 in. in length should be introduced into the liver and its distal end introduced into the jejunum. It should be sutured to the hepatic duct with a single strand of intestinal catgut. The anterior interrupted sutures now are tied.

[Roux-Y anastomosis *continued on page 226.*]

D

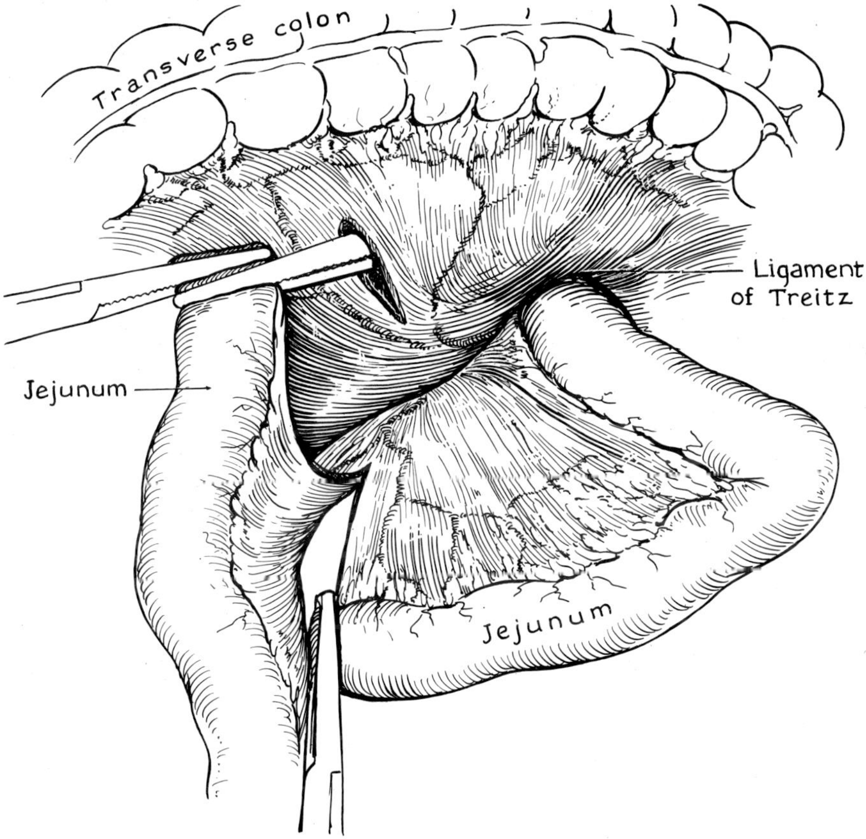
Transverse colon
Ligament of Treitz
Jejunum
Jejunum

E

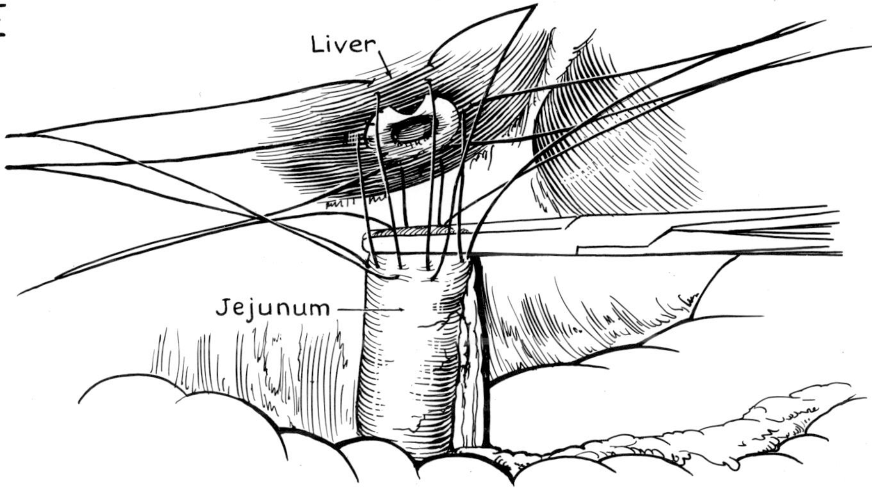
Liver
Jejunum
Transverse colon

F.—After completing the inner row of interrupted cotton sutures between the serosa of the bowel and the capsule of the liver it is well to support the anastomosis further by a continuous outer row of intestinal catgut sutures. A nonabsorbable suture may be used for this row if preferred. The outer row can encompass most of the circumference of the anastomosis but is difficult to place posteriorly without endangering the hepatic artery or portal vein. This omission of posterior sutures is not important since experience has shown that if leakage of the anastomosis occurs, it will invariably cease within one to two weeks.

G.—This figure shows the completed anastomosis. The proximal jejunum has been anastomosed to the distal segment 12–15 in. below the point of division. This is accomplished by an end-to-side anastomosis using two rows of intestinal catgut. The arrows indicate the direction of peristalsis. Bile from the liver is carried downward in the distal jejunal segment to join the stream of intestinal contents at the site of the end-to-side anastomosis. Regurgitation does not occur into the intestinal limb extending to the liver. This prevents an ascending cholangitis and hepatitis. However, bile does not mix with intestinal contents until gastric contents have passed from the stomach through the duodenum and through from 15 to 18 in. of jejunum. This lack of bile in the upper intestinal tract causes a dyspepsia similar to that associated with gallbladder disease.

F

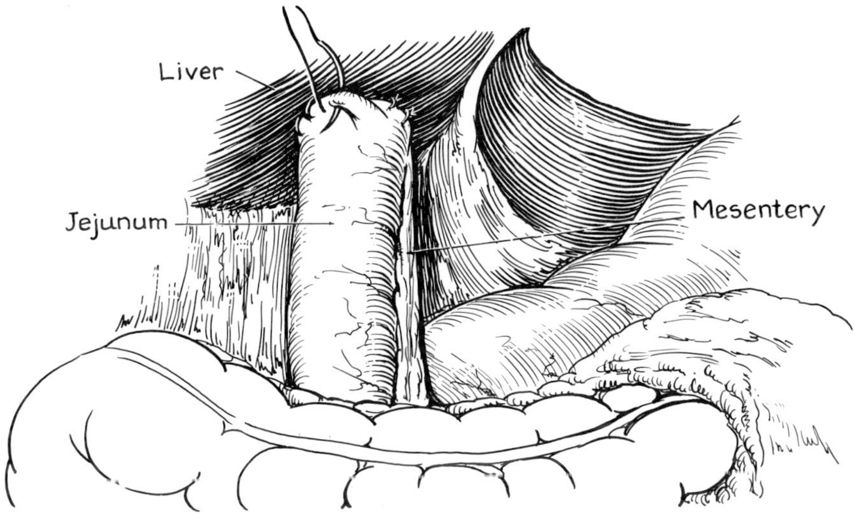
Liver
Jejunum
Mesentery

G

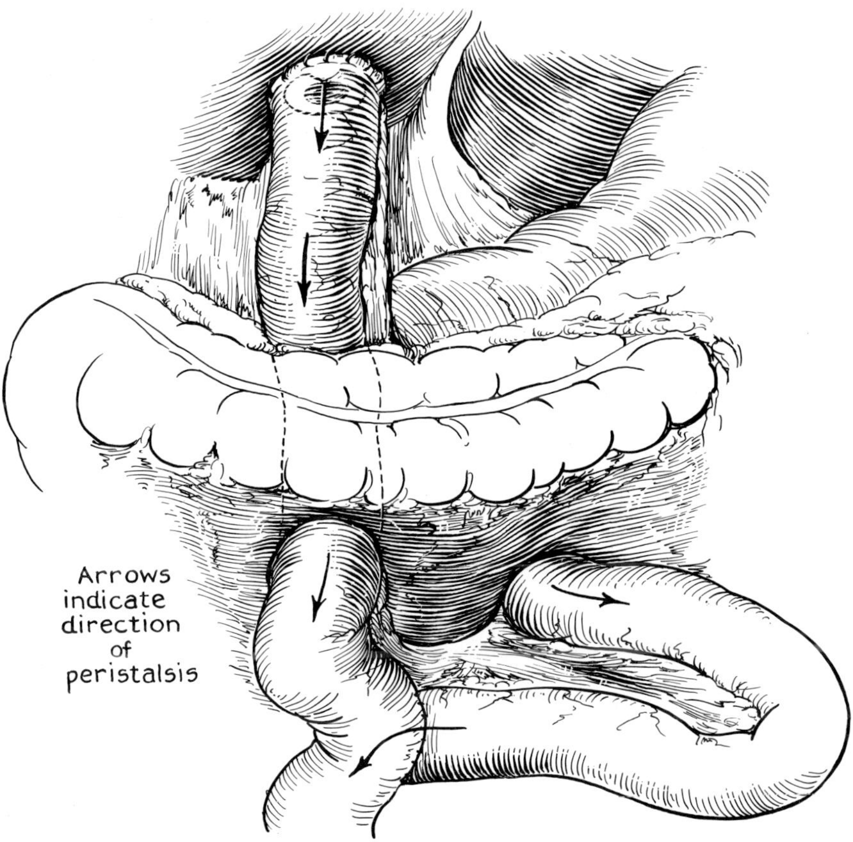
Arrows indicate direction of peristalsis

Strictures Extending into Hilus of Liver: Repair

Strictures of the common duct which extend into the hilus of the liver are difficult to repair and have a high rate of recurrence. Warren Cole has suggested a modification of the Roux-Y operation. Its purpose is to approximate the jejunal mucosa to the wall of an intrahepatic duct.

A.—When no duct can be found external to the liver, the hilus of the liver should be aspirated in an attempt to locate an intrahepatic duct.

B.—When bile is obtained by aspiration, the needle is left in place and the liver substance incised by sharp dissection along the course of the needle.

C.—The opening through the liver to the duct is enlarged by sharp or blunt dissection. The surrounding tissue should be aspirated with a fine needle to locate, and to help avoid entrance into, any large blood vessel.

D.—A Roux-Y arm of jejunum is brought to the hilus of the liver (see Plate 48). The serosa and muscular layers are dissected from the mucosa for a distance of 2–3 cm. at the end of the jejunum.

E.—A section of the bell end of a catheter (shown in *D*) is sutured into the lumen of the mucosal tube and anchored with nonabsorbable sutures. The mucosal cone is trimmed to fit the opening in the liver and must be long enough to reach the bile duct. Nonabsorbable sutures are then passed from the outer surface of the liver to emerge from the opening in the liver as deeply as possible. They then pick up the edge of the mucosal fold and are passed back in the opposite direction. When these are pulled and tied, they anchor the mucosal cone deep in the liver.

F.—The serosa of the jejunum distal to the cone is sutured to the capsule of the liver around the site of anastomosis.

Occasionally, despite repeated aspirations into the hilus of the liver, no bile is obtained. This often occurs when a high stricture is of short duration and the ducts have not had an opportunity to dilate to any great degree. When this condition is encountered and the patient's condition will not warrant more extensive surgery, a catheter should be sutured to the hilus of the liver and brought out through the wound. Frequently, an external biliary fistula will be established and at a later date an internal anastomosis again can be attempted.

PLATE 49

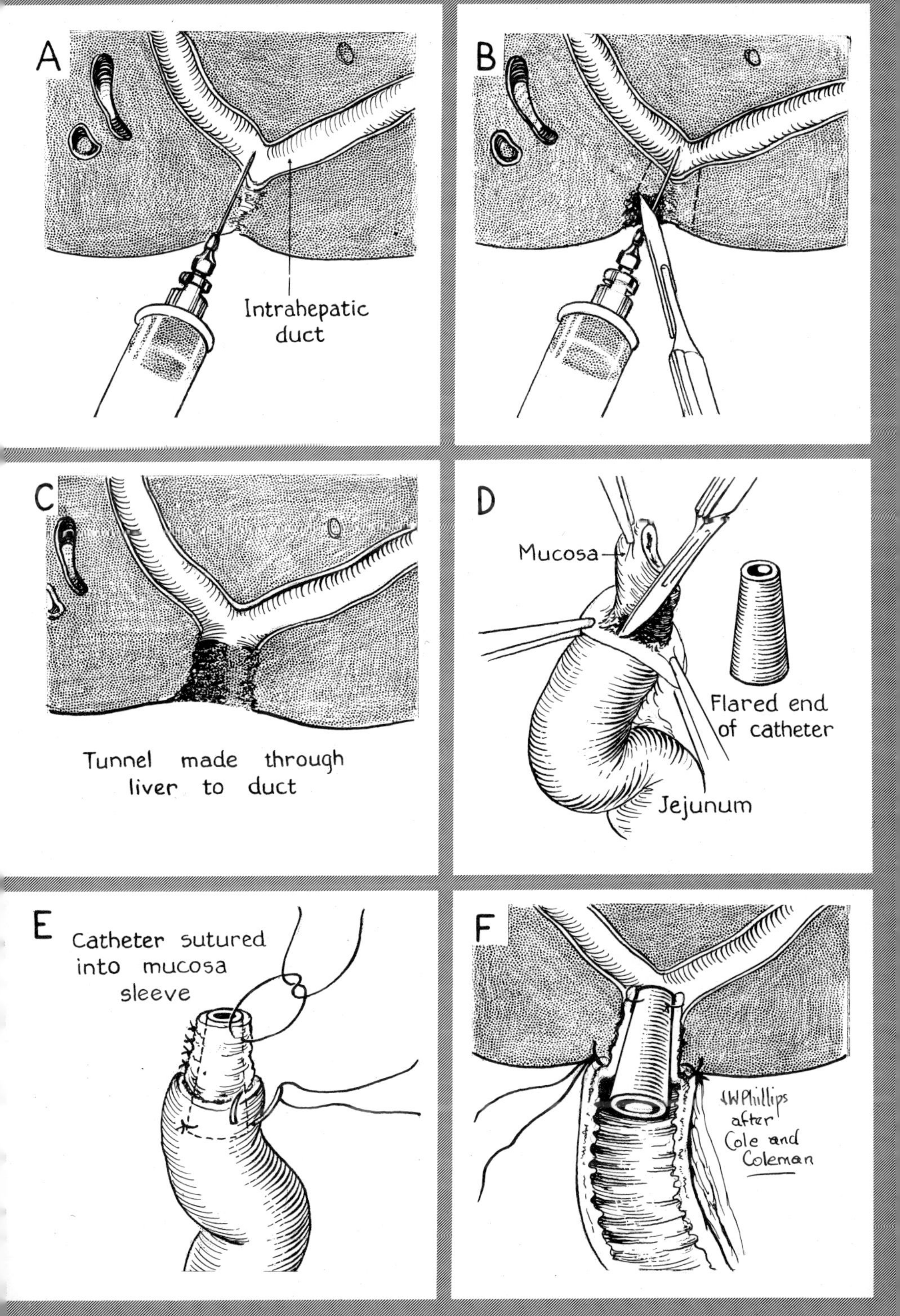
A
Intrahepatic duct
B
C
Tunnel made through liver to duct
D
Mucosa
Flared end of catheter
Jejunum
E
Catheter sutured into mucosa sleeve
F
J.W. Phillips after Cole and Coleman

The inability to locate an extrahepatic bile duct at the hilus of the liver or to find an intrahepatic bile duct by aspiration presents a difficult surgical problem. The anastomosis of an intrahepatic bile duct to the jejunum as described by Longmire may be life-saving. In this operation the left lobe of the liver is resected until a main hepatic duct is encountered. This is anastomosed to the jejunum. The procedure will permit drainage of bile from the left half of the liver if the stricture has extended to a point which occludes the left from the right intrahepatic duct, and it will permit drainage from the entire liver if there is a communication between the left and right hepatic ducts. The Longmire procedure is described with certain modifications.

The left lobe of the liver may be approached through a number of incisions, the approach depending upon the primary purpose of the operation. A long right paramedian, left paramedian or subcostal incision can be used. After ascertaining that bile drainage cannot be established at the hilus of the liver, the left lobe of the liver is mobilized by dividing the falciform ligament.

A.—Beginning at the anterior edge of the left lobe of the liver near the falciform ligament, two rows of locking mattress sutures are placed about 1 cm. apart. The liver is divided between these rows of sutures until the main bile duct is encountered.

B.—An attempt is made to preserve some of the duct beyond the surface of the liver, or the liver is coned out around the duct to leave a small protruding portion. The dissection is carried through the remainder of the left lobe of the liver, curving the incision to the left.

C.—The jejunum is divided below the ligament of Treitz and the distal end brought up through the transverse mesocolon to the cut surface of the left lobe of the liver. A section of rubber tubing is passed into the intrahepatic duct and sutured with a catgut suture. The protruding end of the rubber tube is passed into the jejunal segment. The serosa of the jejunum is then sutured to the capsule of the liver. It may be necessary to oblique the incision in the jejunum for its lumen to equal the cut surface of the liver.

D.—The proximal end of the divided jejunum is then anastomosed to the distal segment below the transverse mesocolon, forming a Roux-Y anastomosis. Such an anastomosis permits drainage from the main bile duct and from any other divided ducts which are not ligated. If the raw surface of the liver is very large, it may be

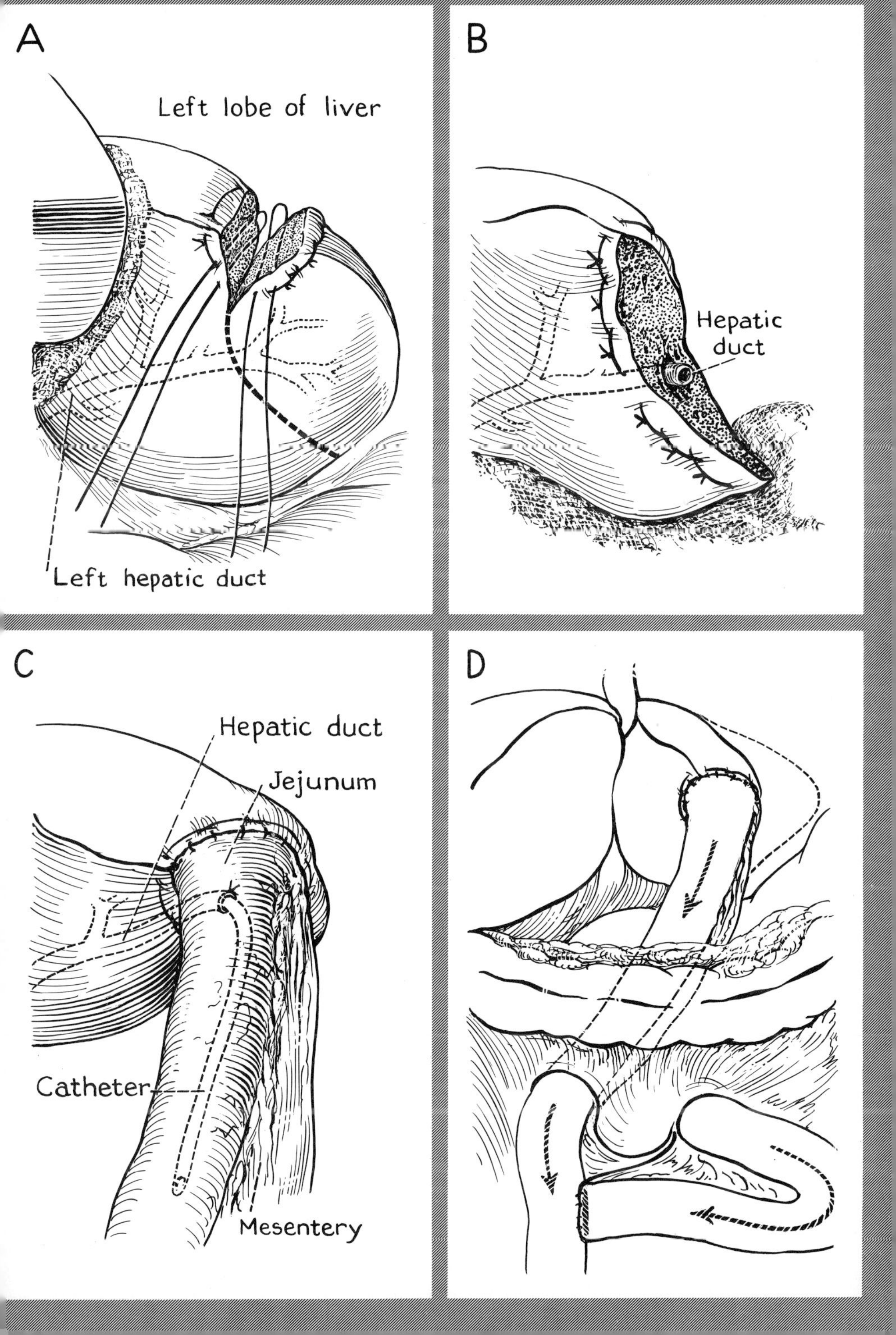
A
Left lobe of liver
Left hepatic duct
B
Hepatic duct
C
Hepatic duct
Jejunum
Catheter
Mesentery
D

advisable to perform a mucosa-to-mucosa anastomosis between the jejunum and bile duct and to cover the remaining surface of the liver with the serosa of the jejunum.

Summary

Benign strictures of the common bile duct constitute one of the greatest catastrophes of surgery. They are easily incurred but difficult to remedy. The most satisfactory procedure of repair is end-to-end anastomosis of the common bile duct, preserving its continuity and the function of its intraduodenal portion and the ampulla of Vater. This method should be utilized whenever possible. When preservation of the distal end of the duct is not possible, it is important to permit drainage of bile into the intestinal tract without regurgitation of intestinal contents into the bile ducts. The Roux-Y procedure accomplishes this aim but diverts bile from the duodenum and proximal segment of the jejunum. The loss of bile in this area has resulted in the development of duodenal ulcers, some of which have been accompanied by severe hemorrhage. The experience of Dragstedt and other investigators has shown the importance of the pyloric antrum as a stimulus to the secretion of gastric acids. The removal of the pyloric antrum may be of some value in diminishing the occurrence of peptic ulcers. These studies and my own experience lead me to conclude that hepaticoduodenostomy with resection of the pyloric antrum and gastrojejunostomy produce a physiologic arrangement least likely to permit regurgitation of intestinal contents into the bile ducts while still permitting bile to flow into the duodenum and to be present at the gastrojejunal anastomosis. For these reasons I believe it the most satisfactory operation for the repair of stricture of the common bile duct when end-to-end anastomosis cannot be accomplished. The use of the Cole and the Longmire procedures should be reserved for intrahepatic obstructions for which other procedures are not applicable.

Benign Tumors of the Bile Ducts

Benign tumors of the extrahepatic bile ducts are rarely found. A variety of types have been reported but papillomas and adenomas have been the most common. In over one third of a million hospital admissions, we have encountered only one benign tumor, an adenoma, exclusive of tumors of the ampulla of Vater. The patient presented symptoms simulating those of common duct stones. At exploration, the adenoma was found and removed.

Benign tumors of the ampulla of Vater likewise are rare. Although various types have been reported, in our experience only benign papillary tumors have been found in this region. The symptomatology is not characteristic, but certain manifestations may suggest this type of lesion. These tumors usually do not completely occlude the passage of bile into the intestine. However, there is some backpressure due to partial obstruction of bile flow which may result in the gradual dilatation of the bile ducts and gallbladder. Occasionally the gallbladder may be palpable. Jaundice frequently develops and may fluctuate to some degree. However, the jaundice is usually not as intense as that associated with obstruction due to stone or to malignant disease, and pruritus is less often an associated symptom. Pain and colic may or may not be noted. Bleeding from the lesions may lead to a rather persistent secondary anemia, the origin of which is difficult to determine. Blood can be found in the stools, but gross bleeding is infrequently noted. Biliary dyspepsia is a common complaint and suggests gallbladder pathology.

The diagnosis of benign tumors of the ampulla of Vater is hard to establish, and jaundice produced by these tumors may be difficult to differentiate from hepatocellular jaundice. X-ray studies are helpful. If there is backpressure on the bile ducts, cholecystograms will reveal a poorly functioning or nonfunctioning gallbladder. Barium studies of the gastrointestinal tract may reveal a filling defect if the tumor protrudes into the duodenum. These lesions seldom produce intestinal obstruction.

We have encountered benign papillary tumors of the ampulla of Vater in three locations.

A.—The tumor shown is limited to the lumen of the distal common duct and ampulla of Vater and does not protrude into the duodenum.

B.—Here the tumor protrudes from the ampulla of Vater into the duodenum. Such tumors frequently can be visualized by radiologic studies of the duodenum.

C.—In this instance, a tumor 5 cm. in diameter was gradually forced by peristalsis to the distal end of the duodenum, pulling with it a pedicle of normal duodenum 10 cm. in length containing the common duct which emptied through the distal end of the tumor.

Treatment

Benign tumors of the distal common duct and ampulla of Vater which do not protrude into the duodenum may require a pancreaticoduodenal resection (see Plate 71) for removal. A more conservative short-circuiting operation such as a cholecystoduodenostomy will relieve the obstructive symptoms but will not prevent further development of the tumor.

D.—Tumor protruding into the duodenum may be locally excised by means of a transduodenal approach. Traction is placed upon the tumor to expose its base, and all tumor tissue is removed. It is important that no tumor tissue remains. If the tumor has a long pedicle, complete removal is facilitated.

E.—After complete removal of the tumor, which usually includes the papilla of Vater and transects the distal common duct, the edges of the cut common duct should be sutured to the cut edge of the posterior wall of the mucosa of the duodenum. If the pancreatic duct can be found, its cut edge should also be sutured to the duodenal mucosa. If the common bile duct has been explored, a T-tube should be sutured into it and brought to the surface for drainage. The duodenum is closed transversely by an inner row of continuous catgut and an outer row of continuous cotton sutures and should be further supported by omentum.

PLATE 51

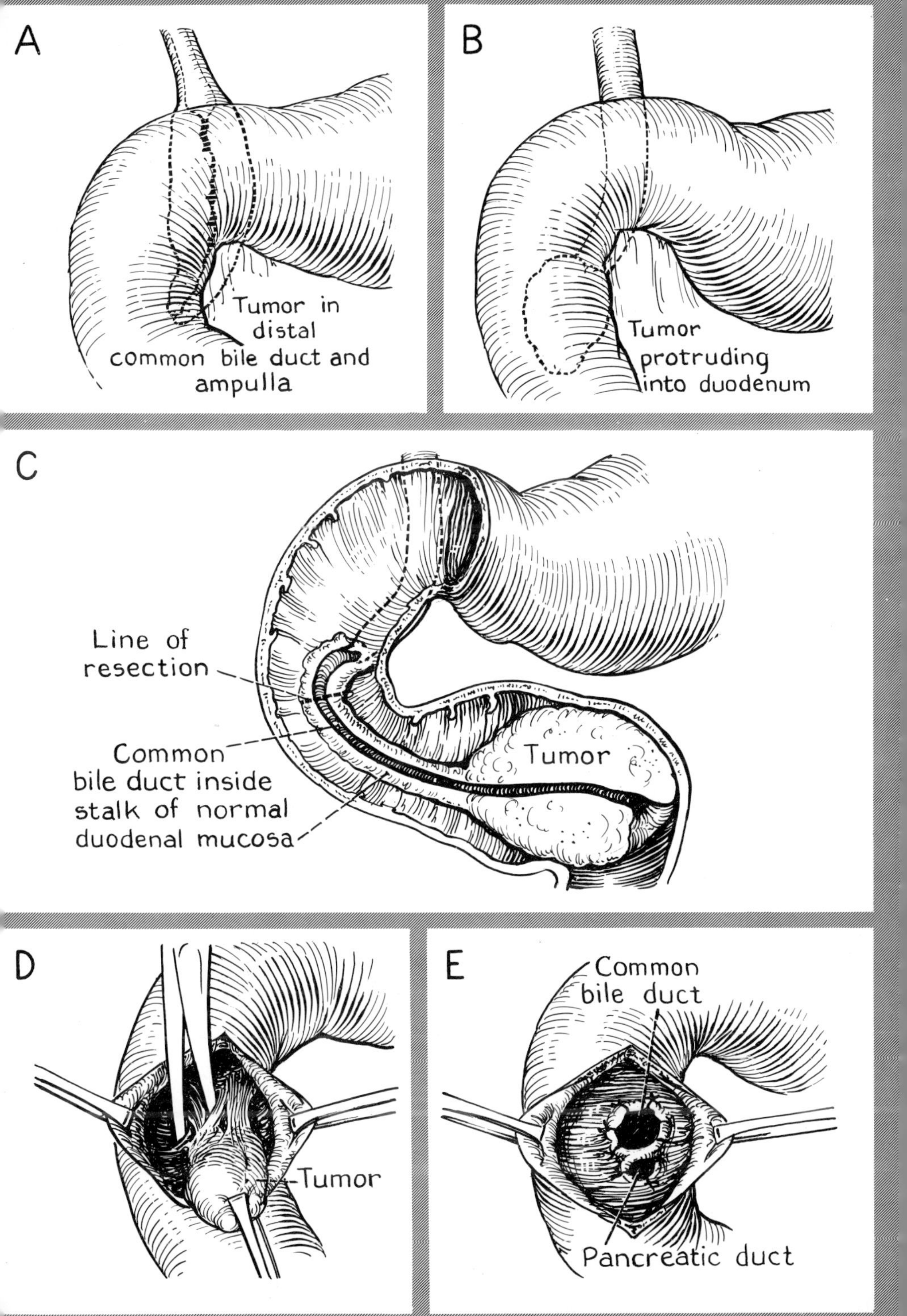

A
Tumor in distal common bile duct and ampulla
B
Tumor protruding into duodenum
C
Line of resection
Common bile duct inside stalk of normal duodenal mucosa
Tumor
D
Tumor
E
Common bile duct
Pancreatic duct

Carcinoma of the Bile Ducts

It is fortunate that carcinoma of the extrahepatic biliary system is an infrequent disease because the results of treatment are most discouraging. Carcinoma of the gallbladder has been discussed in Chapter 7. In a study of approximately 20,000 malignancies, 19 were found to be carcinoma of the bile ducts. The disease was located in the ampulla of Vater in 11 patients and in the bile ducts in eight. Because of some difference in symptomatology and in the theoretical prognosis of early treatment, carcinoma of the ampulla of Vater will be discussed separately.

Carcinoma of the extrahepatic ducts.—Of the eight carcinomas involving the extrahepatic ducts exclusive of the ampulla of Vater, four were located in the hepatic ducts, three at the junction of the hepatic and cystic ducts and one in the common bile duct distal to the entrance of the cystic duct. The symptomatology and progress of the disease were quite similar in all eight patients. The presenting symptoms usually were the result of obstruction of the bile ducts. Jaundice appeared early, became complete and was progressive. Acholic stools, bile in the urine and pruritus were present in all, and all had progressive weight loss, dyspepsia and weakness. Pain as an early symptom was noted less often than in carcinoma of the gallbladder. Likewise, a palpable mass in the epigastrium or right upper quadrant was not an early sign in any patient. Both pain and a palpable mass were later symptoms and findings in these patients. With progress of the disease, the liver became palpable in all patients. Bleeding into the duodenum or gross bleeding from the bowel did not occur.

In the presence of jaundice cholecystograms are of little value. However, all of those taken in these patients revealed a nonfunctioning gallbladder without evidence of stones. In some patients, x-ray studies of the gastrointestinal tract showed evidence of pressure upon the duodenum by an extrinsic mass. Liver function tests revealed a progressive impairment of the functional activity of this organ.

Treatment.—The only satisfactory treatment for carcinoma of the bile ducts is early resection. The incidence of cure by surgery is very low. Difficulty in diagnosis and failure to institute early surgical therapy are factors in the poor results. Despite early treatment, when resection is possible, the survival time usually is not long because of early spread of the disease. Although a cure cannot be anticipated in the presence of evident extension and metastases, it is important to relieve the icterus, if possible, by a short-circuiting operation. Resection of the tumor and an anastomosis of the ducts is the procedure of choice. If the obstruction is below the entrance of the cystic duct, the gallbladder may be anastomosed to the stomach or small bowel. When an anastomosis cannot be established, external biliary drainage will make the patient more comfortable but should not be performed if internal biliary drainage can be established. The technics of these procedures are described in other chapters in this book.

Carcinoma of the Ampulla of Vater.—Carcinoma of the ampulla of Vater theoretically should present a greater opportunity for cure or prolonged relief from symptoms than malignancies of adjacent structures. These tumors tend to grow into the lumen of the duodenum rather than to extend into adjacent structures or to invade the lymphatics. Furthermore, because of the involvement of the distal end of the common bile duct, jaundice is an early symptom. It has been contended that malignancies of the ampulla have a slower rate of growth than neoplasms of adjacent pancreatic tissue. Unfortunately, in our series of 11 malignancies of the ampulla of Vater, 10 of which were adenocarcinomas and one a malignant carcinoid, no patient survived more than two years after radical surgery. Few of these patients, however, presented themselves for treatment in the early stages of the disease.

Symptomatology.—Jaundice is an early symptom. It may be incomplete in its early stages and is more often associated with pain, occasionally of a colicky nature, than is noted in carcinoma of the head of the pancreas. Progressive weight loss usually begins fairly early in the disease. Pruritus, light stools and dark urine are common. Because the gallbladder is not diseased in over 75 per cent of these patients, backpressure upon the bile ducts and the gallbladder causes them to enlarge and often the gallbladder can be palpated. Liver function tests help to establish the obstructive nature of the jaundice and the progression of liver damage. Carcinomas of the ampulla of Vater frequently ulcerate and blood often can be obtained on duodenal aspiration and in the stools. Obstruction of the main pancreatic duct by pressure of the tumor or involvement of the duct by the tumor frequently interferes with pancreatic secretion, causing disturbances which can be determined by blood and stool studies. Barium x-ray studies of the gastrointestinal tract reveal a duodenal deformity in a high percentage of patients. Occasionally the tumor may completely occlude the duodenum and produce symptoms of high intestinal obstruction.

Treatment.—Early and radical surgical excision of malignant tumors of the ampulla of Vater offers the only hope of cure. Early exploration is imperative when such lesions are suspected. Even at the operating table an accurate diagnosis is difficult to establish. If a lesion of the ampulla of Vater is suspected or palpable, the duodenum should be opened on its anterior surface by a longitudinal incision. If a tumor is found, a biopsy should be made with immediate histologic study to determine the nature of the tumor. This is important since a malignant tumor demands more radical therapy than a benign lesion. Careful exploration should be made for metastatic lesions and for lymph node involvement. If the disease proves to be malignant and is localized to the ampulla of Vater, a pancreaticoduodenal resection by the one- or two-stage technic should be performed as shown in Plates 69–71. If spread of the disease prevents its complete removal, a palliative procedure to reestablish the flow of bile into the intestinal tract should be undertaken. Cholecystogastrostomy as shown in Plate 58 is a simple procedure which gives good palliative results. Occasionally it is simpler to anastomose the gallbladder to the duodenum. A Roux-Y type of cholecystojejunostomy is preferred by some surgeons. This is demonstrated in Plate 69. This operation minimizes the danger of the reflux of intestinal contents into the bile ducts but the extent of surgery entailed may not be justified in the presence of malignancy.

EXTRADUCTAL LESIONS INVOLVING THE BILE DUCTS

Inflammatory Lesions

Inflammatory lesions of adjacent organs which may involve the bile ducts most commonly arise in the pancreas. Acute and subacute pancreatitis may produce inflammatory changes in, or compression of, the common duct with resultant biliary dyspepsia and obstructive jaundice. Varying degrees of acute pancreatitis are associated with inflammatory and calculous disease of the gallbladder and bile ducts in a high percentage of cases, and it may be difficult to determine in which structure the primary infection originated. Such differentiation is important because acute inflammatory disease of the bile ducts may be an immediate surgical problem whereas severe inflammatory disease of the pancreas usually should be treated conservatively. Evidences of pancreatic dysfunction with elevation of serum amylase and lipase levels and with disturbances of pancreatic digestion suggest pancreatic involvement. Reference of pain to the back and to the left is commonly associated with pancreatic disease.

Chronic pancreatitis without associated disease of the biliary tract frequently encroaches upon the lumen of the common bile duct. The jaundice may be fluctuant and may be accompanied by colics similar to those produced by stones. Often, however, it is persistent and progressive and may be accompanied by little or no pain or by pain which is dull in character and radiates to the back and to the left. Diminution of the secretion of pancreatic enzymes into the intestinal tract may be manifested by fatty stools. There may be an elevation of serum amylase and serum lipase.

Treatment.—The treatment of obstructive jaundice due to chronic pancreatic disease should be directed to the relief of biliary obstruction and the removal of any existing disease of the extrahepatic biliary system. If the gallbladder is diseased and contains stones and if stones are present in the common bile duct, cholecystectomy and choledochostomy should be performed, with removal of the disease of the extrahepatic biliary tract. The edema of the pancreas usually will subside and patency of the common duct will gradually be restored. Chronic pancreatitis with dilatation of the extrahepatic bile ducts and gallbladder without associated inflammatory change or calculus formation should be treated conservatively. It is difficult to differentiate between chronic pancreatitis and carcinoma of the head of the pancreas. Radical surgery of the pancreas should not be undertaken unless histologic confirmation by biopsy and frozen section can be obtained. Many patients in whom a diagnosis of carcinoma of the head of the pancreas has been made have lived many years after a short-circuiting operation, suggesting an error in diagnosis in most instances. When chronic pancreatitis obstructs the bile ducts, a cholecystogastrostomy (see Plate 58) or cholecystoenterostomy should be performed. Although some surgeons prefer a Roux-Y type of anastomosis between the jejunum and the gallbladder, results of cholecystogastrostomy have been most satisfactory. Upon subsidence of the inflammation of the head of the pancreas and the reestablishment of patency of the common bile duct, the stoma of the anastomosis between the gallbladder and the stomach usually will close and the danger of an ascending cholangitis is minimal. If the common duct has been explored during the course of the operation, a T-tube should be sutured into it in addition to the establishment of an internal anastomosis.

Peptic ulcers, particularly those involving the descending limb of the duodenum, occasionally will cause inflammatory change of the common bile duct with edema and partial or complete obstruction. The symptomatology is that of the primary lesion, occasionally complicated by jaundice and sometimes by cholangitis with chills and fever. If, at operation, the common duct is found to be patent and is adequately drained, surgical treatment of the ulcer will be followed by subsidence of the bile duct involvement.

Lymphadenopathy

Pressure upon the bile duct system by enlarged lymph nodes is a rare cause of obstructive jaundice. It may be associated with inflammatory disease. Occasionally malignancies of the lymphatic system, including lymphosarcoma and Hodgkin's disease and metastatic malignancy from primary lesions of retroperitoneal organs, will produce enlargement of the lymph nodes adjacent to the common duct which will cause partial or complete obstruction.

Malignant Lesions

Malignant lesions of adjacent structures may occlude the common bile duct by external pressure. By far the most common are those which arise in the head of the pancreas. These are discussed in the chapter dealing with pancreatic disease. Carcinoma of the pyloric end of the stomach and the rare malignancies found in the duodenum may likewise obstruct the bile ducts. Jaundice due to metastatic carcinoma most frequently results from intrahepatic metastases.

CHAPTER 13

Factors Causing Symptoms After Biliary Tract Surgery

FEW DISEASES in my opinion respond so satisfactorily and with as low an operative mortality and morbidity as those of the biliary tract which are diagnosed early and treated by adequate surgery. As gallbladder disease originates in an organ which is not essential to life, health or digestive comfort and as the disease usually remains localized for some time after the onset of symptoms, the complete removal of this organ should give excellent results in the great majority of patients. Unfortunately such results are not universally achieved in practice. Delay of treatment is due to the nature of the disease and to the attitude of both patient and physician. Except in an early, acute cholecystitis, attacks of biliary colic do not demand immediate surgical intervention. It is better to let the attack subside and to operate on the patient in a symptom-free period when he can be adequately prepared. However, when the attack is over the patient usually feels very well and both he and his family physician will delay operation in the hope that another attack will not occur. This sequence of events is followed by repeated attacks until finally the disease spreads beyond the confines of the gallbladder and makes surgery more hazardous and difficult, with an outlook of poorer results. Most patients with biliary tract disease know of others who continue to have symptoms after operation and, because of this, fear not only the hazard of the operation but the continuance of biliary distress. Thus a high percentage of patients avoid surgical therapy until a real emergency arises. In our experience, patients have not submitted to biliary tract surgery until they have had symptoms for an average of six years after the first biliary colic. Many submit to surgical therapy only after an emergency complication has arisen, thus greatly increasing the dangers of the operation and diminishing their chance of securing complete relief of symptoms.

Biliary dyskinesia.—Biliary dyskinesia and similar terms have been used to explain the colics, pain and other symptoms which occasionally are encountered following cholecystectomy. These symptoms have been attributed to a physiologic spasm of the sphincter of Oddi. From experimental and clinical evidence, I believe the sphincter of Oddi loses its function after an adequately performed cholecystectomy. The operation must be sufficiently extensive to interrupt the nerve fibers to the sphincter of Oddi. Investigative work has shown that certain drugs can produce an increase in intraductal pressure in the common bile duct after the gallbladder has been removed. It has also been shown that residual disease in the common bile duct, pathologic conditions of the duct wall and contiguous disease involving the ducts can elevate intraductal pressure. Functional disturbances also can produce similar effects. The rise in pressure may result from a spasm of the sphincter of Oddi or may also result from spasm of the duodenum which may compress the intraduodenal portion of the duct. Functional factors should be thoroughly investigated before performing a cholecystectomy to minimize unnecessary biliary tract surgery.

The high incidence of an organic cause of postcholecystectomy symptoms makes it imperative that such factors be thoroughly investigated before attributing symptoms to a purely physiologic disturbance. Careful surgical exploration in patients with postcholecystectomy spasm and pain usually will reveal the etiologic factor and its correction will relieve the symptoms.

The causes of continued distress after surgery on the biliary tract may be listed under three headings: (1) errors in diagnosis; (2) errors in surgical technic, and (3) residual disease.

Errors in Diagnosis

An accurate history is essential to the diagnosis of biliary tract disease. Pain is one of the most important symptoms. When typical and repeated biliary colics have occurred, with radiation of pain around the costal margins or to the right scapula, and when qualitative and quantitative food distress is associated, the diagnosis usually is obvious. If pain is absent or minimal, except in the presence of obstructive jaundice, the diagnosis of biliary tract disease should not be made without careful study.

Cholecystography is a great aid in the diagnosis of gallbladder disease. It is highly accurate in establishing the functional capacity of the gallbladder and often in visualizing calculi. However, a diseased gallbladder does not always produce symptoms and may not be the cause of the patient's complaints. To remove the gallbladder for symptoms due to other causes will not cure the patient. Routine autopsy studies show a high incidence of cholecystitis and cholelithiasis in persons who at no time gave a history of biliary distress. Roentgenographic findings of a nonfunctioning gallbladder are not sufficient justification for cholecystectomy if the history does not support the diagnosis. Contrarily, a normally functioning gallbladder on x-ray does not always exclude cholelithiasis. When the history of biliary colics is typical and examination supports the diagnosis, cholecystectomy may be indicated even though the cholecystogram is normal. Without x-ray confirmation, however, the surgeon should be thoroughly convinced of the diagnosis before operating upon the biliary tract.

A number of other diseases produce symptoms suggestive of biliary tract disease. Cholecystectomy under these circumstances may be followed by persistence of symptoms. Functional dyspepsia is one of the commonest conditions confused with biliary tract disease. Patients with functional disorders may complain of qualitative food distress, indigestion, belching after meals and epigastric discomfort. Their symptoms usually can be differentiated from those of gallbladder disease by the absence of severe pain and tenderness, the indefiniteness of the symptoms and their nervous temperament. This group of patients constitutes the greatest number of cholecystectomized patients with persistence of symptoms postoperatively. So-called spastic colitis is a common functional disease and often is accompanied by indigestion. Cholecystic disease may be coexistent, but if it is not producing typical gallbladder symptoms cholecystectomy is unlikely to relieve that patient's symptoms.

Pancreatic disease can produce symptoms suggestive of biliary tract abnormality. Pancreatic pain may be as severe as that produced by biliary calculi. It is usually located deep in the epigastrium, with radiation to the back and to the left. It may result from pancreatitis, varying in degree from acute to chronic stages. Fortunately, acute inflammation both of the gallbladder and the pancreas can be treated conservatively and, if the patient is carefully observed, surgery may be delayed until the diagnosis is established.

Peptic ulcers usually produce characteristic symptoms which make the diagnosis fairly apparent. Acute perforation or subacute penetration of an ulcer may closely simulate acute biliary disease. If a perforation occurs, evidence of peritonitis and air under the diaphragm shown radiographically are aids in diagnosis.

Diaphragmatic hernias, especially of the hiatus type in which a portion of the stomach is located above the diaphragm, may be responsible for a chronic type of indigestion characterized by distress and belching soon after eating which may simulate biliary tract symptoms. Diaphragmatic hernias may also produce pain similar to that of biliary tract disease. However, true and severe colics are less frequently encountered. The diagnosis of this condition can be made by radiologic studies of the esophagus and stomach. A hiatus hernia and cholelithiasis may coexist. When this occurs, the removal of the gallbladder seldom will be followed by relief of symptoms.

Coronary artery disease may produce pain simulating biliary colic. Differential diagnosis often is difficult, especially when both diseases are present. If the attack is of cardiac origin, epigastric or right upper quadrant pain and tenderness may be present but usually are less severe than those of biliary colic. Other evidences of heart disease may be noted and electrocardiographic confirmation can be obtained.

The most important factor in avoiding surgical procedures on the biliary tract for symptoms produced by other diseases is a carefully taken and evaluated history. Laboratory and x-ray aids are of value in supporting a clinical diagnosis but should not be used as a substitute for careful clinical study and judgment.

Errors in Surgical Technic

It is my belief that biliary distress and indigestion are due largely to the maintenance of the tonus of the sphincter of Oddi in conjunction with a nonfunctioning gallbladder. This deprives the upper intestinal tract of adequate bile in the early stages of digestion. Relief of symptoms after cholecystectomy is due to removal of disease and to a loss of tonus of the sphincter of Oddi. This release of tonus is apparently on a neurogenic basis and is dependent upon adequate surgical treatment. Errors in surgical technic which may be responsible for a continuation of symptoms may be divided into two categories—those based on inadequate surgery and those producing trauma to the bile ducts and vessels.

INADEQUATE SURGICAL THERAPY.—This includes a variety of conditions. Failure to remove the gallbladder, with subsequent reformation of stones, formerly was common. At present, surgeons seldom employ cholecystostomy for chronic biliary tract disease. However, the neck of the gallbladder or a long cystic duct with or without stones can produce severe biliary tract symptoms. In reoperating on patients who had severe colics after cholecystectomy I have found stones embedded in the cystic duct; removal of the stump of the cystic duct and its stones completely relieved the symptoms. In other patients with a persistence of biliary distress, the removal of a long cystic duct stump, even though it contained no stones, has given complete relief.

Residual cystic duct stumps.—There is considerable controversy among surgeons as to whether or not a residual cystic duct stump, not containing stones, can produce postcholecystectomy symptoms. Many surgeons attribute postcholecystectomy pain to neuromas in the region of the cystic duct. Although these have been proved histologically in some cases, I believe they are uncommon. I have operated on many patients for persistent biliary tract symptoms following cholecystectomy and found a long cystic duct stump but no other apparent disease. On removal of the cystic duct stump and negative findings on exploration of the common bile duct, the majority of these patients were relieved of their symptoms. I believe the symptoms were due to a persistence of function of the sphincter of Oddi and that an adequate dissection to remove the cystic duct stump resulted in denervation of the sphincter of Oddi and a drop in intraductal pressure in the choledochus. Intravenous cholangiograms of such patients are shown in Plate 52.

A.—A dentist's wife had had a cholecystectomy three years before being seen by us. During that three years she had severe biliary tract pain, nausea, vomiting, anorexia and a weight loss of 30 lb. She was treated by various medications, diets, steroids, tranquilizers and psychiatrists. At operation we found a cystic duct stump approximately 3 cm. in length and a normal common duct which was explored and contained no stones. The cystic duct stump was removed and histologically showed only a mild, chronic cholangitis. She had complete relief of symptoms and regained weight and a normal digestive capacity.

B.—After cholecystectomy this patient continued to have rather typical biliary tract symptoms. A cholangiogram showed a dilated cystic duct stump. On re-exploration, the stump was removed, the common duct explored and no stones found. She has had no further biliary tract symptoms.

C.—This patient had had a cholecystectomy two years prior to our examination. She continued to have biliary tract symptoms. A cholangiogram revealed a long cystic duct stump. This was removed at operation and revealed no stones and very little chronic disease. The common duct was explored and appeared to be normal. Relief of symptoms followed the second operation.

I do not contend that a persistence of symptoms after cholecystectomy is always the result of a residual cystic duct stump, but I believe it to be a distinct entity which is frequently a factor in the failure of cholecystectomy to relieve patients of their symptoms.

Residual stones in common duct.—Failure to remove gallstones from the common bile duct is often the cause of postcholecystectomy symptoms. This may be due to failure to explore the common duct at the time of cholecystectomy. Intravenous cholangiography has greatly aided in the demonstration of residual stones and other disease following cholecystectomy (Plate 25); the technic of body section radiography has markedly increased the accuracy of intravenous cholangiography. The indications for common duct exploration are discussed under Choledochostomy (Chapter 12). Plate 53 presents cholangiograms showing residual stones in the common bile duct.

PLATE 52

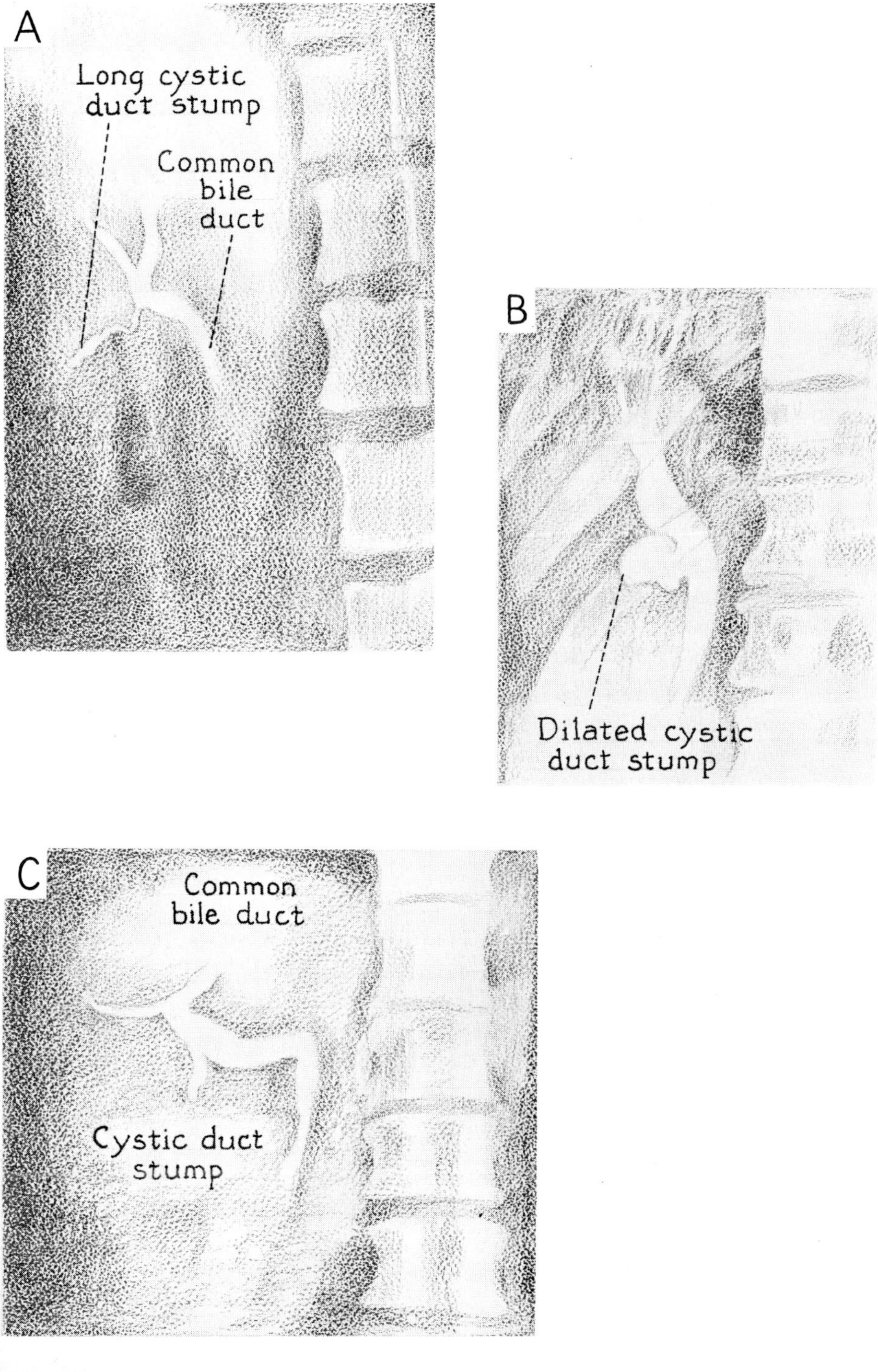
A
Long cystic duct stump
Common bile duct
B
Dilated cystic duct stump
C
Common bile duct
Cystic duct stump

A.—This drawing shows a cholangiogram of a patient whose common duct was explored and a T-tube inserted. A stone is seen which completely occludes the distal end of the common duct.

B.—The common duct was re-explored and the stone removed. A subsequent cholangiogram shows the opaque medium outlining the duct and flowing freely into the duodenum.

C.—This drawing of a cholangiogram of another patient shows a residual stone blocking the distal end of the common bile duct. An anteroposterior view which showed the duct narrowing to a point was interpreted to represent a stricture of the distal common bile duct. This lateral view reveals the outline of the stone with the opaque medium narrowing to a point anterior to it, emphasizing the importance of securing lateral as well as anteroposterior cholangiograms.

Diseases of adjacent organs which have not been remedied at surgery because of failure to recognize or inability to correct them may irritate the extrahepatic biliary tract and produce symptoms. These conditions include duodenal ulcers, chronic pancreatitis and diseases of lymph nodes adjacent to the common bile duct.

Traumatic injury.—Damage to the extrahepatic biliary and arterial system may be the cause of postoperative symptoms. If the hepatic artery or a main branch is ligated or damaged and the patient survives, damage to the liver may be serious. The common duct or hepatic ducts may be damaged by instruments or may be partially or completely ligated, and the resulting symptoms usually are proportionate to the damage done. Gauze packing in the gallbladder bed may press against or damage the ducts or vessels. It is important for all surgeons performing operations upon the biliary tract to have a thorough knowledge of the anatomy and the anomalies of these structures. Damage to them can be avoided if they are carefully dissected at the time of operation and if no structure is clamped, ligated or divided until it is thoroughly identified.

PLATE 53

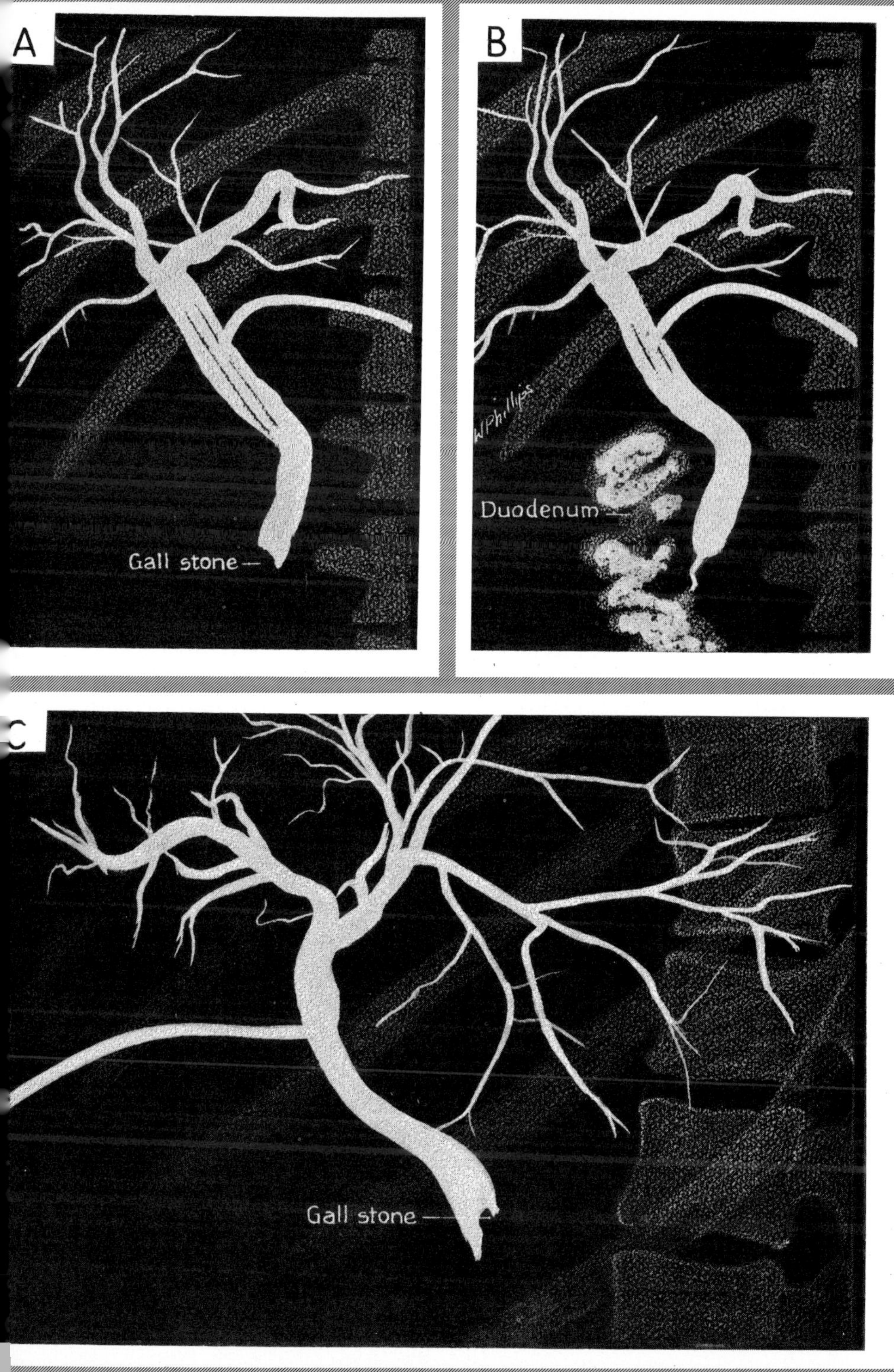

Residual Disease

If disease of the biliary tract has existed for many years and especially if infection has been present, there may be considerable damage to the liver as well as to the gallbladder and bile ducts. Removal of the gallbladder cannot be expected to eradicate such disease. If a suppurative cholangitis has existed, complete removal of stones from the ducts and subsequent drainage will not clear up the infection in the duct walls. Long-standing or intermittent obstruction to the common duct will produce liver damage which may be reflected in the patient's future health. Such damage can be avoided by early diagnosis and treatment.

Reflux from common duct into pancreatic duct.—An anatomic arrangement of the common bile duct and main pancreatic duct which permits regurgitation of bile into the pancreatic duct proximal to the ampulla of Vater is encountered quite commonly. It has been maintained that such regurgitation may produce pancreatitis which in turn is responsible for certain postcholecystectomy symptoms.

A.—This drawing is an exact replica of a cholangiogram of a patient whose common duct had been explored and a T-tube inserted. The opaque medium flows from the common duct into the pancreatic duct proximal to a stone which almost completely occludes the ampulla of Vater.

B.—After re-exploration and removal of the stone, the opaque medium flows freely into the duodenum but continues to regurgitate into the pancreatic duct.

C.—Following a choledochostomy, this cholangiogram reveals gallstones within the common duct and a reflux of opaque medium into the pancreatic duct. This reflux persisted after the stones were removed.

D.—This is a cholangiogram made following a choledochostomy in which there is regurgitation of opaque medium into the pancreatic duct.

The role played by the reflux of bile into the pancreatic duct in the production of chronic pancreatitis is controversial. Likewise, the importance of pancreatic secretion into the biliary system in the production of biliary tract disease has caused considerable speculation. In my experience, patients whose cholangiograms have shown a reflux of opaque medium into the pancreatic ducts from the com-

PLATE 54

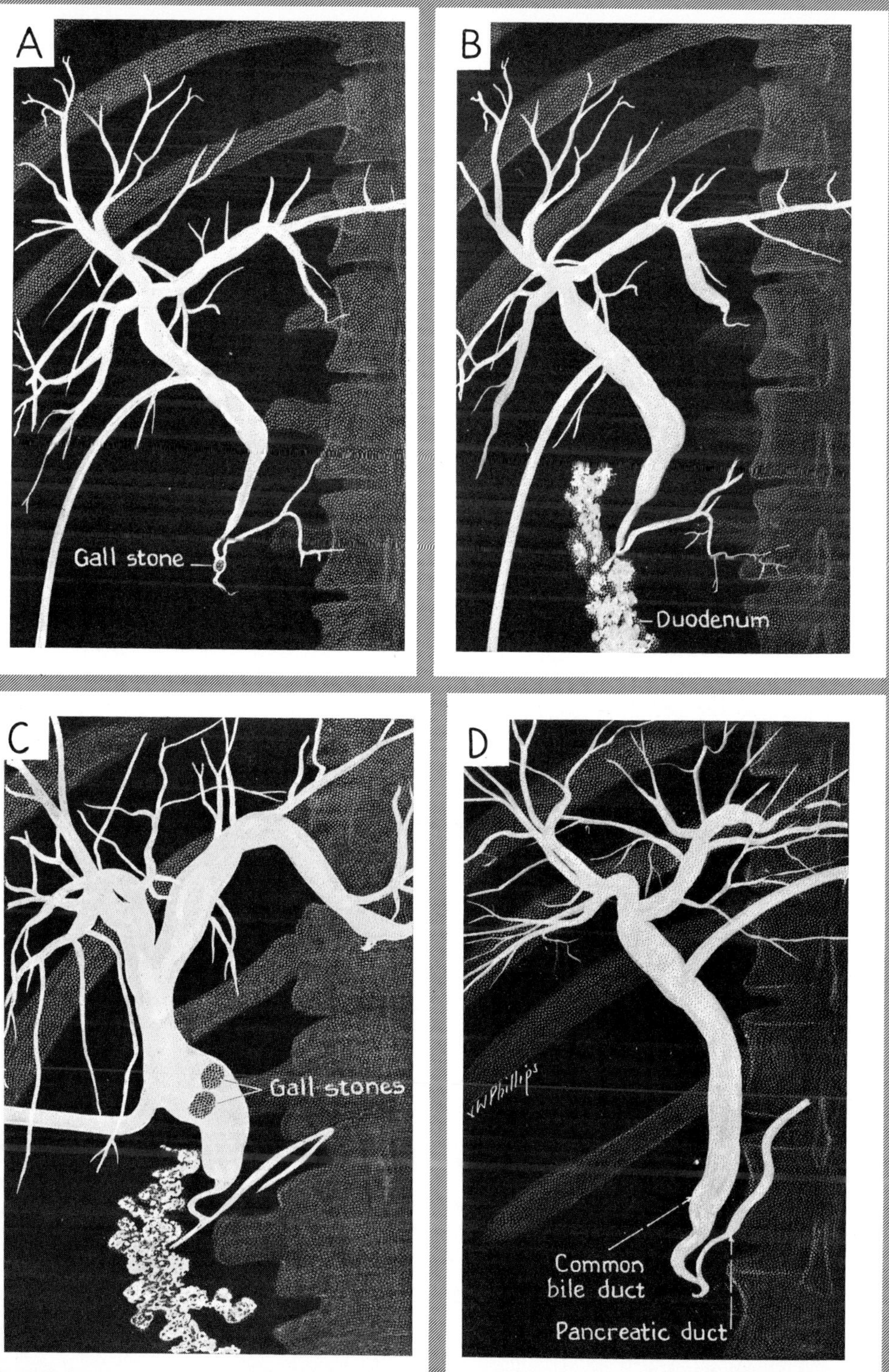
A
Gall stone
B
Duodenum
C
Gall stones
D
Common
bile duct
Pancreatic duct

mon duct have not had symptoms of chronic pancreatitis. For this reason and because I believe that an adequate cholecystectomy with common duct exploration and the establishment of patency of the ampulla of Vater is followed by a loss of tonus of the sphincter of Oddi and the free flow of bile into the duodenum, I doubt the value of sphincterotomy in the treatment of chronic pancreatitis.

Summary

Good results following operation on the biliary tract depend upon correct diagnosis and early and technically correct surgical treatment. A surgeon who undertakes an operation upon the biliary tract has the responsibility of making every effort to get the patient well. He must be sure of the diagnosis, must know the anatomy of the field and must, as far as possible, correct existing disease. Post-cholecystectomy syndromes should not be considered as a purely physiologic abnormality to be referred to an internist for subsequent care. If disease is present only in the gallbladder and the rest of the hepatobiliary system is undamaged, cholecystectomy should give complete relief of symptoms in better than 90 per cent of patients. As the patients are converted physiologically to the type of animal which never possessed a gallbladder, they should be able to live a normal life without dietary or other restrictions directed at the hepatobiliary system.

SECTION III

The Pancreas

CHAPTER 14

Anatomy and Physiology of the Pancreas

ANATOMY

THE DEEPLY SITUATED retroperitoneal position of the pancreas behind the lesser peritoneal sac at the level of the first and second lumbar vertebrae renders it less accessible to surgical approach than most abdominal organs. Its proximity to large blood vessels increases the technical difficulty of surgical therapy. The pancreas is divided into three portions: the right extremity or head which conforms to the concavity of the duodenum, the neck which is the narrowed portion where the organ lies anterior to the portal vein and the body which extends to the left and tapers to form the tail. The uncinate process of the head of the pancreas varies in size and position. It may extend posterior to the superior mesenteric vessels, rendering them vulnerable to injury in removal of the head of the pancreas. The tail terminates close to or in contact with the hilus of the spleen. The superior and inferior pancreaticoduodenal arteries supply the head and neck. The superior mesenteric vessels pass under the neck of the gland. The body crosses the aorta, inferior vena cava and renal vessels. The splenic vessels course along the superior surface of the pancreas, often grooving it and supplying it with branches. The main pancreatic duct enters the duodenum in varying relationship to the common bile duct and the ampulla of Vater (see Plate 22). This relationship may play a role in the association of pancreatic and biliary tract disease.

Various surgical approaches to the pancreas can be used, the choice depending upon the portion of the organ to be explored. The posterior surface of the head of the gland may be reached by elevating the duodenum from the right side. The anterior surface of the head is usually most accessible by division of the gastrocolic omentum overlying it. The body and tail of the pancreas usually are most accessible through the gastrocolic omentum although occasionally they can be approached through the gastrohepatic ligament.

The pancreas is a compound acinotubular gland, each lobule being a ramification of a main duct. It has no true capsule, which makes the organ difficult to oversew when it has been traumatically or surgically incised. For this reason, when operating upon the pancreas, it is important for the surgeon to ligate individually any ducts encountered and to oversew sectioned portions thoroughly. These steps minimize the danger of leakage of pancreatic secretions.

PHYSIOLOGY

The pancreas elaborates both internal and external secretions. The latter contains three enzymes, trypsinogen, amylase and lipase, which serve an important function in the digestion of proteins, carbohydrates and fats. The average daily quantity of external secretion of the pancreas is in excess of 1 L. The quantity and composition varies with food ingestion, the pH of duodenal contents and nerve stimulation. Interference with the flow of pancreatic juice into the intestines may result in a rise of digestive ferments in the blood, especially detectable in the levels of serum amylase and lipase. These rises may be quite pronounced in acute pancreatitis and are of considerable diagnostic aid to the physician. They are of great value in differentiating an acute pancreatitis which demands conservative therapy from certain acute abdominal diseases which present similar symptoms and for which emergency surgery may be necessary.

The islets of Langerhans are responsible for the secretion of insulin. Even after the pancreas is fibrosed with a chronic disease or invaded by tumor tissue, the islets persist in secreting insulin and tend to avoid tumor infiltration. Adenomas of the islets of Langerhans which secrete excessive amounts of insulin are a surgical problem.

CHAPTER 15

Benign Surgical Lesions of the Pancreas

PANCREATIC TRAUMA

THE POSITION of the pancreas within the upper abdomen offers it excellent protection from injury. However, like all other organs of the body, it is not protected from penetrating wounds. Its fixed position in front of the spine, with only soft tissues anterior to it, renders the pancreas vulnerable to any injury which applies great force to the anterior abdominal wall.

Symptomatology and diagnosis.—In evaluating the symptoms produced by injury to the pancreas one must be aware of the variations in intensity, which depend upon the degree of injury to this organ, and must differentiate symptoms produced by injuries to adjacent structures. Mild injury to the pancreas may result in pain which varies in intensity from minimal to severe and which is usually located in the epigastric or lumbar region. The pain may become severe and then subside, to recur with gradual development of inflammation. If diaphragmatic irritation occurs, the pain may be referred to the shoulder or subscapular area. Nausea and hiccups are common but vomiting usually is a late symptom. In severe injury to the pancreas the patient may manifest symptoms of shock varying in degree according to the amount of tissue destruction, blood loss and the extravasation of pancreatic secretion. Traumatic pancreatitis may soon produce an elevation of blood serum amylase, glycosuria and hyperglycemia as well as leukocytosis. A decrease in the erythrocyte count and hematocrit value is dependent upon associated hemorrhage. Roentgenographic examination of the abdomen may reveal an absence of the psoas shadow due to hemorrhage. Elevation of the diaphragm and displacement of the stomach and colon can result from hemorrhage and the accumulation of fluids. Gas under the diaphragm usually indicates injury to a hollow viscus.

The pathology of pancreatic injury usually consists of incomplete or complete rupture of the organ. If the rupture is incomplete, edema and hemorrhage result in traumatic pancreatitis. This may be accompanied by hemorrhage and peritonitis in the lesser or greater omental cavity. Complete rupture usually produces hemorrhage, loss of pancreatic fluid and peritonitis. Either of these conditions may result later in the formation of pseudocysts.

Treatment.—Mild and uncomplicated injury of the pancreas responds best to conservative therapy. In the absence of evidence of injury to adjacent organs or of hemorrhage and shock, nonsurgical treatment is indicated. This consists of gastric suction, supportive therapy, adequate intravenous administration of fluids and careful observation. Shock must be anticipated and prevented or treated vigorously when it occurs. The administration of whole blood and plasma expanders in adequate quantities may be essential.

If there are evidences of injury to adjacent organs, such as the stomach, intestines, liver or spleen, early exploration is indicated. During such operations, hemorrhage must be controlled and the indicated surgery on abdominal viscera performed. The pancreas should be examined. Exposure is usually best obtained by dividing the gastrocolic omentum and elevating the stomach. If the coverings of the pancreas are not ruptured and if there is no active bleeding or hematoma formation, it is inadvisable to incise the gland and insert drains to its surface because of the danger of subsequent pancreatic fistula. If the pancreas is ruptured and bleeding, hemorrhage should be controlled by adequate ligatures and sutures. When pancreatic ducts are ruptured, it has been recommended that repair by suture be attempted and the gland then oversewn and drains placed in its proximity. Because of the small size of the ducts and the damage to adjacent pancreatic tissue, it is usually impossible to repair the ducts so that they will drain adequately into the duodenum and, as a result, there will be extravasation of pancreatic secretion into the surrounding tissues or to the surface of the abdomen.

When an injury transects the pancreas near the head of the organ, internal drainage may be established by anastomosing a defunctionalized limb of jejunum to the surface of the pancreas, suturing the edge of the bowel a considerable distance beyond the traumatized area. If the transsection occurs to the left of the spine and the proximal portion of the pancreas is not badly damaged, it may be feasible to remove the distal segment, ligate any recognizable pancreatic ducts, and oversew the distal end of the remaining portion of the pancreas. However, a caudal pancreaticojejunostomy, if the condition of the patient permits, will give added assurance that a pancreatic fistula will not result. With the distal pancreas removed, splenectomy may be necessary. After such surgical procedures, it is well to drain the area by Penrose or sump drains. The latter are preferable because of their efficiency in removing serum, blood and pancreatic secretions.

Trauma to the pancreas may be followed by the development of cysts, abscesses or fistulas. The treatment of these is discussed in the section on Pancreatic Cysts.

PANCREATITIS

Inflammatory disease of the pancreas has been attributed to a number of etiologic factors. Partial or complete obstruction of the pancreatic ducts with interference of the free flow of pancreatic juice into the duodenum is often followed by this disease. Such obstructions can result from disease within the pancreas itself due to fibrous tissue, metaplasia of intraductal cells, occlusion by malignant disease or ligation of the ducts during an operative procedure in the vicinity. Occlusion of the pancreatic ducts may also result from disease of adjacent structures such as duodenal ulcer, tumor of the ampulla of Vater and disease of the biliary tract. The frequent association of stones within the common bile duct with pancreatic disease suggests the possible occlusion of the pancreatic duct by such calculi. The reflux of bile into the pancreatic ducts is considered by some investigators to be a cause of pancreatitis. Such reflux can be demonstrated on cholangiograms. It may result from the anatomic arrangement of the ducts which establish a common channel proximal to the ampulla of Vater. Obstruction of the ampulla of Vater by stones may force bile into the pancreatic ducts. Spasm of the sphincter of Oddi as the cause of pancreatitis is controversial. The transmission of bacteria from adjacent diseased structures, particularly the biliary tract, as a cause is supported by the frequently occurring coexistence of inflammation of the two systems.

The frequency with which acute pancreatitis follows the ingestion of a large meal or an excessive amount of alcohol suggests a dietary factor. The mental characteristics and behavior of many patients who have pancreatitis intimate a psychologic factor. Trauma to the upper abdomen occasionally is followed by this disease.

Varying degrees of inflammation of the pancreas may occur. These range from acute fulminating disease to chronic progressive changes. The intensity of the disease may fluctuate, producing symptoms of what is termed *chronic relapsing pancreatitis.* Pancreatitis will be discussed under the acute and chronic forms.

Acute Pancreatitis

Acute pancreatitis may be divided into three categories, depending upon the intensity of the disease. These are the acute edematous form, in which the patient usually survives, and the acute hemorrhagic and acute suppurative forms, which are more severe and in which there is a high mortality rate.

The symptoms begin with pain, usually severe, which is located in the epigastrium, the right upper quadrant or occasionally the lower abdomen and frequently extends to the back. Nausea and vomiting invariably occur. The rapid development of prostration or shock indicates a progressive and serious form of the disease. Abdominal examination usually elicits tenderness, the location roughly corresponding to that of the pain. It is most common in the epigastrium; if in the right upper quadrant, it suggests the possible coexistence of acute biliary tract disease. Abdominal distention develops due to paralytic ileus. Jaundice may often be detected.

The leukocyte count may range from 10,000 to 45,000. In our series most patients who recovered from this disease had a leukocyte count below 20,000. The concentration of serum amylase increases rapidly, often to a very high level, but usually returns to normal in two to four days if the disease subsides. Serum lipase concentration is increased and returns to normal more slowly than that of serum amylase. Albuminuria is invariably found.

Diagnosis.—Acute pancreatitis may produce symptoms similar to those of other acute abdominal conditions and a correct diagnosis often is hard to establish. An increase of serum amylase and lipase and the presence of albuminuria are very suggestive of acute pancreatitis but are not diagnostic as they are seen in many acute abdominal diseases. Roentgenograms are of value in differentiating perforations of peptic ulcer or of other hollow viscera from this disease by the demonstration of air in the peritoneal cavity. Diseases which may simulate acute pancreatitis include acute cholecystitis, perforated peptic ulcer, intestinal obstruction, mesenteric thrombosis, acute diverticulitis and severe inflammation in a high-lying appendix.

Treatment.—Surgical intervention in acute pancreatitis is followed by a considerably higher mortality than conservative management. For this reason diagnostic accuracy is important. To avoid surgical neglect of a disease which should receive early operative therapy, conservative management demands constant and critical observation of the patient. It includes bed rest and relief of pain. Various types of opiates in fairly large doses are sometimes used for the relief of pain. If their use is prolonged, there is danger of drug addiction. Splanchnic block has proved fairly satisfactory for relief of pancreatic pain (Plate 59). Its effects may be only temporary, but occasionally the pain relief will be permanent. The continuous epidural administration of various anesthetic agents is a simple method of securing analgesia and is believed to relax the sphincter of Oddi. The stomach should be kept empty by continuous gastric suction. Fluid and chemical balance should be maintained by intravenous infusion and blood administered when indicated. A careful record of fluid intake and output should be maintained, and frequent studies of blood chemistry should guide the amount and nature of fluids administered. Blood sugar levels will indicate the need for insulin. Serum amylase levels should be followed closely in order to estimate the progress of the disease.

Subsequent care will depend upon the response of the patient. If the disease subsides, careful studies should be made to determine if it is secondary to disease of the biliary tract or other systems. The primary cause of the disease should not be treated surgically until the patient has thoroughly recovered from the acute attack unless progression of symptoms and findings make immediate surgery mandatory. If a pancreatic abscess develops, it should be subsequently drained. Presence of an abscess will be indicated by persistence of fever, leukocytosis and frequently a tender midabdominal mass. Such symptoms should suggest this complication even though the serum amylase concentration has returned to normal or below.

When, because of an error in diagnosis, a patient with acute pancreatitis is operated on, a minimal amount of surgery should be performed. The pancreas should not be incised or widely exposed. We have recently incised the pancreas and covered it with a defunctionalized jejunal segment when this was technically feasible. Although this operation has been successful, our series is too small to prove the merits of this procedure. If no other disease exists, the abdominal cavity should be drained and closed. If disease of the biliary tract is present, minimal procedures such as cholecystostomy or choledochostomy should be used to establish external biliary drainage. A perforation of the gastrointestinal tract must of course be closed.

Chronic Pancreatitis

Following an attack of acute pancreatitis, there is frequently a gradual progression of disease of this organ. It mav be manifested by remissions and exacerbations of the inflammatory process. Such a course is called "chronic relapsing pancreatitis." During exacerbations of the disease, the symptoms are similar to those of acute pancreatitis. Pain is a predominant symptom and is associated with nausea, vomiting, disturbance of bowel habits and occasionally fever and jaundice. The pain is noted most frequently in the epigastrium or left upper quadrant, slightly above the umbilicus, and often radiates directly through to the back. Pain in the right upper quadrant, especially when biliary tract surgery has been performed, is often believed to be due to pancreatitis but is far more frequently due to residual biliary tract disease. Careful studies including intravenous cholangiography will help establish the true diagnosis. The pain of chronic relapsing pancreatitis varies in character, intensity and duration. Attacks may recur at short or long intervals. Abdominal examination may reveal epigastric tenderness during an attack, and a mass may be felt in the region of the pancreas owing to enlargement of the gland or formation of a pseudocyst. Elevation of serum amylase and serum lipase levels may accompany early attacks, but with gradual destruction of the gland such changes may not be detectable. With progressive damage to the acinar cells, digestive disturbances are manifested by progressive weight loss in spite of an adequate diet and by steatorrhea. As the islet cells become involved, disturbances of carbohydrate metabolism are revealed by the development of diabetes.

Complications.—Involvement of the head of the pancreas may cause occlusion of the common bile duct with development of a progressive obstructive jaundice. Differential diagnosis of obstructive jaundice due to carcinoma of the head of the pancreas from chronic pancreatitis may be difficult to establish. Chronic pancreatitis usually is accompanied by pain, whereas in carcinoma pain may be absent or, if present, is less severe. Calcification may occur within the pancreatic ducts or throughout the gland. This is demonstrable by roentgenograms. Pancreatic lithiasis may occur in isolated areas of the pancreas or throughout the entire gland. Pancreatic cysts are not infrequent complications.

The frequent recurrence of pain may cause the patient to become a narcotic addict or a chronic alcoholic. Unfortunately, former methods of therapy for chronic pancreatitis seldom cured the disease. There is frequently gradual progression with subsequent death from malnutrition, intercurrent infection, hemorrhage from peptic ulcer or peritonitis from pancreatic infection.

Treatment of chronic pancreatitis and its complications.—Nonsurgical treatment is designed for relief of symptoms and as supportive therapy. A diet low in fats and high in carbohydrates with easily digestible or predigested proteins is supplemented by pancreatic ferments. Alcohol should be avoided. Vitamins and bile salts should be administered early. Diabetes should be controlled.

Every effort should be made to eradicate diseases which may contribute to the persistence or progression of chronic pancreatitis. Chronic cholecystitis and cholelithiasis as well as calculi within the common duct are so frequently associated with pancreatitis that it is justifiable to assume that they contribute to the disease. In diagnosing cholecystic disease, it must be remembered that cholecystograms taken during a relapse of pancreatitis may suggest gallbladder disease. Repeated cholecystograms during a remission may show a normally functioning gallbladder. Therefore, it is important to repeat the examination during a quiescent stage to ascertain the true status of biliary tract function. Cholecystectomy and choledochostomy should be performed when diseases of the extrahepatic biliary tract exist. If the gallbladder is not diseased and stones are not present, it is well to preserve this organ for a subsquent anastomotic procedure. In the absence of a history of jaundice, if there is a grossly normal biliary tract, external drainage of the common duct should be utilized if this structure has been explored. Prolonged drainage of the common duct has been advocated in chronic pancreatitis. The T-tube may remain clamped except for hourly periods daily. Long, cross-limbed T-tubes extending into the duodenum have also been advocated for such drainage. Although some good results have been reported with both of these methods, discouraging results have also been recorded. A number of patients in whom a long-limbed T-tube was used have had exacerbations of pancreatitis and even fatal hemorrhagic pancreatitis, presumably due to pressure on the pancreatic duct and varying degrees of obstruction.

Various surgical procedures have been devised for the treatment of chronic pancreatitis, some based on the theory of etiology, some designed to relieve complications or symptoms and others to remove the disease. Having become discouraged with the results of operations which did not attack the pancreas itself and with frequent failure of various types of nerve sections to relieve pain, we again tried the retrograde pancreaticojejunostomy. By removing the tail of the pancreas for a short distance, splitting the main pancreatic duct for 0.5–1 cm. and inserting the tail of the pancreas in a defunctionalized limb of jejunum, we had some good results, but many patients continued to have symptoms or subsequently had recurrences. To determine the reason for these failures, we inserted a small polyethylene catheter in the caudal end of the main pancreatic duct, bringing it through the jejunal and abdominal walls for the purpose of making pancreatograms. Plate 55 reveals the results of these studies.

A is a lateral x-ray taken after injection of opaque medium through the polyethylene tube. *B* is an anteroposterior view of a similar pancreatogram. Both reveal a long stricture extending from the papilla of Vater distalward for several centimeters. Beyond this stricture the pancreatic duct is markedly dilated, but a number of intervening strictures can be seen. Alternate pockets and strictures suggest a chain-of-lakes effect. They also explain why caudal drainage of the pancreas alone did not give relief. Residual, undrained pockets continued the patient's symptoms. These pancreatograms show the need for incision of the pancreatic duct as far to the right as necessary to drain all pockets. The operation was then modified to what we now term longitudinal pancreaticojejunostomy (Plate 56).

In A_1 and B_1 the surrounding viscera have been sketched in to allow better orientation.

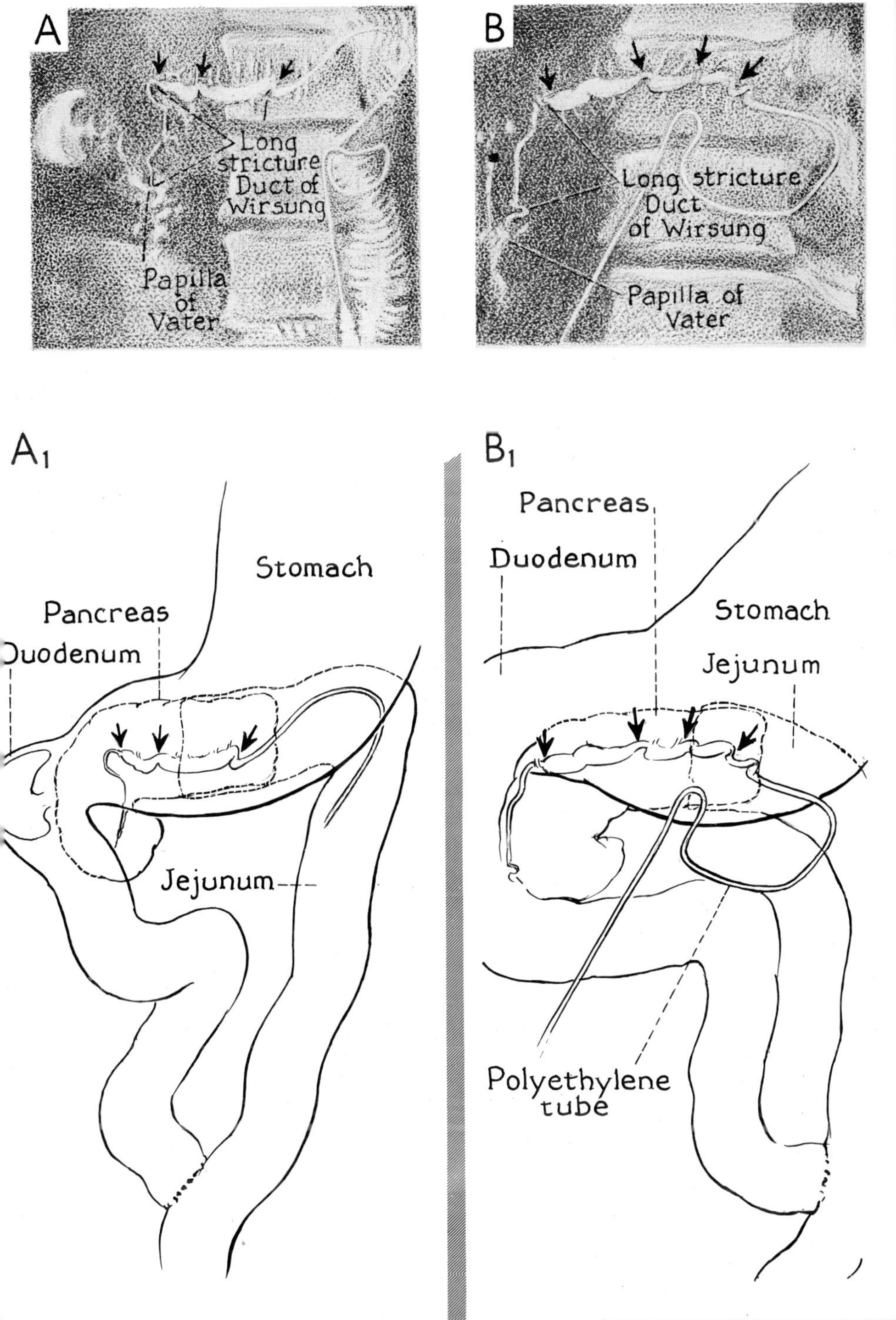
A
Long stricture Duct of Wirsung
Papilla of Vater
B
Long stricture Duct of Wirsung
Papilla of Vater
A1
Stomach
Pancreas
Duodenum
Jejunum
B1
Pancreas
Duodenum
Stomach
Jejunum
Polyethylene tube

Longitudinal pancreaticojejunostomy was devised to permit a free flow of pancreatic secretions from the entire pancreas into the jejunum.

A.—The abdomen is opened through a vertical or a transverse incision. The vertical incision, if used, should be a left paramedian or a left rectus incision. The transverse incision should be made above the umbilicus, extending farther to the left than to the right. Either permits access to the pancreas and spleen. We usually prefer to remove the spleen, although the decision to do so is made after the pancreas is exposed and the degree of pathology determined. With splenectomy, greater mobilization of the pancreas can be obtained.

Pancreaticojejunostomy with Splenectomy

The pancreas is exposed by dividing the gastrocolic omentum sufficiently far to the left to give free access to the tail of the pancreas. If surgery on the pancreas is warranted by inspection and possible aspiration, the spleen is then removed by the technic of Plate 74.

B.—The tail of the pancreas with the splenic vessels is mobilized from its bed, the dissection beginning on the inferior surface. Bleeding is seldom disturbing except in the presence of portal hypertension. The pancreas can readily be elevated to the right as far as the superior mesenteric vessels. From 0.5 to 1 cm. of the tip of the pancreas is then transected by sharp dissection. This usually divides a dilated pancreatic duct, and pancreatic secretion often will emerge under pressure. If no duct is encountered, a transection is made 0.5 cm. to the right and similar resections repeated once or twice until a dilated duct is encountered.

C.—A probe is passed to determine the length of the dilated duct and the existence of multiple strictures.

D.—With one blade of a scissors in the duct and the other anterior to the pancreas, the duct and pancreatic tissue are incised to the point of the next stricture. Sharp dissection may then be necessary to cut through the stricture into the next pocket, whereupon the scissors is again introduced. This process is continued until a probe can be passed well into the head of the pancreas. No effort is made to incise the long strictures encountered between the ampulla of Vater and the approximation of the ducts of Santorini and Wirsung.

[Longitudinal Roux-Y pancreaticojejunostomy *continued on page 268.*]

PLATE 56

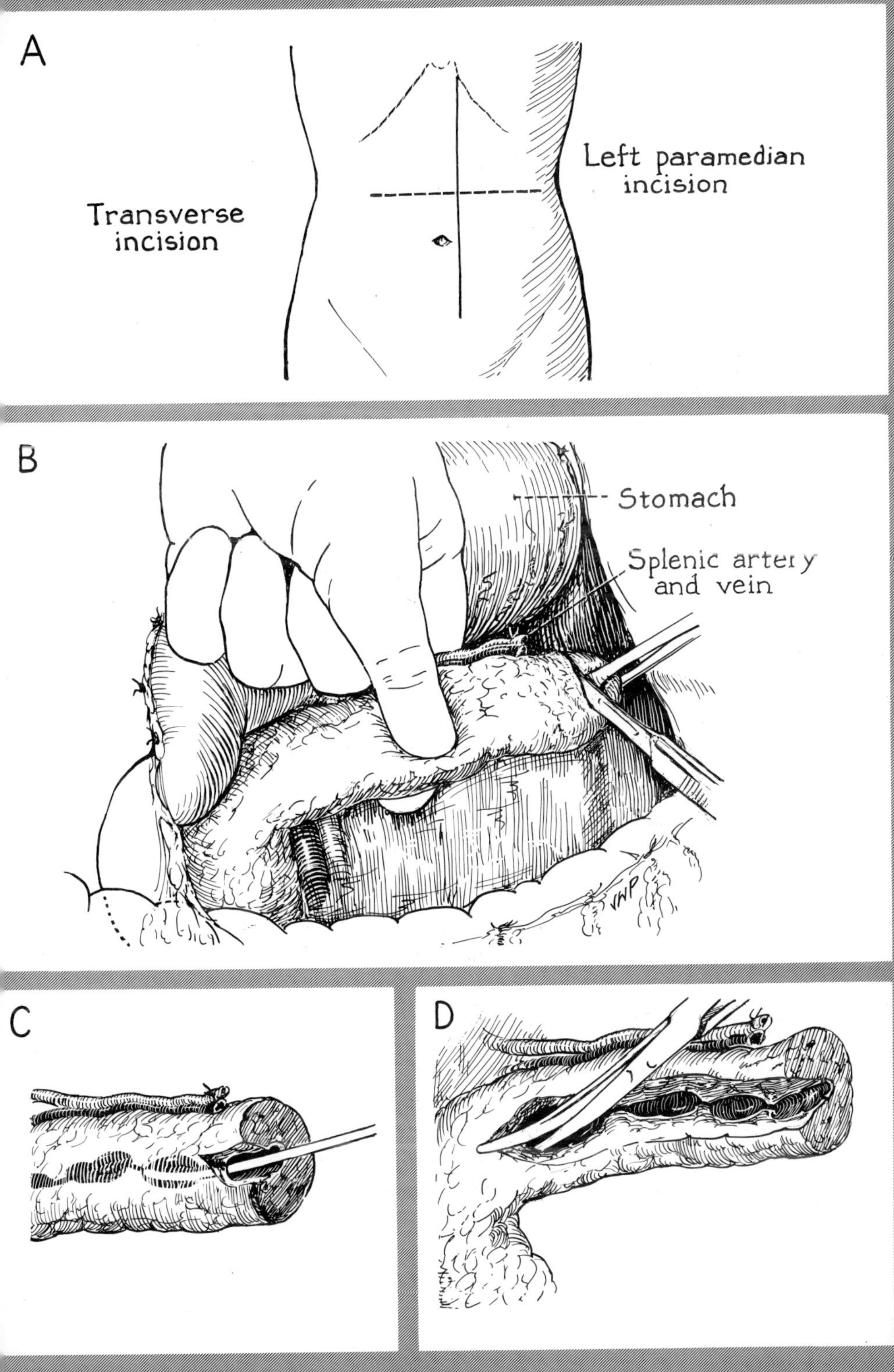

A
Left paramedian incision
Transverse incision
B
Stomach
Splenic artery and vein
C
D

Occasionally, in a patient with chronic relapsing pancreatitis no dilated ducts or pockets can be found. Under these circumstances, three or four parallel longitudinal incisions may be made through the pancreas to more than half its depth to open the smaller channels. The pancreas is then embedded in a Roux-Y jejunostomy.

The chronically diseased pancreas seldom has a troublesome blood supply. With the pancreas mobilized, the surgeon may grasp it with his index finger posterior and his thumb anterior to the gland and compress it at the time he makes the incisions (*B*). This will control bleeding, and on release of pressure any bleeding vessels can be controlled with Allis forceps. Occasionally, mattress sutures may be necessary. It is not advisable to oversew the entire cut edge of the pancreas, for this could occlude divided contributory ducts.

The pancreaticojejunostomy is then performed. The jejunum is explored for an area 10–15 cm. below the ligament of Treitz where the vascular arcades will permit division with the greatest mobility of the distal segment. The mesentery and bowel are divided and the distal end brought through a rent in the transverse mesocolon. No attempt should be made to bring the jejunum anterior to the colon, for tension on the anastomosis may result in its disruption.

E.—The clamp is removed and the edges of the bowel are grasped with Allis forceps. To secure the pancreas at the desired distance within the bowel, a suture is placed in the distal end of the pancreas and a needle holder, carrying a curved intestinal needle with the point held toward the open end of the bowel, is passed 3–5 in. into the bowel. The needle is turned and brought out. The pancreas is pulled into the bowel and anchored at the desired position.

F.—The serosa of the cut edge of the bowel is sutured to the surface of the pancreas with interrupted cotton sutures. This is difficult in a normal pancreas, but the fibrosis of a chronically inflamed pancreas results in tissue that will hold sutures well. The suture line should be well to the right of the cut edge of the pancreas. After completion of the pancreaticojejunostomy, the proximal end of the jejunum is anastomosed to the distal limb, forming an enteroanastomosis.

G.—The posterior aspect of the anastomosis is shown. Here the anastomosis can be brought to the right only as far as the superior mesenteric vessels. As the anterior surface frequently must be brought much farther to the right, it is necessary to cut the bowel obliquely.

PLATE 56

E

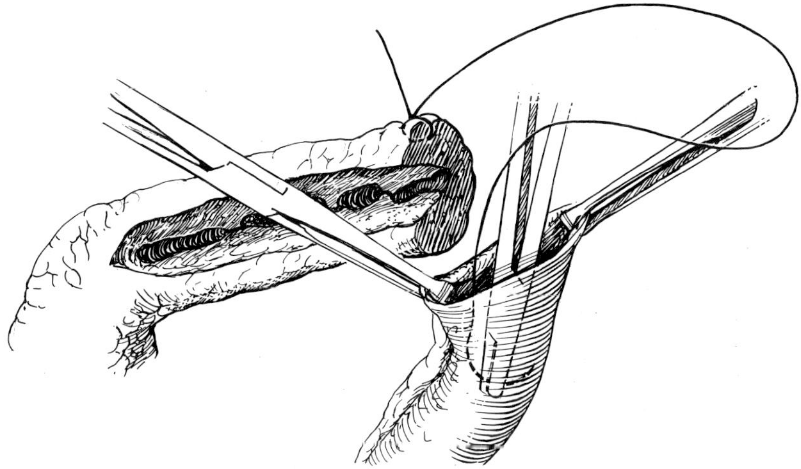

F

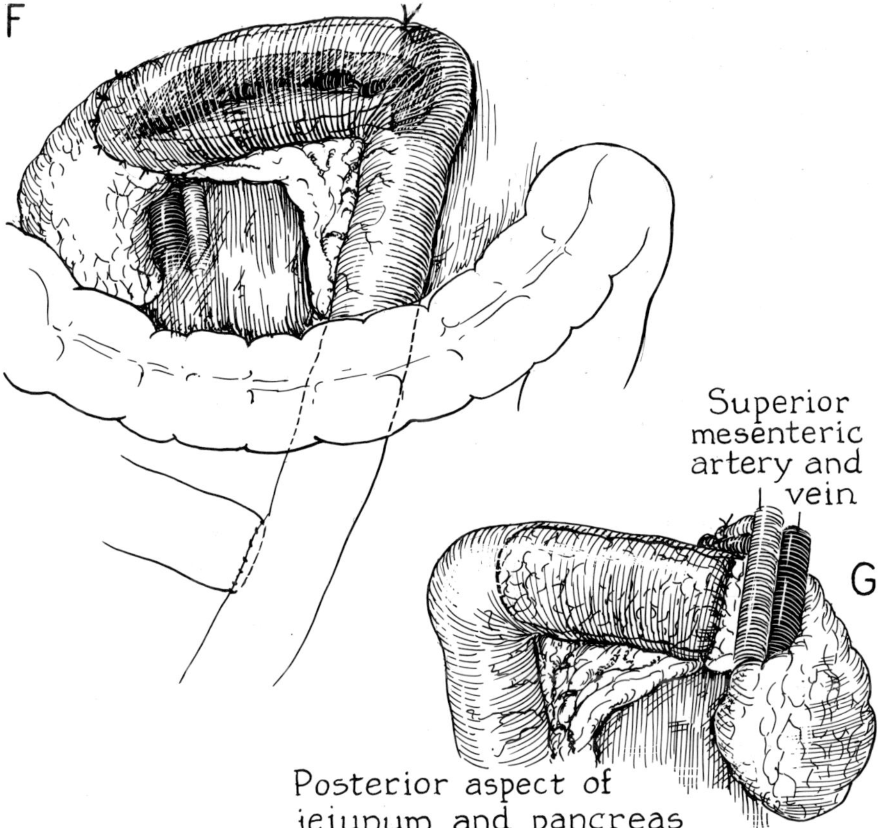
Superior mesenteric artery and vein
G
Posterior aspect of jejunum and pancreas

Pancreaticojejunostomy without Splenectomy

Removal of the spleen and mobilization of the pancreas affords the best opportunity to do a satisfactory pancreaticojejunostomy. In less advanced cases of chronic pancreatitis, in which the ducts are not markedly dilated, it is difficult to perform a well-functioning anastomosis without removal of the spleen. However, in certain chronic cases in which, by use of a needle, one can demonstrate dilated pockets within the pancreatic duct with pancreatic secretions under pressure, and in which surgical trauma and the duration of the operation must be minimized, a satisfactory pancreaticojejunostomy may be done without splenectomy.

A.—After exposure of the pancreas as described in Plate 56, *A* and *B*, needles are inserted to determine whether pockets exist, with fluid under pressure. If any are found, the needle is left in place and an incision is made longitudinal to the pancreas and adjacent to the needle to open the immediate pocket.

B.—The incision is then extended both to the right and to the left until all pockets within the pancreas are adequately opened. When it is certain that there are no undrained areas of the pancreas, the pancreaticojejunostomy can be performed.

C.—The pancreaticojejunostomy is the same as that in Plate 56 except that the pancreas is not embedded into the jejunum, for this cannot be done without splenectomy. Instead, the distal end of the divided jejunum is sutured to the anterior wall of the pancreas from 0.5 to 1 cm. away from the cut edges of the pancreas. Because a larger opening in the bowel is needed for a side-to-side anastomosis, it is advisable to divide the jejunum obliquely.

D.—If a still larger opening is needed, the jejunum may be incised on its antimesenteric border.

This procedure works well in advanced disease in which there is marked dilatation within the duct. If marked dilatation is not encountered, it may be necessary to remove the spleen and inspect the pancreas more thoroughly.

Essentials of surgery.—Infallible rules and dictums generally are not good surgical teaching. However, there are certain dictums in surgery of chronic pancreatitis which we believe are essential.

1. Be sure all obstructed pockets within the pancreas are adequately opened.

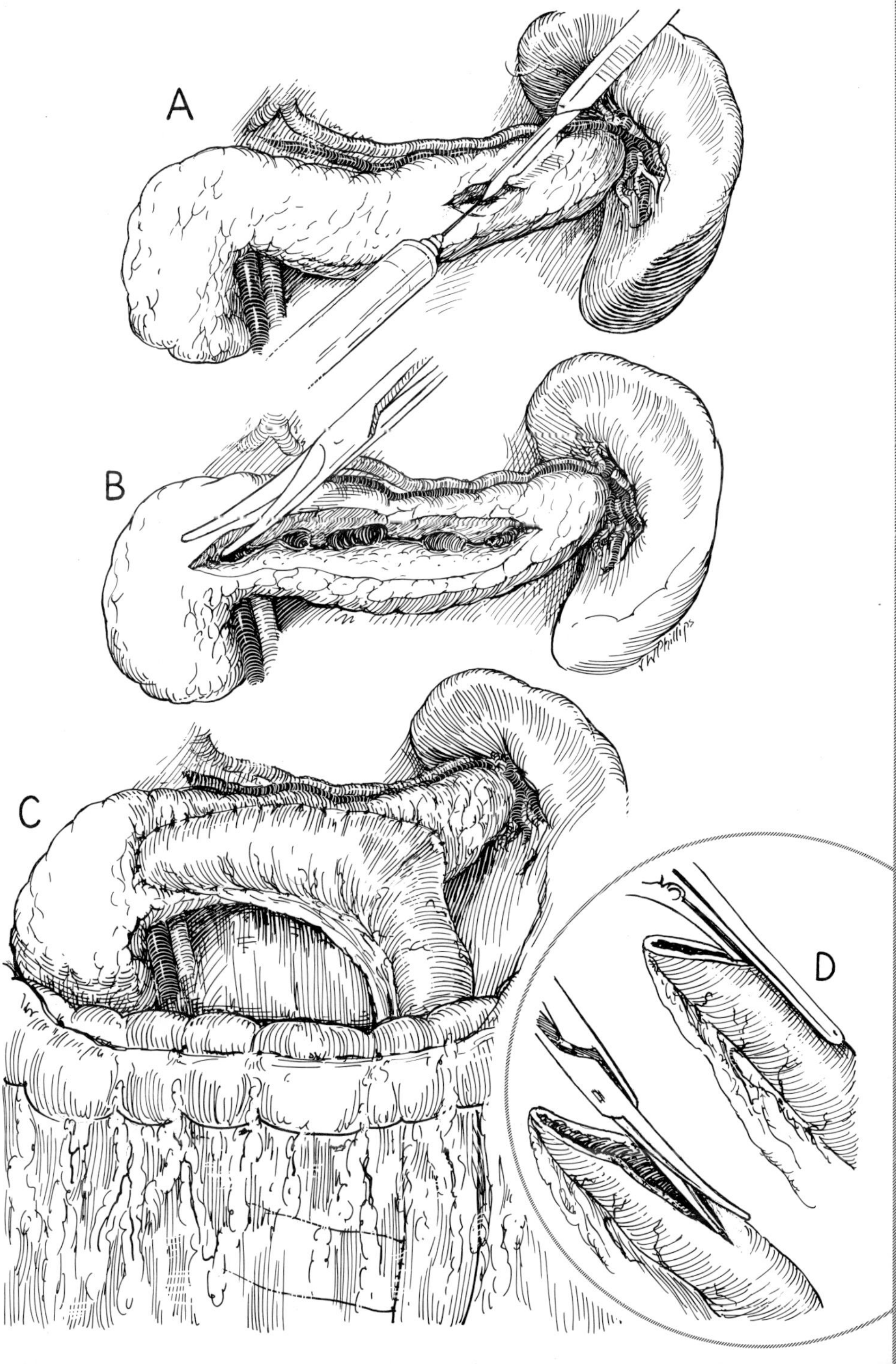
A
B
C
D

2. Never perform a mucosa-to-mucosa anastomosis between the pancreatic duct and the jejunum. To open the pancreatic duct, it is necessary to divide tributary ducts and these will drain into the peritoneal cavity with a mucosa-to-mucosa anastomosis.

3. Always suture the serosa of the bowel to the outer surface of the pancreas well beyond its incised area.

4. Never anastomose the pancreas to the bowel in continuity. Always use a defunctionalized loop of bowel. Properly used, a defunctionalized loop of bowel prevents intestinal contents from coming in contact with the pancreas. If intestinal contents come in contact with the pancreas, the organ may be destroyed.

5. Always perform a retrocolic pancreaticojejunostomy. Antecolic anastomoses may put tension on the suture line.

Results.—The results of longitudinal pancreaticojejunostomy have been far better than we had anticipated, and results reported to us by other surgeons have been better than our own. More than 75 per cent of our patients were immediately and completely relieved of pain and have had a gradual restoration of pancreatic function, manifested by a return to normal stools, a gain in weight and no laboratory evidences of pancreatic insufficiency. Immediate relief of pain, as expressed by the patient on recovery from anesthesia, signifies the success of the operation. Continuance of pain immediately after surgery usually means that the operation has been inadequate and that obstructive pockets remain. Patients who have become narcotic addicts because of the pain of pancreatitis may be rapidly withdrawn from the drugs and cured of addiction. Pancreaticojejunostomy is a primary surgical attack on the disease itself and is not designed merely to relieve symptoms.

Needle biopsies and aspiration of the pancreas carry with them a considerable danger. Often they result in pancreatic fistulas and sometimes in acute hemorrhagic pancreatitis. If on exploration of the pancreas a needle aspiration is felt to be advisable, it may be well also to perform a pancreaticojejunostomy. Then if a fistula develops, it will drain into the bowel and not into the peritoneal cavity.

We have used longitudinal pancreaticojejunostomy in patients with carcinoma of the head or body of the pancreas which has obstructed the main pancreatic ducts with resultant pancreatic pain. This operation has relieved the pain and, we believe, has maintained the nutrition of the patient for a longer period by permitting pancreatic secretion to enter the intestinal tract.

Partial Resection of the Pancreas

Occasionally chronic pancreatitis involves only the tail and/or a portion of the body of the gland, and the disease in the head of the pancreas may be minimal or absent. Under such circumstances, resection of the tail and the involved portion of the body of the gland, with ligation of the end of the duct and oversewing of the cut surface of the gland, may give considerable relief (Plate 64, *C*). One must determine that no proximal strictures of the duct exist. If the duct is not completely patent, a retrograde pancreaticojejunostomy should be established.

When pancreatitis is confined to the head and varying amounts of the body of the pancreas, the involved portion of the gland and the adjacent duodenum may be resected (Plate 70). The duct in the remaining pancreas usually is dilated and can be anastomosed to the mucosa of the jejunum (Plate 70, *K*). Since one is not dealing with malignancy, the resection need only include the involved portion of the pancreas and the first and second portions of the duodenum.

Partial proximal pancreatectomy and duodenectomy has the advantage of removing the diseased tissue while preserving the uninvolved portion of the pancreas and re-establishing continuity between the remaining pancreatic duct and the jejunum. It is a formidable procedure, carrying with it a considerable operative risk. In addition, some pancreatic tissue is sacrificed which could conceivably regain functional capacity when pressure on the pancreatic ducts and the pancreatic cells is relieved. For these reasons, we prefer the less extensive procedure of a retrograde pancreaticojejunostomy.

Total Pancreatectomy

Occasionally in a "burned-out pancreas," in which the organ has been extensively destroyed by repeated recurrences of pancreatitis, removal of the entire pancreas and the adjacent duodenum may be justified if the patient has a great deal of pain. Some surgeons have recommended the removal of all of the pancreas except a small portion of the head adjacent to the lesser curvature of the duodenum. This preserves the blood supply to the duodenum and avoids the necessity of a partial duodenectomy. At this stage of the disease most patients have become drug addicts and no therapeutic measure has much to offer. The operation then carries with it a rather high mortality rate. It may leave the patient a permanent pancreatic invalid who will need pancreatic therapy for the rest of his life. It seldom is justifiable in view of the relief of pain and restoration of pancreatic function which usually follows a longitudinal pancreaticojejunostomy.

Sphincterotomy

It has been theorized that chronic pancreatitis is due to a reflux of bile into the pancreatic ducts produced by spasm of the sphincter of Oddi. If this hypothesis is correct, surgical division of the sphincter muscles should prevent such reflux when it is anatomically possible for a single channel to be established proximal to the sphincter. One may be justified in trying this procedure before attempting more radical surgery if no definite cause of disease is apparent on abdominal exploration and if gross findings do not substantiate the diagnosis of a rather diffuse chronic pancreatitis. Two technics have been described. In one, the common bile duct is opened and a special instrument is inserted distally and passed through the ampulla of Vater into the duodenum. A blade on the end of the instrument is then elevated, the instrument retracted until the blade becomes wedged against the papilla of Vater and the blade then drawn down to incise the papilla and sphincter muscles. The second method consists of a transduodenal approach to the ampulla of Vater. When the ampulla of Vater has been located, its anterior wall and the sphincter of Oddi are incised under direct vision.

The success of this operation has varied in the hands of different surgeons. Some have reported very satisfactory results, others are less enthusiastic.

Pancreatograms we have made following retrograde pancreaticojejunostomy for chronic pancreatitis (Plate 55) indicate that stenosis of the pancreatic duct usually extends several centimeters distalward from the ampulla of Vater. Since sphincterotomy would not relieve this obstruction, we believe it would be of little benefit.

Choledochoenterostomy

Division of the common bile duct and anastomosis of the proximal end to the duodenum or to a Roux-Y limb of jejunum has been advocated as a form of treatment for chronic pancreatitis. Its principle is to divert the flow of bile from the distal common duct and thus to prevent it from entering the pancreatic duct; its use is based on the premise that the bile entering the pancreatic duct may be an etiologic factor in the disease. One disadvantage is the removal of the sphincter, permitting regurgitation of intestinal contents into the common duct, possibly to produce a cholangitis and hepatitis when anastomosis is made to the duodenum. When the common duct is anastomosed to a Roux-Y limb of jejunum, bile enters the intestine some distance below the ligament of Treitz, and symptoms of biliary dyspepsia or a duodenal ulcer may develop.

Relief of Complications

The treatment of chronic pancreatitis must at times be directed to the relief of complications or symptoms of the disease. Important among these are jaundice and pain (Plates 59–61). Calcification may also be a complication (Plate 62).

Jaundice.—Jaundice produced by pancreatitis should be treated by some form of biliary tract drainage. As the common duct should always be explored, external drainage can readily be instituted by the use of a T-tube. Internal drainage may be established when obstruction to the flow of bile into the duodenum exists. If the cystic duct is patent and the gallbladder is comparatively healthy, anastomosis between the gallbladder and some portion of the gastrointestinal tract will establish adequate internal drainage. Cholecystogastrostomy (Plate 58) is usually satisfactory. Many patients in whom biliary obstruction has been thought to be due to carcinoma of the pancreas have lived a normal life span after internal biliary drainage. This suggests an error in diagnosis which is understandable because of the difficulty in differentiating chronic pancreatitis from carcinoma without a satisfactory biopsy.

The gallbladder may be anastomosed to the duodenum or to the jejunum, depending upon the ease of approximation and the preference of the surgeon. If a cholecystojejunostomy is performed, the Roux-Y technic minimizes the danger of ascending cholangitis.

When the cystic duct is obstructed or the gallbladder has been removed or is diseased, the common duct may be anastomosed to the intestine. A side-to-side anastomosis may be performed with the duodenum (Plate 44). Some surgeons divide the common duct and anastomose its proximal end to the duodenum by an end-to-side technic or use an end-to-end anastomosis with a Roux-Y limb of jejunum.

A.—The abdomen is opened through an upper right rectus incision. The round ligaments should be divided to permit elevation of the hepatic end for better exposure of the gallbladder and bile ducts. Frequently there will be considerable enlargement of the liver and its anterior edge must be elevated for adequate exposure. The upper abdomen should be carefully explored and an effort made to determine the nature of the primary disease and the existence and location of metastatic lesions. Any dissection should be carefully accomplished because of the increased tendency toward bleeding in jaundiced patients. The duodenum should be inspected and palpated for existing or impending obstruction to determine the possible need for gastroenterostomy. The extrahepatic biliary tract should be examined for primary disease and to ascertain that the obstruction of the biliary tract is below the junction of the cystic and common bile ducts.

B.—The anterior wall of the stomach should be grasped with Allis or Babcock forceps 1–3 in. proximal to the pylorus to determine if it can be approximated to the gallbladder without undue tension.

C.—Two Allis forceps are placed on the fundus of the gallbladder about 1 in. from the undersurface of the liver and 1–2 in. apart. The gallbladder is opened midway between them by a trocar connected to suction or by a knife incision parallel to the undersurface of the liver. The contents of the gallbladder are aspirated.

D.—The opening in the gallbladder is lengthened to a total of about 1½ in. to insure an adequate stoma. The gallbladder is explored with scoops and with the finger to be sure no stones remain. A probe should be passed through the cystic duct into the common duct to determine their patency and to aid in the detection of stones within them.

[Cholecystogastrostomy *continued on page 278.*]

PLATE 58

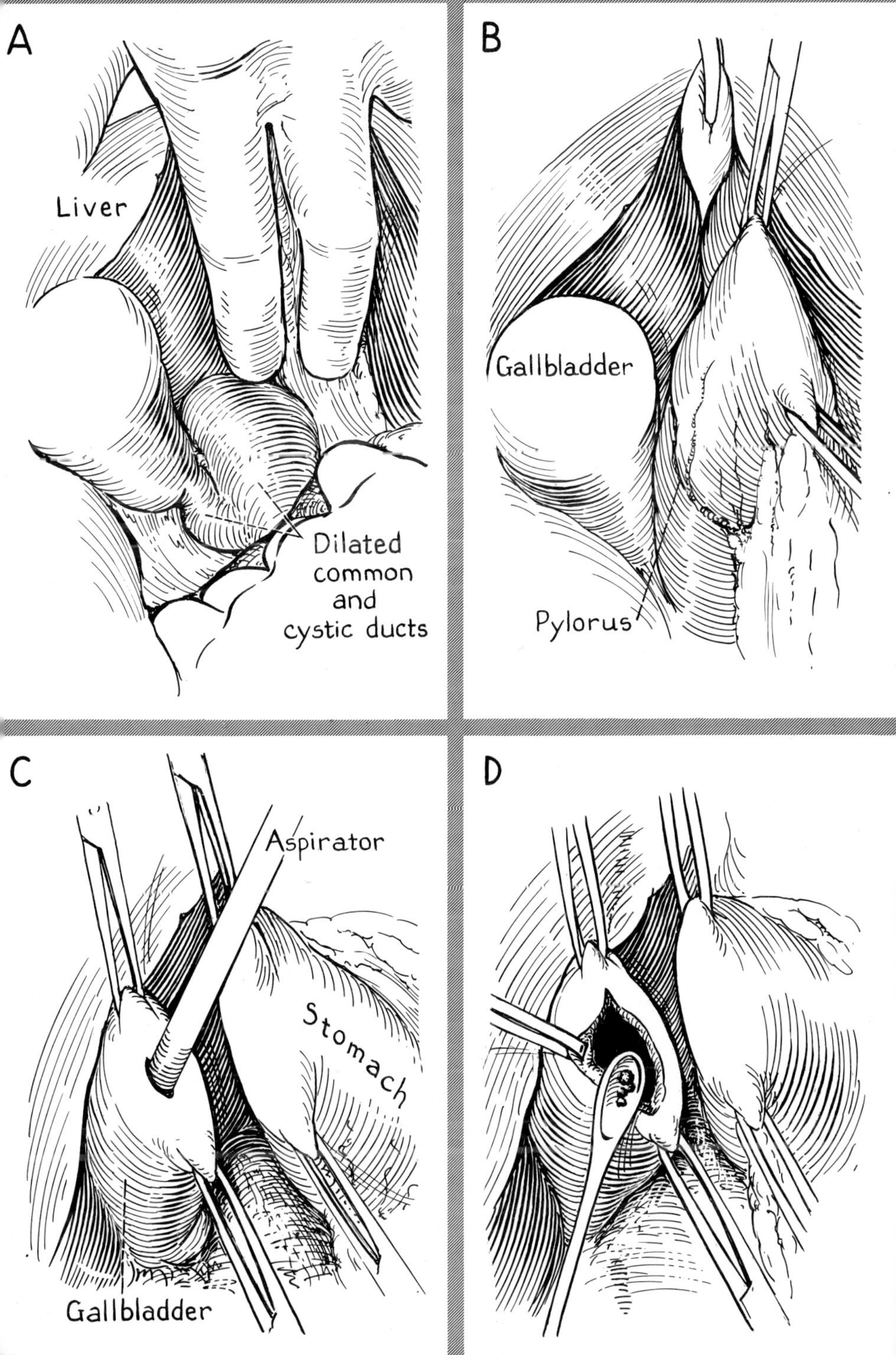
A
Liver
Dilated common and cystic ducts
B
Gallbladder
Pylorus
C
Aspirator
Stomach
Gallbladder
D

E.—The posterior outer row of sutures is now placed between the anterior wall of the stomach and the gallbladder 5 mm. below the incision in the latter. Because of the poor nutritional state of these patients, it is well to use a nonabsorbable suture and cotton has proved very satisfactory. This row may be made with a continuous or with interrupted sutures.

F.—An incision is made in the anterior wall of the stomach an equal distance proximal to the posterior row of sutures and equal in length to the incision in the gallbladder. This incision is carried to the mucosa of the stomach where existing blood vessels are doubly clamped, after which the mucosa and blood vessels are divided between the opposing clamps. The blood vessels should be ligated on both sides of the incision. It is well to aspirate the stomach contents to minimize contamination.

G.—The posterior inner row of sutures consists of an over-and-over catgut suture and includes the entire thickness of the walls of the stomach and gallbladder.

H.—This row of sutures is continued to form the anterior inner row of the anastomosis.

I.—The anterior outer row consists of interrupted cotton sutures, inverting the inner row.

J.—The entire suture line, both on the posterior and anterior surfaces, should be protected by a layer of omentum sutured both to the stomach and to the gallbladder. The abdominal wall is closed in layers without drainage.

PLATE 58

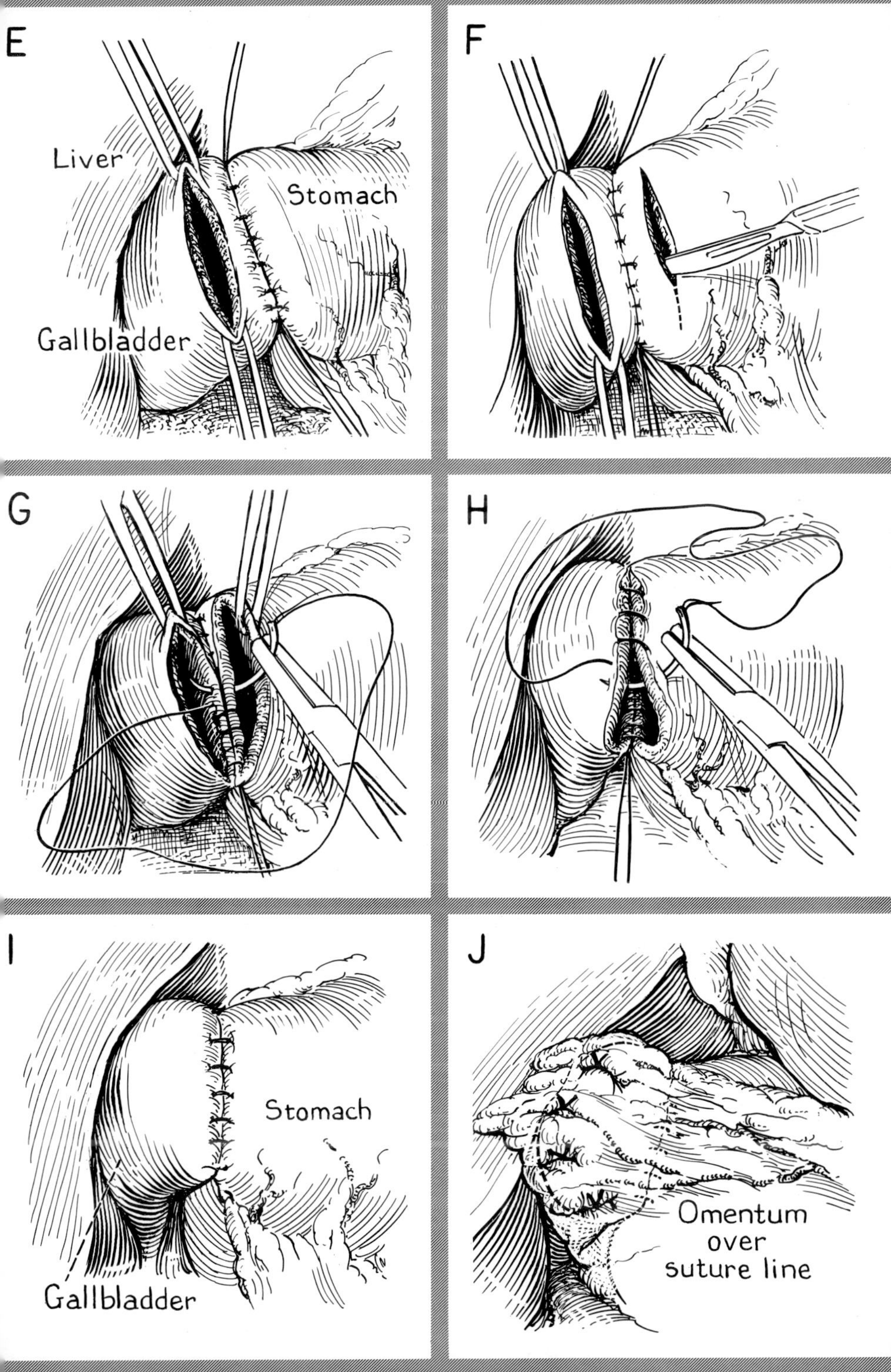
E
Liver
Stomach
Gallbladder
F
G
H
I
Stomach
Gallbladder
J
Omentum
over
suture line

Pancreatic pain.—Pain may be severe and is difficult to control by conservative therapy. If surgical therapy directed at removal of the cause of the disease fails to relieve the pain, interruption of the nerve pathways from the pancreas is sometimes successful. In our hands, however, these operations have been unsatisfactory in providing complete and permanent pain relief. They also have the disadvantage of not attacking the diseased pancreas and thus do not restore pancreatic drainage to the intestinal tract or permit pancreatic regeneration. We rely on the far superior results of longitudinal pancreaticojejunostomy.

A.—It is believed that pancreatic pain is transmitted through nerve fibers leading to the sympathetic chain, the splanchnic nerves and possibly the vagus nerves or may accompany blood vessels to the organ. These pathways may be interrupted by a nerve block or by resection of the sympathetic or splanchnic nerves.

Splanchnic Block

B and *C*.—With the patient in the lateral position, the side to be blocked uppermost, the skin is prepared and draped. A skin wheal is raised opposite the spine of the first lumbar vertebra, 7 cm. lateral to the midline. A 20 gauge, 15 cm. needle is introduced through the skin wheal and advanced at an angle of 30 degrees from the perpendicular, pointed medially. The twelfth rib should be encountered at a depth of 2–3 cm. from the skin edge. The needle is then partly withdrawn and advanced at about a 45 degree angle from the perpendicular until the vertebral body is encountered, ordinarily at a depth of 5–8 cm. The needle is again partly withdrawn and redirected until it just clears the vertebral body anterolaterally. This is ordinarily at a point somewhere between the first two angles described. No resistance to the needle's progression should be encountered. It should be advanced to a depth of 10–12 cm., at which position the tip of the needle should lie just anterolateral to the body of the twelfth thoracic vertebra. After careful aspiration in several planes, 15–20 cc. of anesthetic solution is injected.

The anesthetic agent of choice for diagnostic block is procaine 2 per cent or Xylocaine 1 per cent without epinephrine. When therapeutic block is desired, a longer acting agent such as 6 per cent aqueous phenol is preferred. This gives a satisfactory block for from one week to one month or longer, with minimal side effects.

PLATE 59

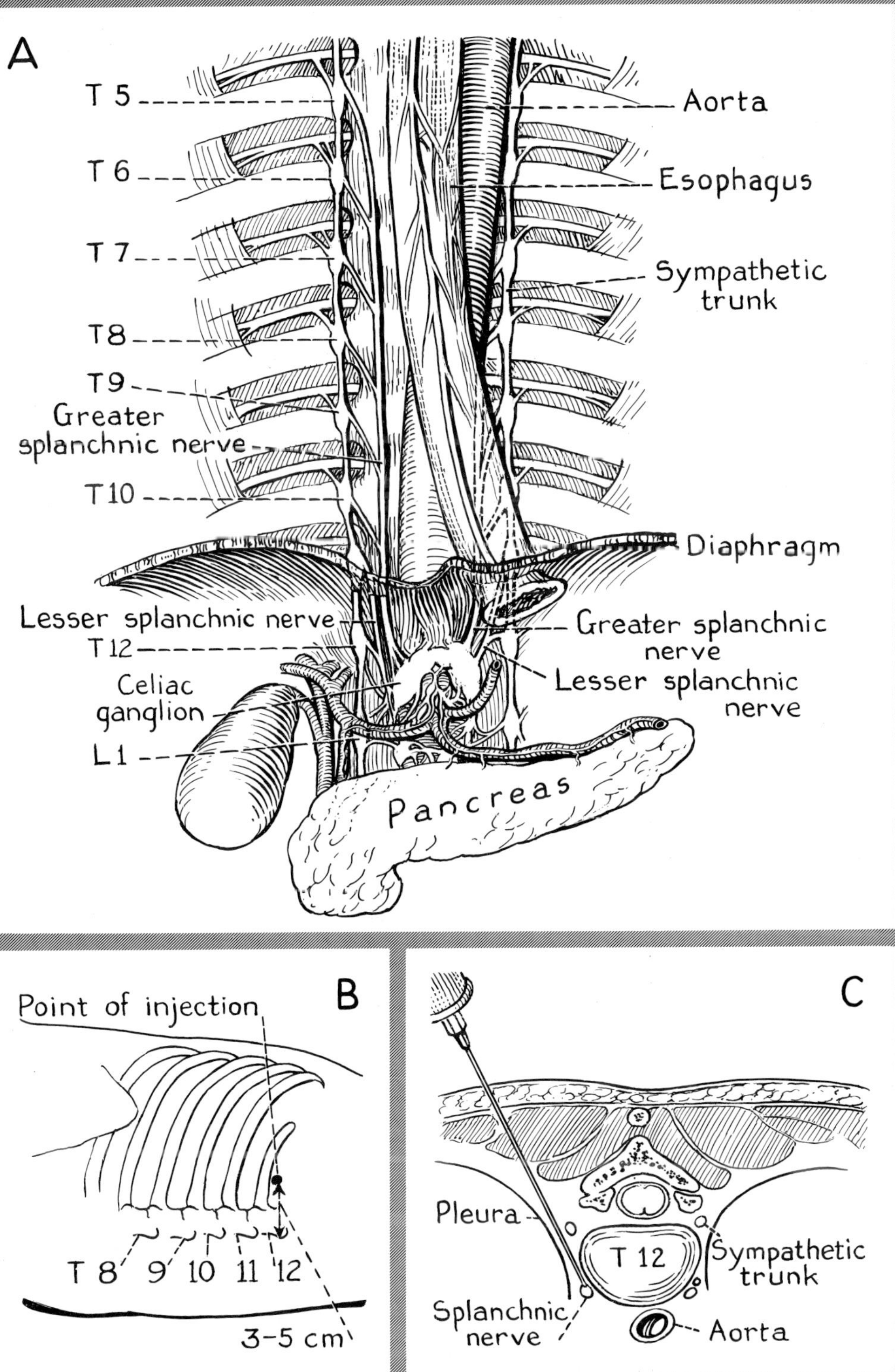
A
T 5
T 6
T 7
T8
T9
Greater splanchnic nerve
T10
Lesser splanchnic nerve
T12
Celiac ganglion
L1
Aorta
Esophagus
Sympathetic trunk
Diaphragm
Greater splanchnic nerve
Lesser splanchnic nerve
Pancreas
B
Point of injection
T 8
9
10
11
12
3–5 cm
C
Pleura
T 12
Sympathetic trunk
Splanchnic nerve
Aorta

As the bulk of the pancreas is in the left half of the abdominal cavity, it is believed that resection of the left splanchnic and sympathetic nerves will relieve pancreatic pain in a higher percentage of patients than will resection on the right side alone. If resection on the left is followed by recurrence of pain, a right lumbodorsal sympathectomy and splanchnic neurectomy may subsequently be performed.

A.—Endotracheal anesthesia is the technic of choice for this operation. The patient is positioned on the right side with the left arm supported on a Mayo stand in front of the patient. The hips are rendered immobile by strapping with a broad band of adhesive tape attached to the sides of the table. The patient is prepared and draped, with the left lower chest posteriorly and the upper lumbar area exposed. An incision 4–6 in. in length is made parallel to and about 2 in. to the left of the spinous processes and centered at the eleventh interspace. This incision is carried through the skin and subcutaneous tissues. After hemostasis is secured, the skin edges are protected by wound towels.

B.—A longitudinal incision is made through the latissimus dorsi muscle parallel to and directly below the skin incision. It should be equal in length to the skin incision to provide adequate exposure. The divided muscle is separated from the lumbodorsal fascia by blunt dissection for a considerable distance on each side of the incision. A longitudinal incision is then made in the lumbodorsal fascia directly beneath and of equal length to the incision in the latissimus dorsi muscle. The lateral edge of the incised lumbodorsal fascia is dissected from the sacrospinalis muscle group to expose its lateral border.

C.—The sacrospinalis muscles are retracted medially and the attachments to the tenth, eleventh and twelfth ribs divided.

[Lumbodorsal sympathectomy and splanchnicectomy *continued on page 284.*]

PLATE 60

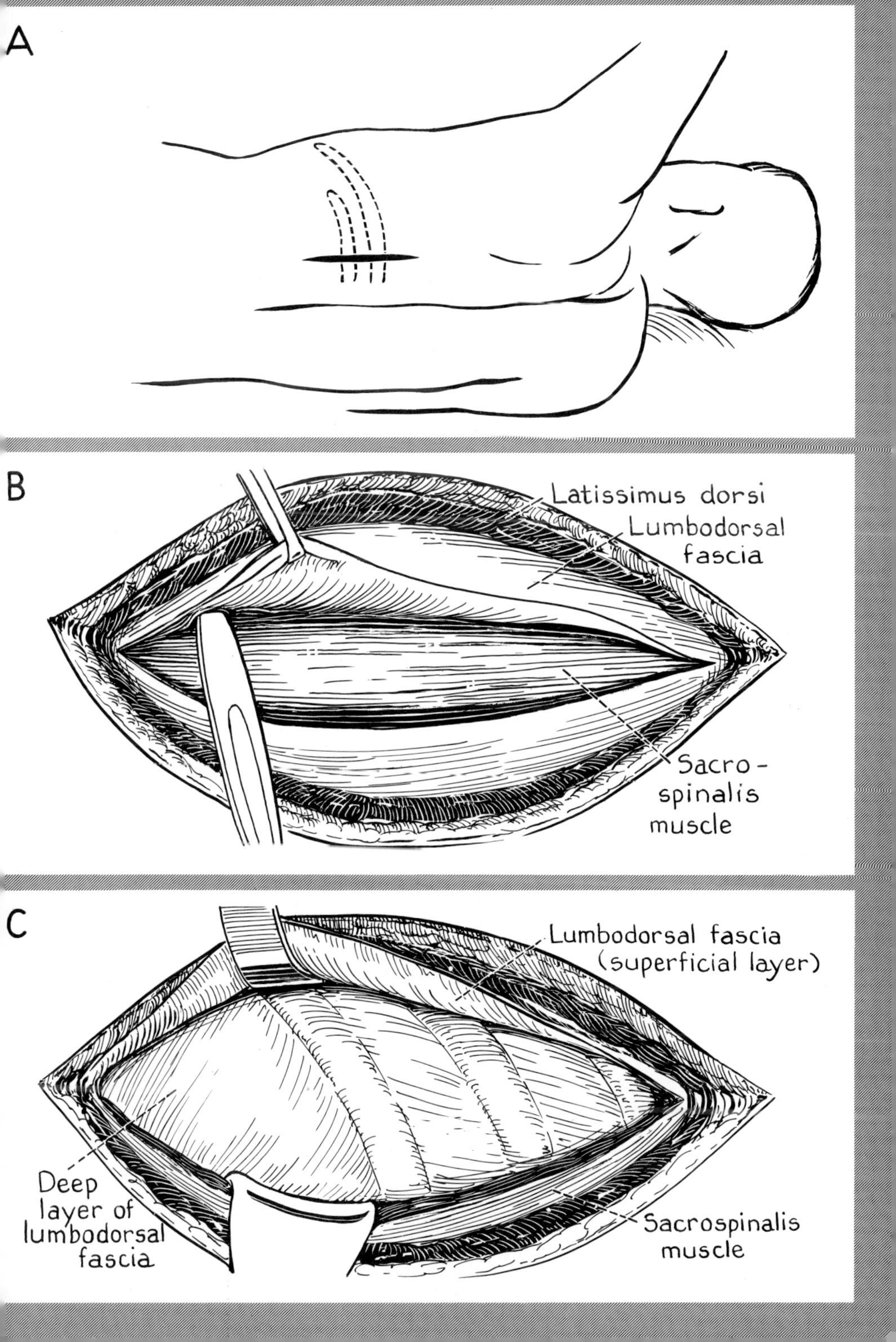

A
B
Latissimus dorsi
Lumbodorsal fascia
Sacro-spinalis muscle
C
Lumbodorsal fascia (superficial layer)
Deep layer of lumbodorsal fascia
Sacrospinalis muscle

D.—The periosteum overlying the eleventh and twelfth ribs is incised and dissected from the ribs. The twelfth rib is removed from its tip to a point close to the lateral process of the spine. The eleventh rib is removed from a point close to the spine laterally for a distance of about 3 in. The parietal pleura is exposed in the bed of the resected eleventh rib. The eleventh intercostal bundle is retracted downward and the parietal pleura separated from the endothoracic fascia to the lower pleural margin. The dissection is continued, separating the lateral portion of the pleura from the chest wall for a distance sufficient to expose the superior and lateral surface of the diaphragm to the left crus. The parietal pleura is finally dissected from the posterior chest wall and the anterior surface of the vertebral bodies, exposing the lower intrathoracic portion of the splanchnic nerves.

E.—The diaphragm is incised parallel to and about 1 in. from its costal attachments. The incision is carried through the muscle and the underlying perirenal fascia.

F.—The perirenal fat is separated from the undersurface of the diaphragm. The incision in the diaphragm is then continued medially until the crus is reached. Through the incision in the diaphragm, the perirenal and retroperitoneal fat is dissected from the inferior surface of the diaphragm, exposing the diaphragm completely to the vertebral bodies and visualizing the upper end of the psoas muscle. This opens a retroperitoneal space below the diaphragm and a retropleural space above, the two being separated by the remainder of the body of the diaphragm and by its crus. One or two phrenic arteries are usually cut and must be ligated.

[Lumbodorsal sympathectomy and splanchnicectomy *continued on page 286.*]

PLATE 60

D

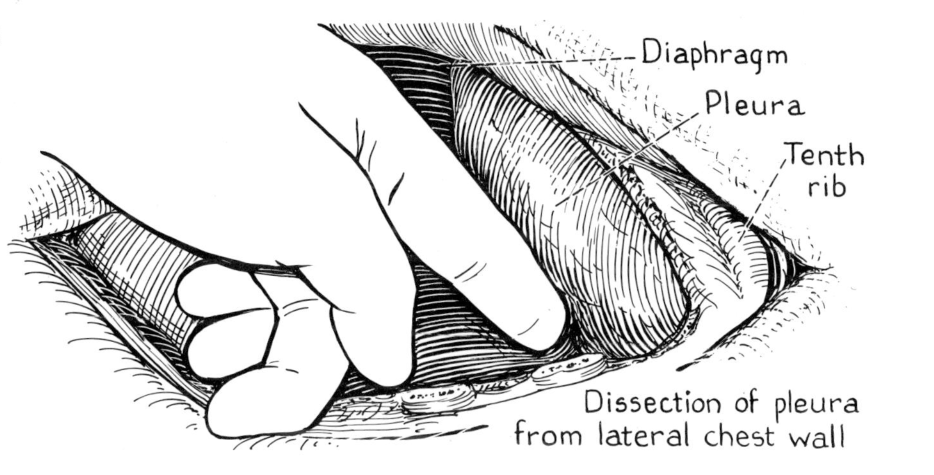

Dissection of pleura from lateral chest wall

E

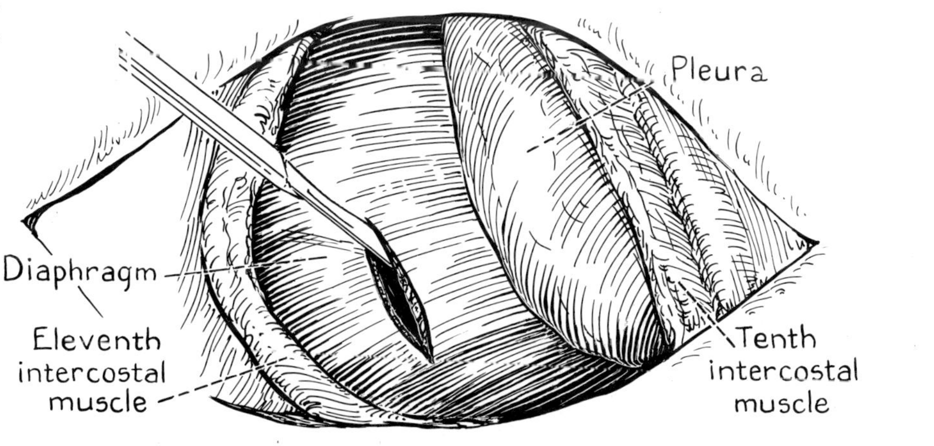

F

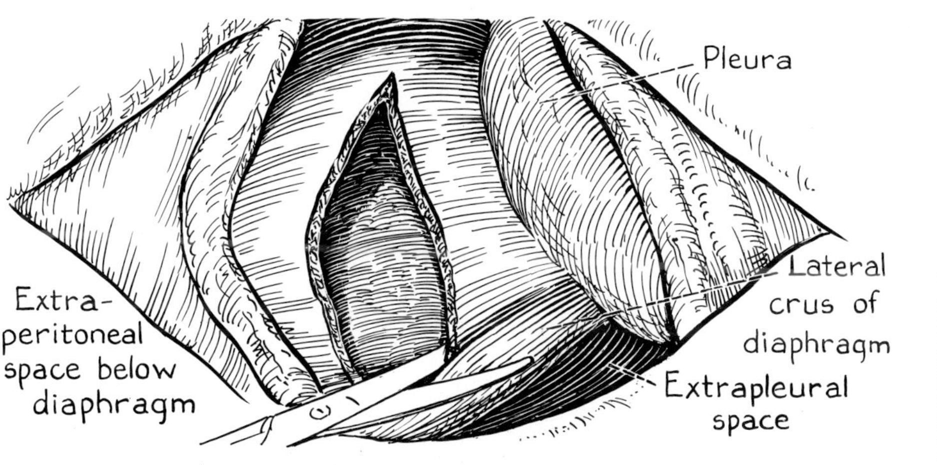

G.—By blunt dissection, the retroperitoneal fat is dissected from the lateral surface of the splanchnic nerve, visualizing the nerve to its entrance into the celiac ganglion. After the nerve is exposed, it should be injected with procaine to obviate harmful reflexes.

H.—At this point the left crus intermedius is dissected from the underlying splanchnic nerve and is divided. This exposes the splanchnic nerve from the celiac ganglion upward and into the retropleural space. The nerve is isolated by blunt dissection upward beyond the eleventh sympathetic ganglion. The splanchnic nerve and dorsal sympathetic chain above the diaphragm can then be elevated and cut at a level above the eleventh dorsal ganglion. By following the sympathetic chain downward, the first lumbar ganglion is exposed, freed from its attachments and the sympathetic chain divided below it.

The resected specimen contains the sympathetic nerve with the eleventh and twelfth dorsal and first lumbar sympathetic ganglions, together with the greater, lesser and least splanchnic nerves as they enter the celiac ganglion.

I.—The incision in the diaphragm is then closed by a continuous catgut suture, beginning at the crus and continuing laterally to the lateral end of the incision. The incisions through the muscles, fascia and skin are closed in layers without drainage.

PLATE 60

G

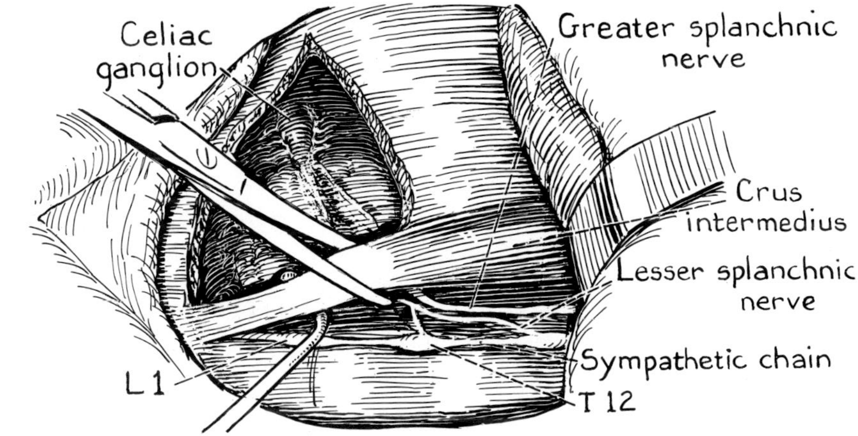

Celiac ganglion
Greater splanchnic nerve
Crus intermedius
Lesser splanchnic nerve
Sympathetic chain
L1
T 12

H

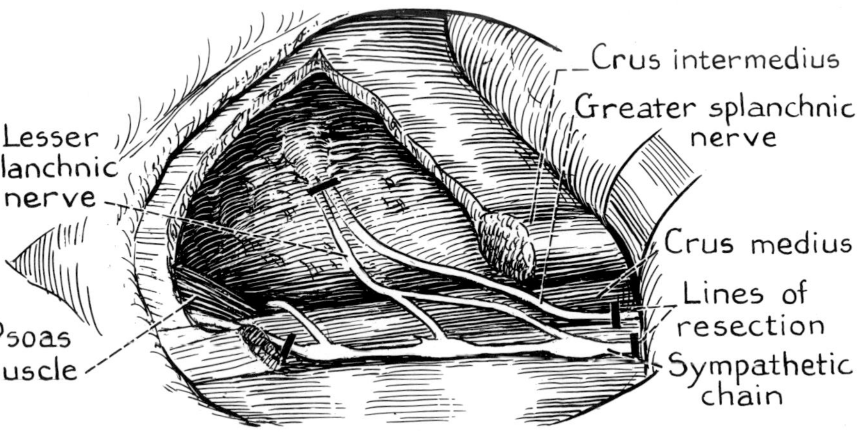

Crus intermedius
Greater splanchnic nerve
Lesser splanchnic nerve
Crus medius
Lines of resection
Psoas muscle
Sympathetic chain

I

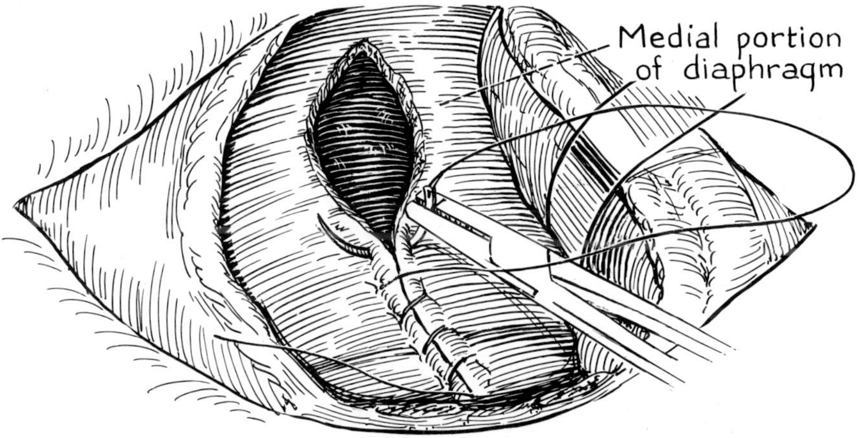

Medial portion of diaphragm

Transpleural Lumbodorsal Sympathectomy

Many surgeons believe a more extensive resection of the sympathetic chain more successfully relieves pancreatic pain.

A.—In this operation the dorsal sympathetic chain is removed from above the fourth dorsal ganglion to and including the first lumbar ganglion and the associated splanchnic nerves are excised. The patient is placed in the lateral position and the seventh or eighth rib is resected. The pleural cavity is opened and the chest cavity widely exposed with a rib spreader. The left lung is retracted medially. The sympathetic chain can be seen through the parietal pleura close to the vertebral bodies. The overlying pleura is incised from the third dorsal ganglion to the diaphragm. The sympathetic chain and splanchnic nerves are carefully dissected from above the fourth dorsal ganglion to the diaphragm. The diaphragm is elevated or incised where the nerves pass through it to permit exposure of the first lumbar sympathetic ganglion, beyond which the chain is divided. The splanchnic nerves are divided close to their entrance into the celiac ganglion.

Some surgeons believe it advantageous to remove a segment of the vagus nerves which course along the esophagus to permit a more complete denervation. If a left thoracolumbar sympathectomy does not relieve pain, the same procedure may later be carried out on the right.

Subphrenic Splanchnicectomy

B.—It is well to explore the pancreas and adjacent organs for correctible disease before attempting to interrupt the nerve pathways. During such a procedure, a subdiaphragmatic splanchnicectomy may be performed with the hope of diminishing pancreatic pain. The abdomen is opened through a vertical upper abdominal incision. The gastrocolic omentum is divided and the stomach elevated. By careful dissection above the pancreas, the celiac axis is located. The celiac ganglions usually lie on both sides of the celiac axis. The greater and lesser splanchnic nerves are isolated as they enter the ganglions on each side and are freed. A small segment of each nerve is removed. There is considerable doubt as to the efficacy of this operation, but it is an additional form of treatment for a difficult therapeutic problem.

PLATE 61

A

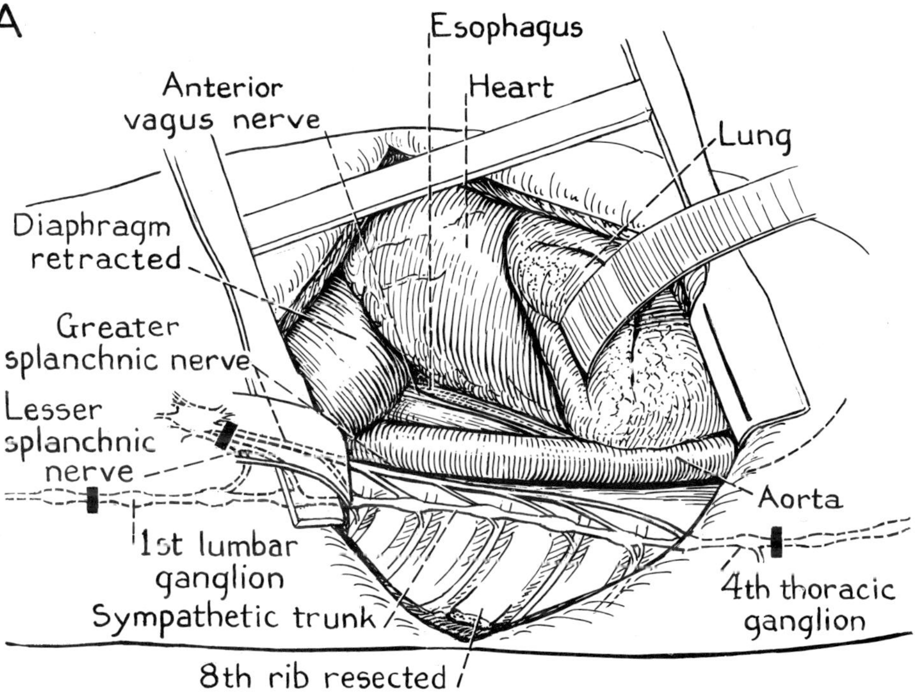

Esophagus
Anterior vagus nerve
Heart
Lung
Diaphragm retracted
Greater splanchnic nerve
Lesser splanchnic nerve
Aorta
1st lumbar ganglion
4th thoracic ganglion
Sympathetic trunk
8th rib resected

B

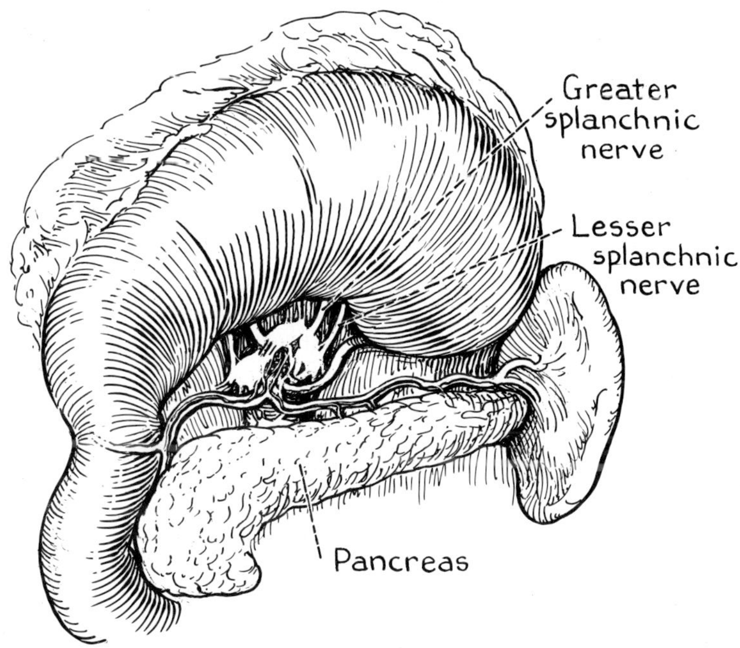

Greater splanchnic nerve
Lesser splanchnic nerve
Pancreas

PANCREATIC LITHIASIS.—Calcification may be a complication of chronic pancreatitis. Calcium may be deposited in the glandular tissue and may be localized to any portion of the gland or found throughout the entire organ. Occasionally, stones will form within the ducts and cause partial or complete obstruction. Roentgenograms will demonstrate the existence of calcification in a high percentage of patients and will denote its character and distribution. Solitary calculi in the pancreas must be differentiated from gallstones, renal calculi and calcified retroperitoneal nodes.

A.—This anteroposterior roentgenogram shows diffuse calcification throughout the entire pancreas.

B.—Lateral x-rays demonstrate the calcification in the pancreas and help to differentiate it from calculi of other structures.

C.—Calcification may be demonstrated in the tail of the pancreas alone. Such findings may indicate a partial pancreatectomy.

D.—In this patient a large pancreatic cyst was explored, a calculus was removed from the main pancreatic duct near the ampulla of Vater and external drainage established. A persisting sinus was injected with opaque medium and this roentgenogram obtained. It shows dilatation of the pancreatic duct from which the stone had been removed and the free flow of medium through the duct and into the duodenum.

Treatment.—Solitary calculi within the ducts of the pancreas may be removed by making a longitudinal incision over the duct and exploring for the stone. If a single stone is located near the ampulla, it may be removed by a transduodenal approach and incision of the wall of the ampulla. Occasionally, multiple incisions over isolated calculi may be necessary. If calculi are removed from the pancreatic ducts in this manner, one should not attempt to close the duct by suture because of the danger of subsequent formation of pseudocysts or external pancreatic fistulas. It is better to suture a defunctionalized limb of jejunum over the incised duct or to incise the duct adequately and perform a longitudinal pancreaticojejunostomy. Calculi in the tail of the pancreas may be removed by partial distal pancreatectomy. If this is performed, the patency of the pancreatic duct throughout its length must be determined, and retrograde pancreaticojejunostomy should be performed. Total pancreatectomy or pancreaticoduodenectomy should be reserved as a final procedure when all other forms of surgical therapy have failed.

PLATE 62

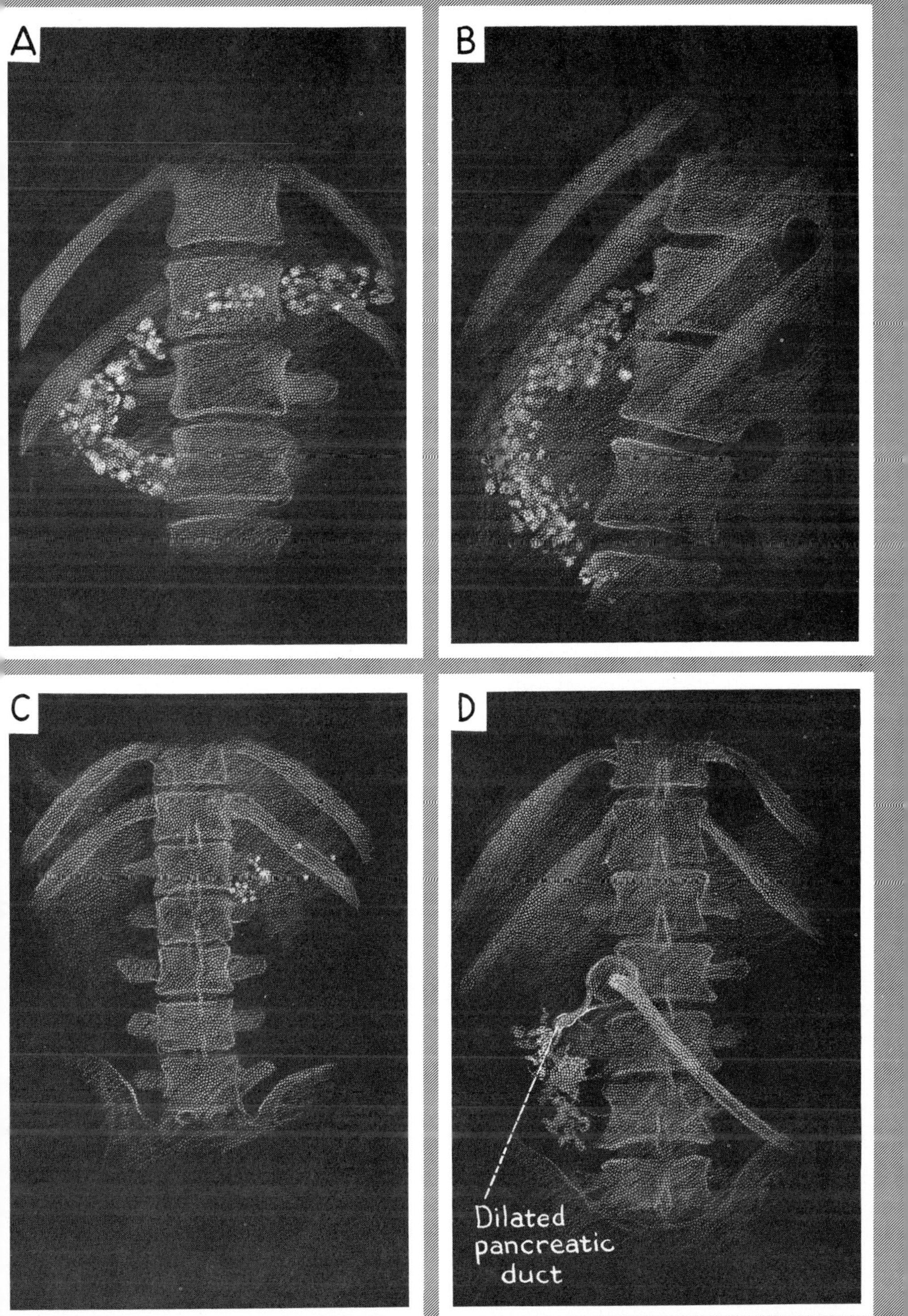

PANCREATIC CYSTS

Pancreatic cysts constitute one of the rarer forms of disease of this organ. The various types and locations of these lesions and the variety of symptoms produced demand individual consideration of each case and present an interesting challenge to the surgeon.

Classification.—Pancreatic cysts have been classified in various ways, largely on the basis of pathology and etiology. Although extensive classifications have been made, we believe that, for the purposes of this book, a simple one will suffice. The rarer types include congenital cysts, such as those associated with fibrocystic disease, polycystic disease or dermoid cysts, parasitic cysts and neoplastic cysts; the commonest of the last group are cystadenomas and cystadenocarcinomas. The more common types are retention cysts and pseudocysts. Retention cysts form as the result of partial or gradual obstruction of a main pancreatic duct, usually due to calculi, tumor, inflammation or fibrosis. These cysts have an epithelial lining and a true cyst wall. It may be difficult to differentiate them preoperatively or at the time of abdominal exploration from pseudocysts although they frequently can be more readily mobilized and totally excised. At operation, their contents may be dark in color and may contain considerable necrotic material. If they are marsupialized and drained, the nature of the drainage may gradually change until it becomes clear and colorless and is composed of pure pancreatic juice. Pseudocysts are not true cysts since they do not have an epithelial lining. The wall is composed of fibrous tissue. The commonest etiologic factors are trauma and inflammatory disease of the pancreas. Pseudocysts may arise from any portion of the pancreas but are not limited to this organ and may extend in any direction. They are far more common than any other type.

Pancreatic cysts usually originate in the retroperitoneal tissues in or adjacent to the pancreas. They extend in the direction of least resistance and their location is determined largely by the portion of the pancreas in which they arise. Cysts originating in the head of the pancreas may present largely to the right of the midline. Those arising in the body and tail of the pancreas have their greatest volume to the left of the midline. They usually remain retroperitoneal but occasionally will rupture into the lesser peritoneal sac. In one of our patients the cyst ruptured into the peritoneal cavity, the parietal peritoneum forming the boundary and containing over a gallon of cystic fluid. The size of pancreatic cysts varies from a few millimeters to many centimeters in diameter. The contents may vary from a clear fluid to a brown or greenish brown, thick liquid containing necrotic debris.

Symptomatology and diagnosis.—The history of symptoms of pancreatitis can often be elicited. Pain, the most common symptom, is located in the epigastrium or in the right or left upper quadrant and frequently radiates to the back. Dyspepsia and gradual weight loss are common complaints. When the cyst is of adequate size, a mass can be palpated in the abdomen. It is usually smooth, rounded, nontender and firm. It may be so tense as to present the feel of a solid tumor. Jaundice is noted in a moderate number of patients, especially when the cyst is located to the right of the midline. Laboratory studies may reveal an increase in serum amylase and lipase levels during acute exacerbations of pancreatitis, but between attacks these values return to normal. Blood sugar levels may be elevated if there is extensive destruction of islet tissue. Stool studies may indicate impaired pancreatic digestion.

Roentgenology is most helpful in the diagnosis of pancreatic cysts. A plain film may delineate the tumor. Barium studies of the stomach and colon may show displacement or distortion.

A.—This anteroposterior roentgenogram shows the stomach displaced upward by a midline pancreatic cyst which presented between the stomach and transverse colon.

B.—A cyst presenting behind the stomach is seen to displace the proximal portion of the stomach anteriorly in a lateral roentgenogram.

C.—A large cyst high in the midportion of the abdomen displaces the stomach downward and increases the arc of the lesser curvature.

D.—The duodenal sweep is markedly widened by a cyst of the head of the pancreas.

E.—It is important to rule out tumors of the kidney. This patient had a large mass in the upper abdomen. An intravenous pyelogram showed relatively normal kidney pelves and ureters and helped to establish the diagnosis of pancreatic cyst. Gas in the colon showed a downward displacement of the midtransverse colon. Roentgenograms taken after a barium enema confirmed the downward displacement of the transverse colon.

F.—This patient had fluid in the left pleural cavity. Thoracentesis produced a cloudy fluid containing a high concentration of amylase. The needle had been passed through the diaphragm into a previously unrecognized cyst. This roentgenogram shows the cyst under the left diaphragm and partly filled with air. The stomach is displaced downward and toward the midline.

Treatment

Pancreatic cysts which produce symptoms should be treated surgically. The objective of surgery is to establish internal or external drainage or to remove the cyst and adjacent portions of the pancreas. Internal drainage of pancreatic cysts shortens convalescence and permits most patients to leave the hospital in 10–14 days. It restores all pancreatic juice to the intestinal tract to aid digestion. This is most important in the presence of pancreatic damage.

No one procedure is satisfactory for all types of cysts. The size, location and accessibility of the cyst and its place of origin from the pancreas play an important role in the technic to be employed.

PLATE 63

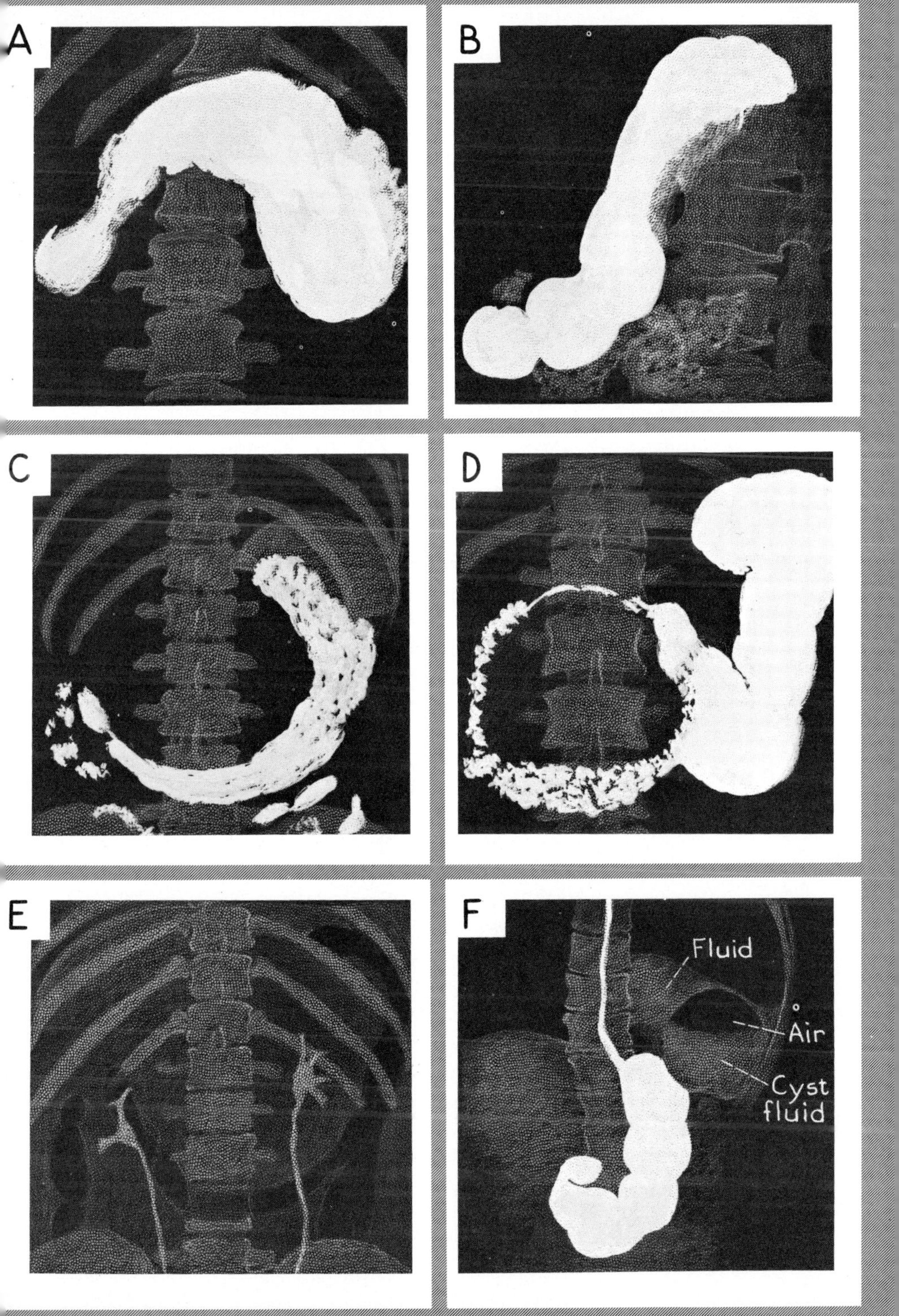

Marsupialization and drainage carries with it a low operative risk and is easily accomplished. Its disadvantage is that it drains most or all pancreatic secretions to the surface, thus depriving the body of adequate nutrition and recuperative powers. When this operation is used, nearly one fourth of the patients require subsequent pancreatic surgery.

A.—The abdomen is opened through an incision over the dome of the cyst. If the cyst lies behind the stomach or colon, these structures should be separated from it to expose the cyst wall. The cyst should be aspirated to determine the nature of its contents. The wall is then incised for 1–2 in. and the cyst evacuated. The cyst cavity should be inspected and the wall palpated to be sure that no additional cysts are left undrained. If any are encountered, they should be incised and drained into the main cyst cavity.

B.—The edges of the cut cyst wall are sutured to the edges of the parietal peritoneum. Several Penrose drains should be placed in the cyst cavity and the remainder of the abdominal wall closed around them.

C.—In most pseudocysts and retention cysts, the walls will collapse and the cavity will eventually be obliterated; however, an external pancreatic fistula is apt to result, which may continue indefinitely and may result in progressive weight loss and debility. These complications may be less serious if the fistula leads to the tail of the pancreas. This diagram shows a draining sinus leading to the distal pancreas. Under such circumstances, the pancreas may be divided to the right of the fistula and the tail removed. The divided pancreas should not be oversewn but should be anastomosed to a defunctionalized limb of jejunum.

When the fistula leads to the head of the pancreas or the body near the neck, it is better not to resect the pancreas to the right of the fistula because of the dangers of creating pancreatic insufficiency. Such fistulous tracts can be dissected free and transplanted into the stomach or intestine. I prefer to transplant the fistula into the upper jejunum, using a Roux-Y technic similar to that described in Plate 65. If a definite fistulous tract cannot be identified, a pancreaticojejunostomy should be performed.

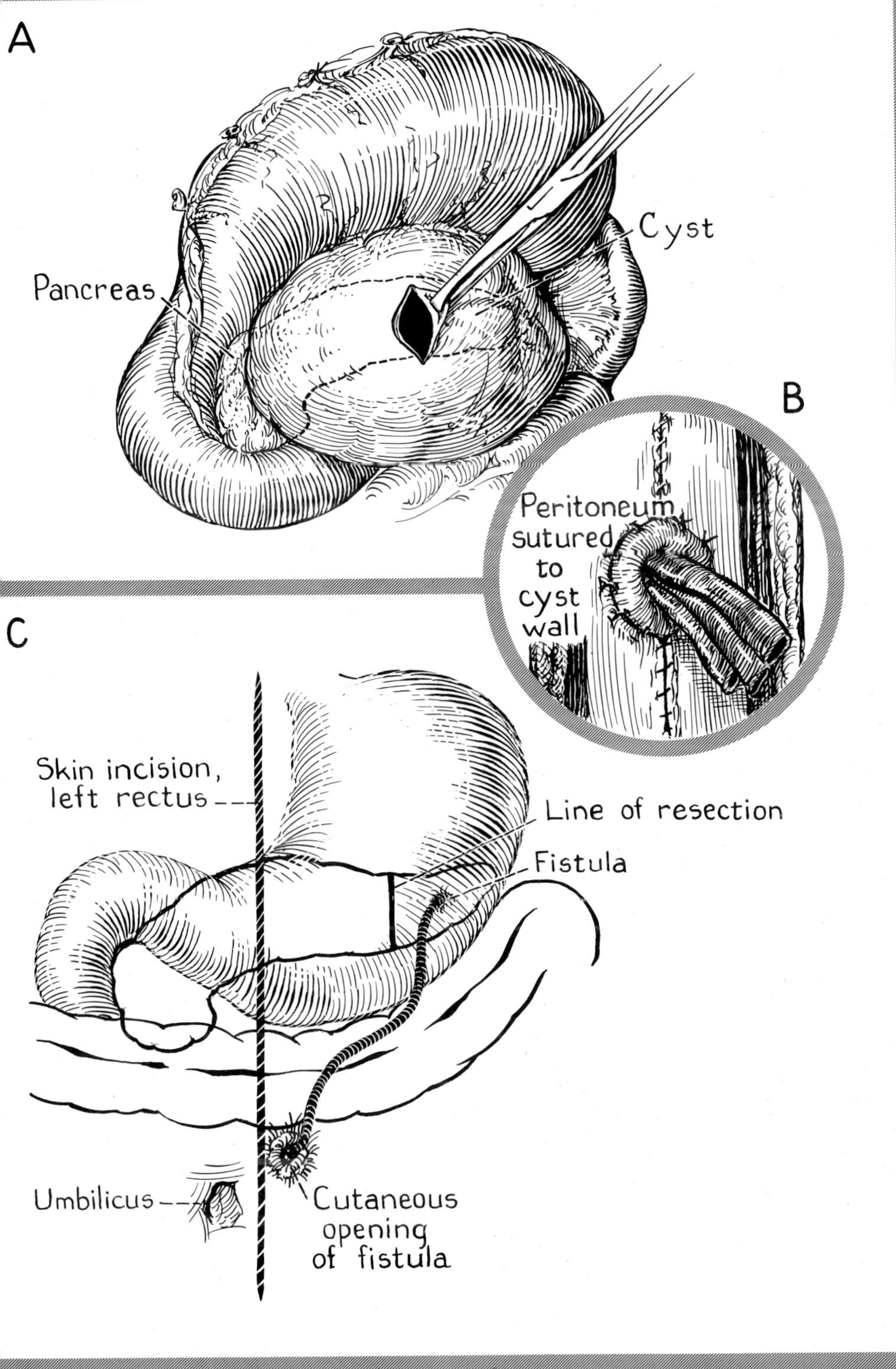
A
Cyst
Pancreas
B
Peritoneum sutured to cyst wall
C
Skin incision, left rectus
Line of resection
Fistula
Umbilicus
Cutaneous opening of fistula

A pancreatic cystojejunostomy is an excellent form of internal drainage. The abdomen should be opened through a vertical incision centered over the cyst. This may be a midline, right or left paramedian or a right or left rectus incision.

A.—The gastrocolic omentum is divided for a sufficient distance to expose completely the anterior surface of the cyst.

B.—The stomach is elevated and its posterior wall freed from the cyst. It is well to free as much of the surface of the cyst on all sides as can be done without too great dissection and without danger of cutting into the cyst. This permits a better evaluation of its size and position. From its anterior surface, the cyst is then aspirated with a syringe and needle to determine the nature of the contents and to cause partial decompression.

C.—A transverse incision 2–4 cm. long is made in the cyst wall and the cavity is evacuated by suction and sponging. The lesion demonstrated in this figure had a second isolated cavity to the right of the main cyst cavity. This was aspirated and a portion of septum removed to establish a single cavity.

D.—The jejunum is divided between clamps about 10–12 in. distal to the ligament of Treitz. A point of division is selected which will permit the mesentery to be divided between main arterial arcades to its root.

E.—The distal end of the divided jejunum is brought through an opening in the midportion of the transverse mesocolon and is approximated to the opening in the cyst wall. It is important to establish a large anastomosis and it is better to utilize the entire opening in the cyst for the anastomosis than to partially close it. The end of the jejunum may be cut obliquely to make the lumen equal in size to the opening in the cyst. A posterior outer row of continuous cotton sutures approximates the jejunum to the outer surface of cyst about 5 mm. from its posterior cut edge.

F.—The jejunum is incised an equal distance anterior to the first line of sutures. The posterior inner suture line consists of a continuous catgut stitch which includes all layers of the bowel wall and cyst wall. The triangular piece of jejunum is excised.

[Pancreatic cystojejunostomy *continued on page 300.*]

PLATE 65

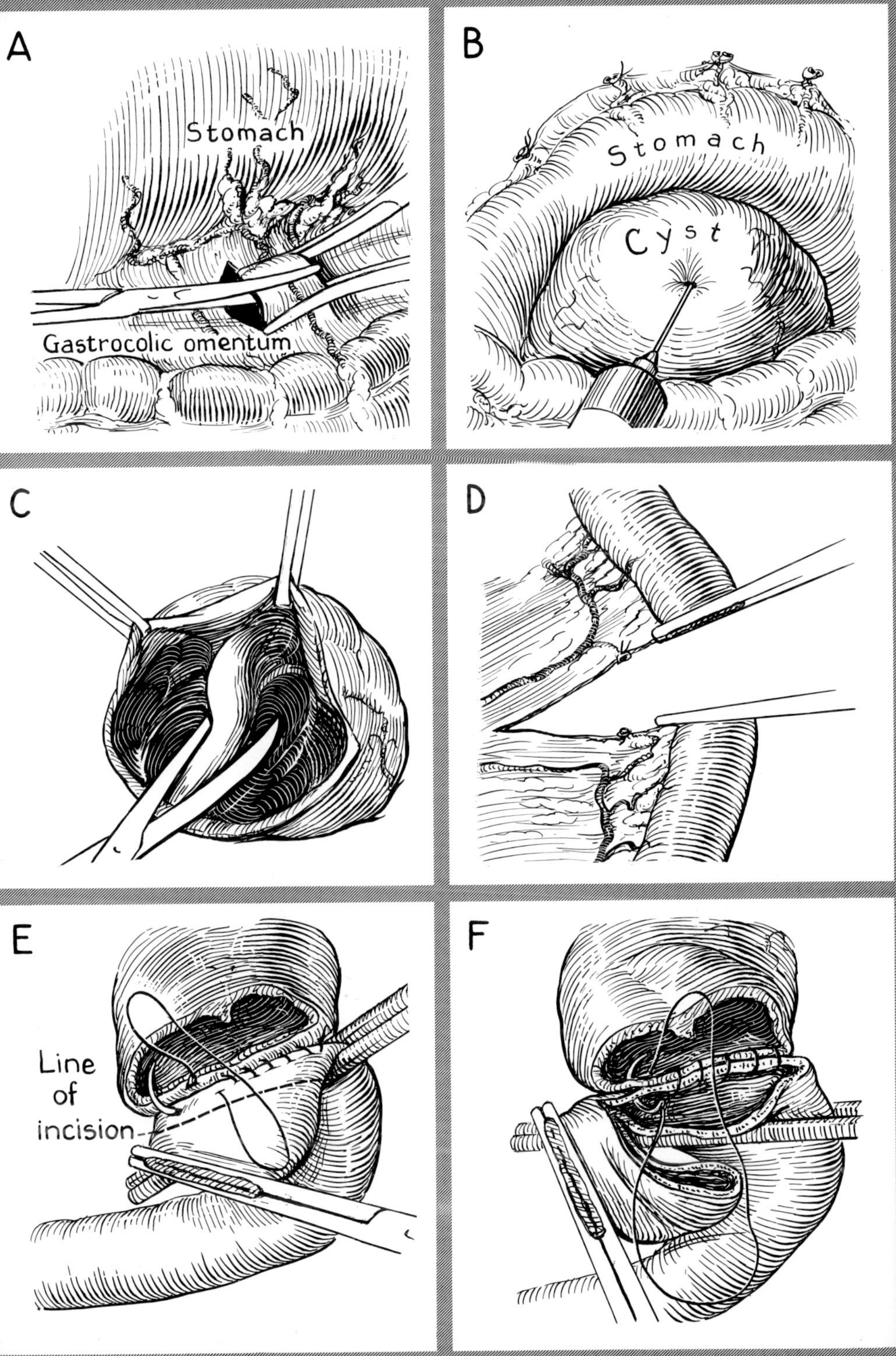
A
Stomach
Gastrocolic omentum
B
Stomach
Cyst
C
D
E
Line of incision
F

G.—The catgut suture is continued to form the anterior inner row and approximates the obliquely cut anterior edge of the jejunum to the anterior edge of the cyst.

H.—An anterior outer inverting row of continuous cotton sutures completes the anastomosis.

I.—The proximal end of divided jejunum is anastomosed to the distal limb 10–12 in. below the pancreatic cystojejunostomy. An oblique end-to-side anastomosis is performed, using two rows of continuous intestinal catgut. The technic is similar to that described in Plate 48. After completion of the anastomosis it is important to suture the free edge of the divided mesentery of the proximal end to the mesentery of the distal segment. This obliterates an opening which could be a site for an internal hernia.

This drawing shows the completed anastomosis. The cyst contents drain into the jejunal limb in the direction of peristalsis. Gastrointestinal continuity is established by the enteroanastomosis. If the opening through the transverse mesocolon is large, it may be well to close it around the jejunal limb. The abdominal wound should be closed in layers without drainage.

Pancreatic Cystogastrostomy

The drainage of pancreatic cysts into the stomach has proved a satisfactory form of internal drainage. Theoretically, the passage of gastric contents into the cysts may result in chemical irritation or infection and interfere with the obliteration of the cavity. However, in practice this has not occurred. We have found that, within two weeks of the establishment of the fistulous opening between the stomach and the cyst, barium given by mouth will not demonstrate the cyst cavity or the anastomosis. It is our belief that if pancreatic secretions continue to enter the area of the cyst, a small fistula usually will persist, permitting the secretions to escape into the stomach. This belief is based on the fact that we have not encountered the re-formation of cysts and that patients have been relieved of pancreatic symptoms. Reports in the medical literature indicate that only 2–4 per cent of patients with internal drainage of pancreatic cysts require subsequent pancreatic surgery.

Two technics for the establishment of pancreatic cystogastrostomy are described in Plate 66.

PLATE 65

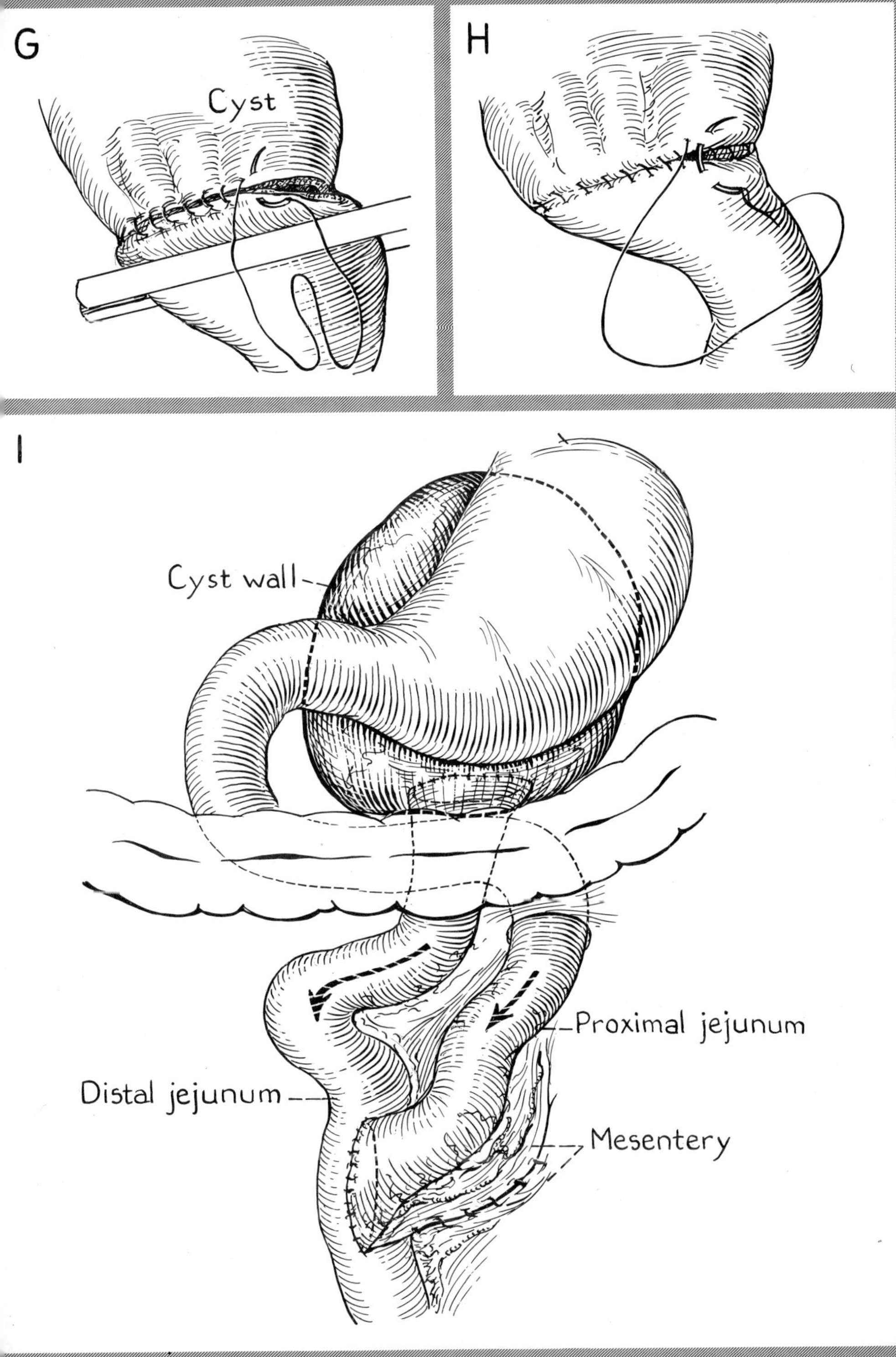
G
Cyst
H
I
Cyst wall
Proximal jejunum
Distal jejunum
Mesentery

A.—Pancreatic cysts which lie behind the stomach may be drained through its posterior wall. Usually the cyst is most easily exposed by division of the gastrocolic omentum and elevation of the stomach. The anterior surface of the cyst is freed and its contents aspirated. A two-row anastomosis is then made between the anterior wall of the cyst and the posterior wall of the approximated stomach, using an outer row of cotton and an inner row of intestinal catgut. The stoma of the anastomosis should be 2–4 cm. long. All blood vessels encountered in the incision through the posterior wall of the stomach should be carefully ligated.

TRANSGASTRIC APPROACH.—*B.*—Occasionally retrogastric pancreatic cysts will be encountered which are densely adherent to the posterior wall of the stomach and other overlying structures, making exposure of the cyst difficult. A transgastric approach will minimize the amount of surgery necessary for a satisfactory anastomosis. A longitudinal incision is made through the anterior wall of the stomach. It should be centered over the cyst unless this would place the incision close to the pylorus; an incision several centimeters above the pylorus is preferable. Before the posterior wall of the stomach and the anterior wall of the cyst are incised, aspiration through a needle inserted in the contemplated line of incision is carried out to confirm the diagnosis of pancreatic cyst. A longitudinal incision at least 2–4 cm. long is then made through the posterior wall of the stomach and anterior wall of the cyst. The firm union between the cyst and the stomach makes two rows of sutures unnecessary. However, a single row of continuous intestinal catgut will not only assure union of the cyst and stomach walls but will also be of hemostatic value. After complete evacuation of the cyst contents and conversion of any additional cysts into a single cavity, the anterior wall of the stomach is closed, usually with two rows of continuous intestinal catgut sutures. The abdominal wall is closed in layers without drainage. It is well to maintain gastric suction for a few days after operation.

PLATE 66

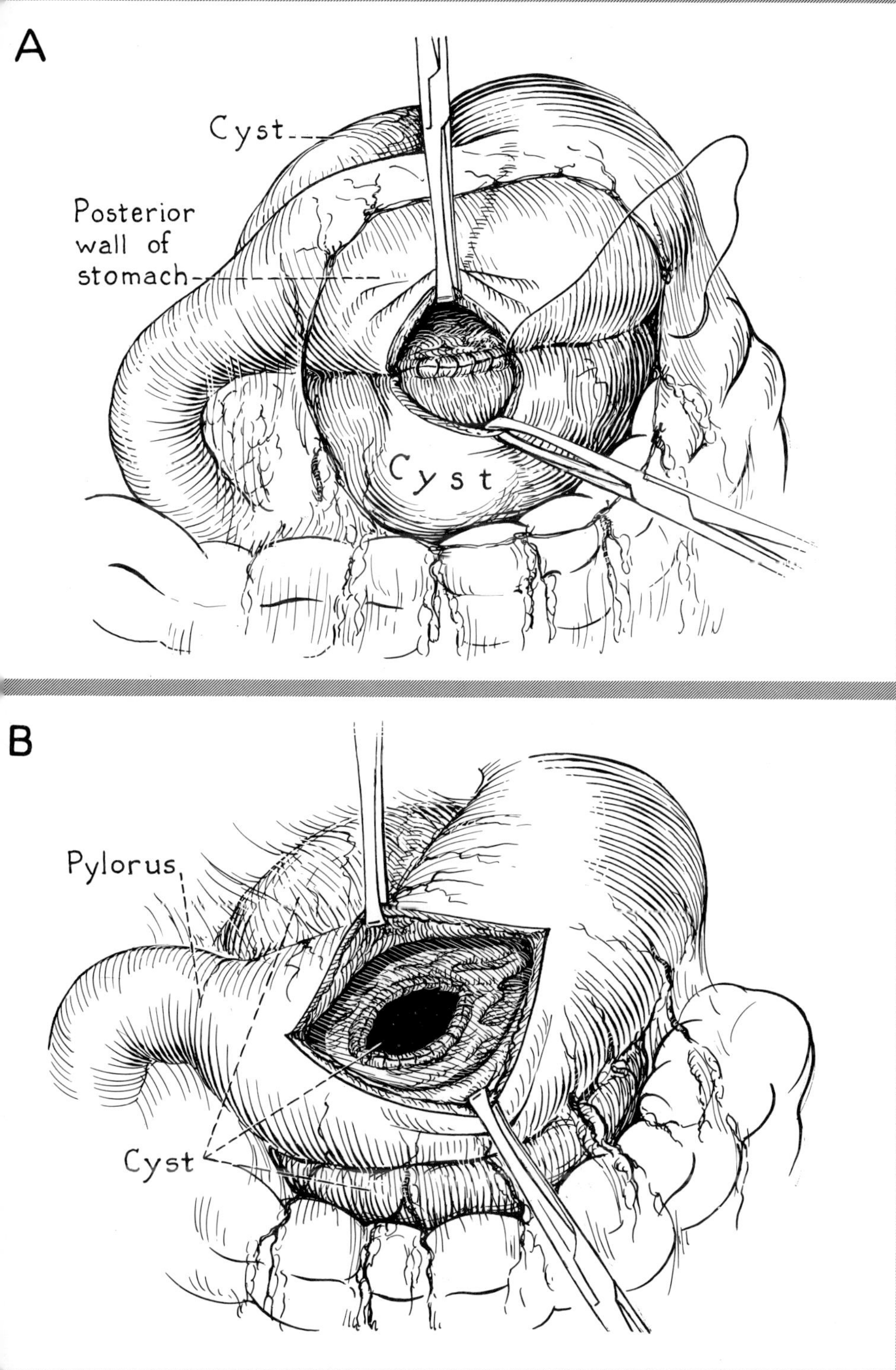

Gastric Resection with Internal Drainage

The many variations in pancreatic cysts and associated pathology should cause each case to be an individual problem which may demand variations in technic. Plate 67, *A*, shows a pancreatic cyst arising from the head of the pancreas and elevating the pyloric end of the stomach and duodenum. The patient also had a duodenal ulcer producing partial obstruction. Pressure upon the common duct resulted in jaundice. Thus, this patient presented a duodenal ulcer with obstruction, obstructive jaundice and a cyst, all of which needed surgical therapy.

B.—The distal portion of the stomach was resected at the levels indicated in *A*. The pancreatic cyst was incised close to the open end of the duodenum and, after aspiration, an anastomosis was made between the open end of the duodenum and the cyst wall. A cholecystoduodenostomy was then performed to relieve the obstructive jaundice. A posterior Polya type of anastomosis was made between the jejunum and stomach. This patient had an uneventful convalescence and was completely relieved of all symptoms.

Excision of Pancreatic Cysts

Total excision of benign pancreatic cysts rarely is feasible. Cysts arising from the head of the pancreas may underlie portions of the stomach, duodenum and common bile duct. It may be dangerous to remove them because of damage to adjacent structures. Cysts arising from the tail of the pancreas occasionally may be totally extirpated.

C illustrates a large pseudocyst lying anterior to the pancreas and extending into the hilus of the spleen. The stomach and colon were separated from the cyst wall. It was possible to remove the cyst, spleen and distal one fourth of the pancreas. The main pancreatic duct was ligated and the proximal end of the pancreas oversewn. The remainder of the pancreas showed little disease. Although this operation was successful, I believe a longitudinal pancreaticojejunostomy a safer procedure because of the possibility of proximal ductal obstruction.

PLATE 67

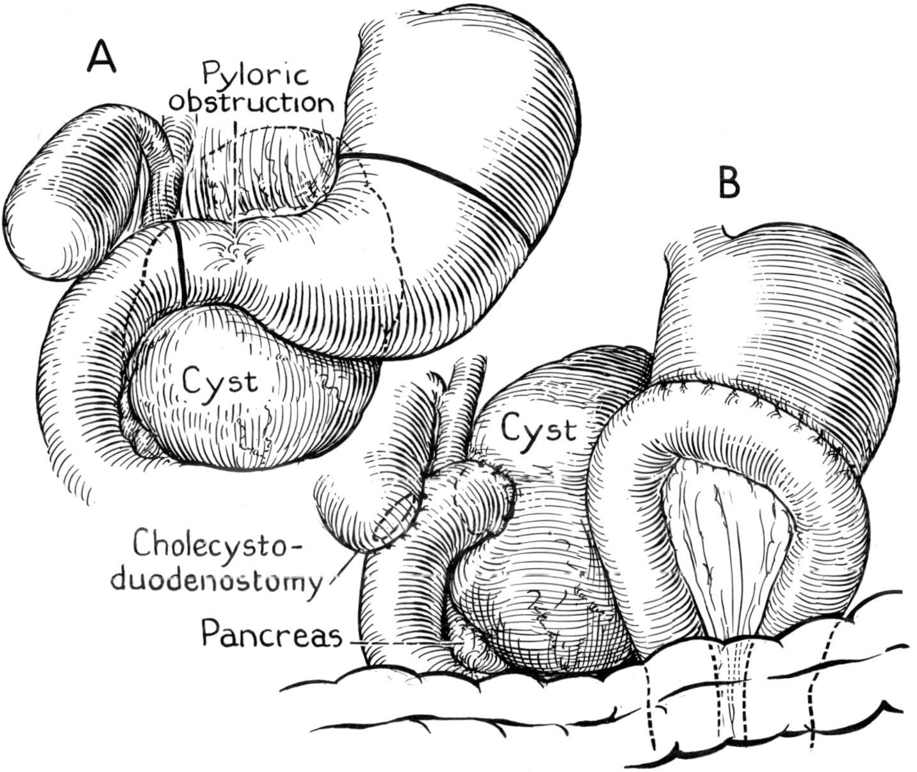
A
Pyloric obstruction
Cyst
B
Cyst
Cholecysto-duodenostomy
Pancreas

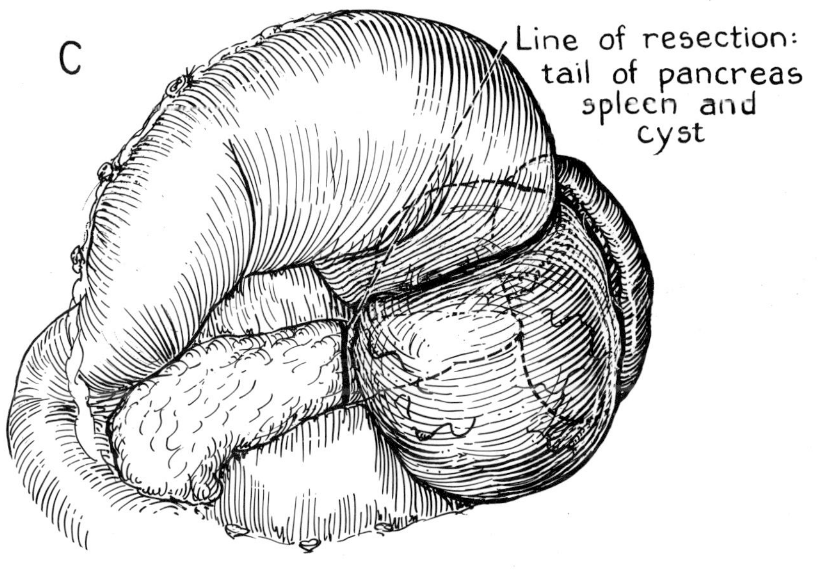
C
Line of resection: tail of pancreas spleen and cyst

TUMORS OF THE ISLETS OF LANGERHANS

Tumors of the islets of Langerhans are usually located in the tail or body of the pancreas. They will rarely become larger than 2 cm. in diameter. Those which produce hyperinsulinism are easily recognized because of the characteristic syndrome which consists of attacks similar to insulin reactions with sweating, nervousness, increasing mental confusion, drowsiness and finally unconsciousness. The fasting blood sugar level often drops below 50 mg. Treatment consists in removal of the tumors by enucleation or by resection of the distal pancreas.

A.—The abdomen is opened either through a high left rectus incision or through a transverse incision. The gastrocolic omentum is divided and the stomach elevated. The anterior surface of the pancreas is exposed to the tip of the tail.

B.—The entire pancreas is palpated for tumors. If a tumor is felt within the substance of the pancreas, a longitudinal incision may be made over it to expose the tumor and permit its enucleation. One should avoid, if possible, opening the main pancreatic duct. If pancreatic ducts are opened, no attempt should be made to oversew them but an anastomosis of the surrounding pancreas to a defunctionalized limb of jejunum should be carried out.

C.—If a decision is made to resect the distal pancreas, the inferior surface of the gland is carefully dissected from surrounding structures. This must be carefully done to avoid injury to the inferior mesenteric vein. The dissection is continued, freeing the posterior surface of the gland. The tip of the pancreas is freed from the hilus of the spleen. It is usually necessary to ligate the splenic vessels at this point. When this is done, the spleen should be removed because its blood supply has been interrupted.

D.—The pancreas is elevated and dissection gradually carried to the right, a little beyond the decided point of resection. If a large portion of the pancreas is to be removed, the gland may be elevated from the superior mesenteric vessels and portal vein. It is usually necessary to religate the splenic artery and vein near the point of resection. The pancreas is divided by sharp dissection and the end closed as shown in Plate 64.

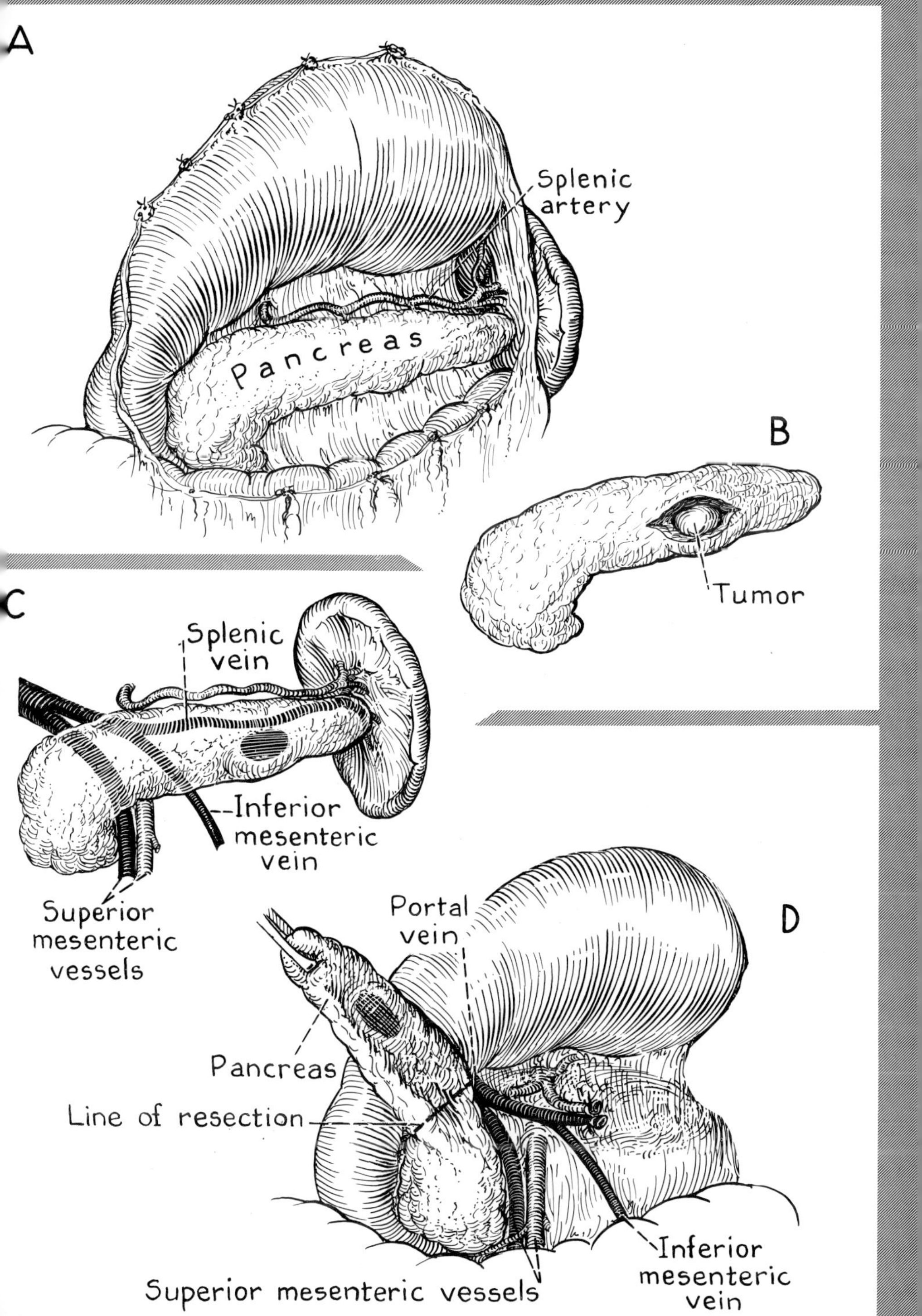
A
Splenic artery
Pancreas
B
Tumor
C
Splenic vein
Inferior mesenteric vein
Superior mesenteric vessels
D
Portal vein
Pancreas
Line of resection
Superior mesenteric vessels
Inferior mesenteric vein

CHAPTER 16

Carcinoma of the Head of the Pancreas

UNTIL RECENT YEARS treatment of carcinoma of the head of the pancreas has consisted of palliative procedures designed to relieve complications of the disease and not for its cure. An anastomosis between the extrahepatic biliary tract and stomach or small intestine or external drainage of the gallbladder or common duct was performed to relieve jaundice resulting from common bile duct obstruction. If the tumor obstructed the duodenum, some form of gastroenterostomy was performed. More recently, in an effort to cure the disease, the removal of a part or all of the duodenum and head of the pancreas has been attempted. Mortality following these resections has been high and the cures have been discouragingly few. Many surgeons have abandoned such radical resections for carcinoma of the head of the pancreas and are limiting surgical treatment to short-circuiting operations.

It is frequently difficult to diagnose carcinoma of the head of the pancreas without histologic studies. Pancreatitis and benign tumors may simulate both the clinical picture and gross findings of a malignant lesion. Many patients who have had short-circuiting operations for obstructive jaundice thought to be due to carcinoma of the pancreas have survived many years, indicating that there probably was an error in diagnosis. In view of the high mortality from pancreaticoduodenectomy and the infrequent cures obtained by it, I do not believe the procedure justifiable unless the diagnosis has been confirmed by biopsy. The operation is not justifiable if metastases are present in adjacent or distant lymph nodes or other organs. When these exist, surgical treatment should be designed only for the relief of obstructive symptoms. In addition to other dangers, a radical resection may leave the patient a pancreatic invalid.

Many patients with tumors of the head of the pancreas which have not metastasized and which meet the criteria justifying resection are poor surgical risks. If prolonged jaundice, heart enlargement and damage to the liver manifested by disturbed liver function and a poor nutritional state exist, the patient may not be able to tolerate a one-stage radical resection. Under such circumstances, it is preferable to perform a two-stage operation, the first stage having for its purpose the relief of biliary obstruction. There will usually be sufficient improvement in the patient's nutritional state for him to withstand a radical resection several weeks later at a minimal risk.

Technics for both the radical and palliative procedures are described in the following pages. A careful evaluation of the patient must be made before deciding upon the technic to be used.

Two-Stage Pancreaticoduodenal Resection

The two-stage operation for removal of the duodenum and varying amounts of pancreas is of particular value in the poor risk surgical patient with disturbed nutrition and impaired physiologic function of one or more vital organs of the body. It is also of value in the patient with obstruction of the common bile duct and its resultant jaundice. The first stage of the procedure relieves the obstruction of the biliary tract and permits a free flow of bile into the intestinal tract. It can be accomplished with a minimum of anesthetic and surgical trauma and is much safer than more radical procedures. It permits recovery from jaundice and improvement in the nutritional state. Liver and kidney function increases and thus the risk of the more extensive second stage is lessened. Preoperative preparation (Chapter 9) is most important to minimize the risk of operation. The time lapse between the first and second stage should be adequate to permit maximal improvement of the patient.

First Stage

A.—The abdomen is opened through a high right rectus incision extending from the angle between the xiphoid cartilage and costal margin to the umbilicus. The contents of the abdomen should be carefully examined and a search made for metastatic lesions. The gallbladder and common duct are exposed and examined. Usually they are considerably dilated. The pancreas should be palpated and exposed for visual examination. However, one should not be misled by the feel or appearance of the pancreas, as the nature of the diseases of this organ is very difficult to determine by such examination.

B.—If metastases do not preclude the possibility of a radical resection and it is believed that a tumor exists in the pancreas, biopsy specimens should be obtained. If by palpation the tumor mass is determined to be on the anterior surface of the head of the pancreas, it should be approached by a small incision in the gastrocolic omentum. Satisfactory biopsy specimens can be obtained with a Silverman needle. (See liver biopsy, Plate 2.) Frozen sections should be examined immediately and repeated biopsies should be made until a satisfactory diagnosis is established.

C.—If the surgeon believes the tumor to present on the posterior surface of the head of the pancreas, the peritoneum is incised along the right border of the duodenum.

D.—The duodenum and head of the pancreas are freed on their posterior surfaces and rotated to the left to expose the undersurface of the head of the pancreas. Suspicious areas should be biopsied by a suitable method. In this drawing a specimen is procured by knife biopsy. This is a satisfactory method for superficial biopsies but may produce troublesome bleeding in deeper lesions.

[First stage *continued on page 312.*]

PLATE 69

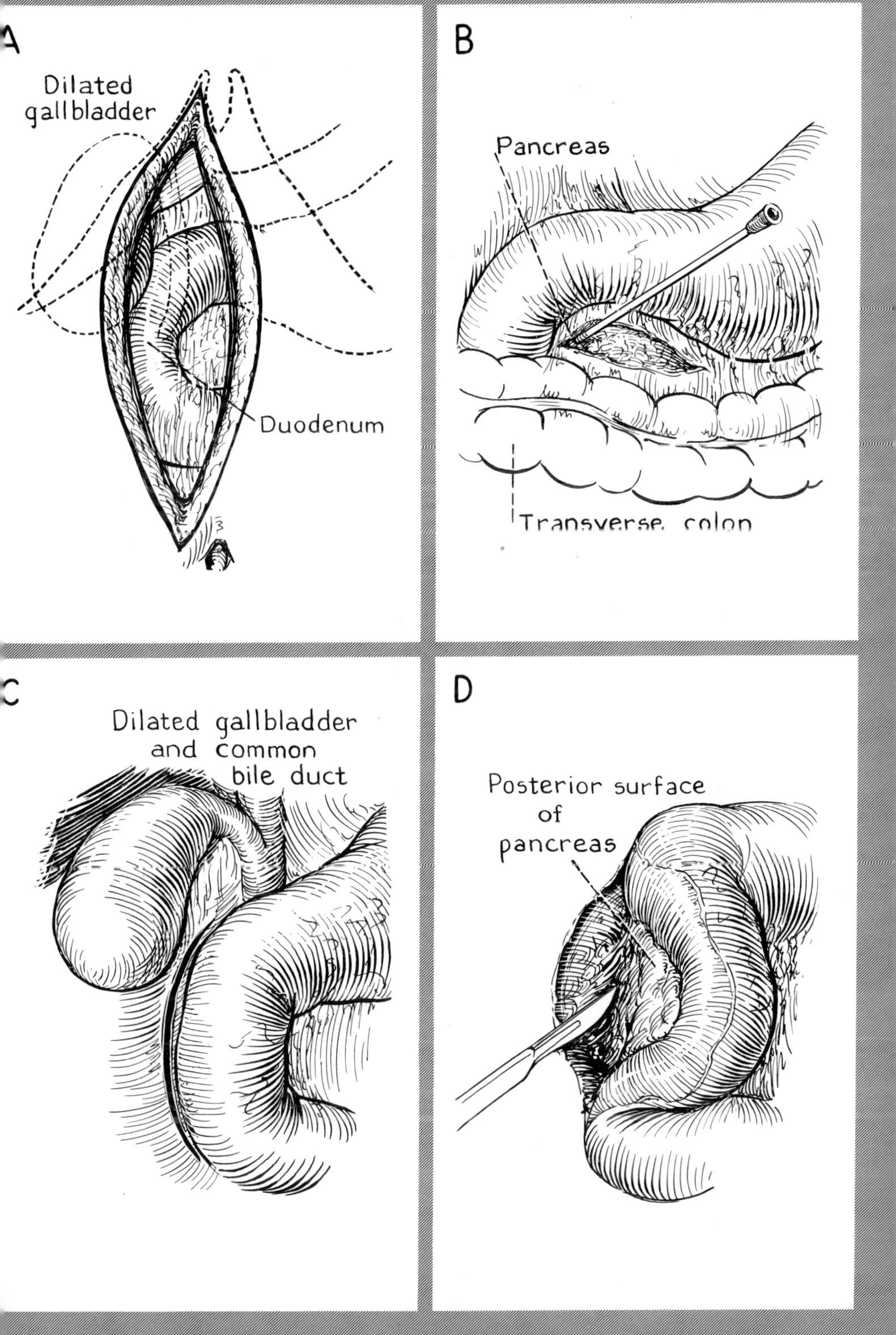
A
Dilated gallbladder
Duodenum
B
Pancreas
Transverse colon
C
Dilated gallbladder and common bile duct
D
Posterior surface of pancreas

E.—If palpation reveals that the tumor extends into the duodenum in the region of the ampulla of Vater, the duodenum should be incised longitudinally to permit a transduodenal examination of the tumor and the procurement of a biopsy specimen.

F.—If the specimen is obtained by a transduodenal incision, the opening in the duodenum should be closed in a transverse direction to minimize the danger of decreasing the caliber of the duodenal lumen. The closure is made with an inner row of continuous catgut and an outer row of interrupted cotton sutures.

G.—The fundus of the gallbladder is grasped with two Allis forceps preliminary to opening the organ and removing its contents. The contents may be removed by plunging a trocar and cannula attached to a suction tube into the fundus of the gallbladder. This may also be accomplished by making a small knife incision and inserting a glass rod attached to suction. After removal of as much of the contents from the gallbladder as is possible, the opening into the organ should be enlarged to permit exploration with the finger and with scoops.

H.—The upper jejunum is located and a site of division selected about 12–14 in. distal to the ligament of Treitz. The point of division should be midway between two arteries forming a primary arcade. This assures a good blood supply to the ends of the bowel and permits division of the mesentery to its root. The latter is important since it enables the distal jejunal segment to be brought to the gallbladder with the least possible tension. The mesentery and its arcades are divided from the root to the mesenteric edge of the jejunum and all severed blood vessels are ligated. Two Kocher type clamps are placed side by side across the bowel and the bowel divided between them.

I.—The distal end of the divided jejunum is brought anterior to the transverse colon. The mesenteric edge is placed to the left, as that is the shortest distance between its root and the gallbladder. The end of the jejunum is anastomosed to the fundus of the gallbladder by first placing an outer posterior row of continuous cotton sutures. This should be placed in the jejunum about 5 mm. distal to the edge of the clamp.

[First stage *continued on page 314.*]

PLATE 69

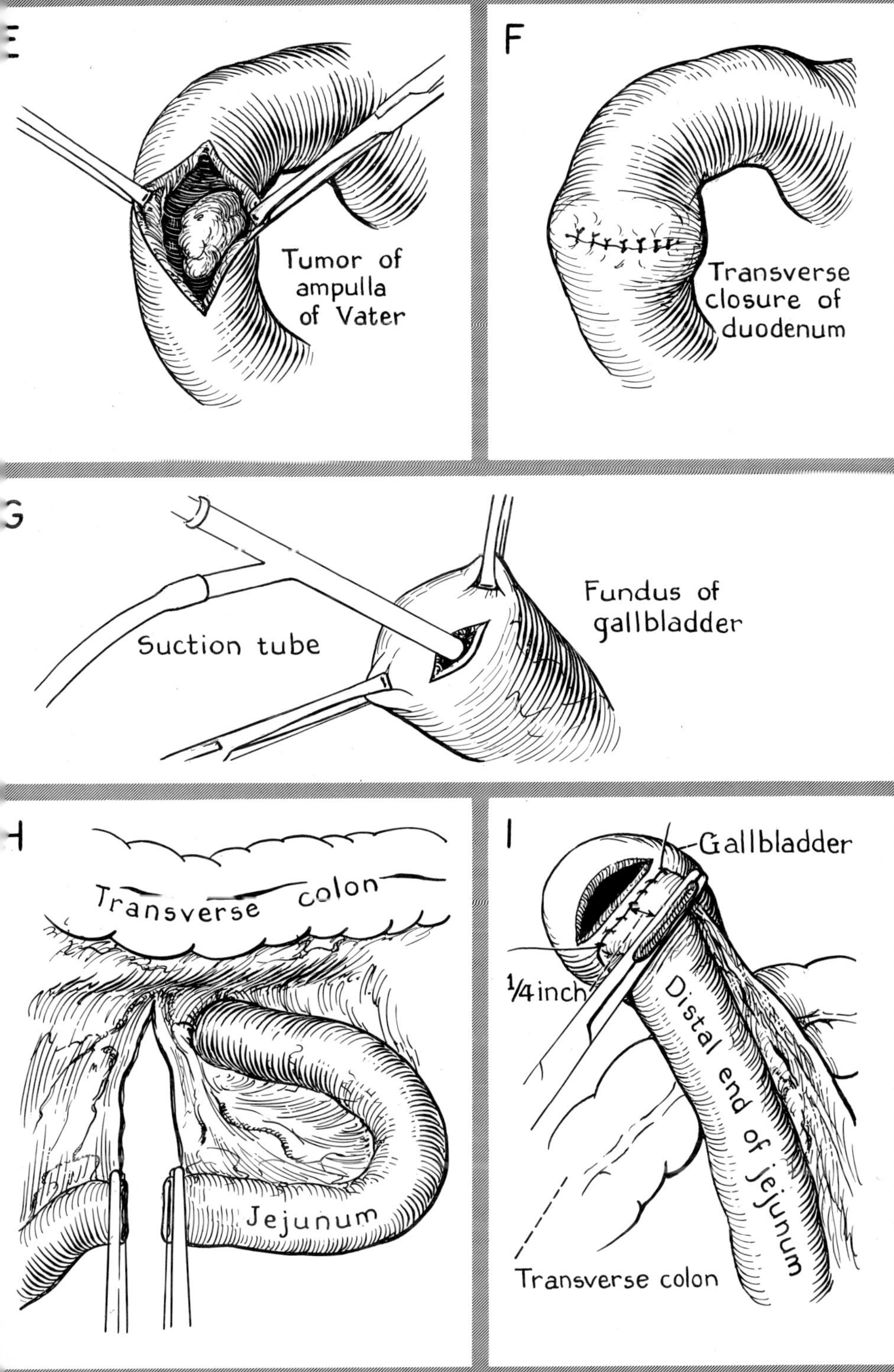
E
Tumor of ampulla of Vater
F
Transverse closure of duodenum
G
Suction tube
Fundus of gallbladder
H
Transverse colon
Jejunum
I
Gallbladder
1/4 inch
Distal end of jejunum
Transverse colon

J.—A rubber- or shoestring-covered clamp is placed across the jejunum about 2 in. distal to the site of anastomosis to minimize gross contamination by bowel content. The Kocher clamp is removed from the end of the jejunum and the crushed segment of bowel is removed by sharp dissection.

K.—The posterior inner row of sutures is placed, using a continuous over-and-over stitch of intestinal catgut. This should include all layers of the wall of the jejunum and of the gallbladder. Traction should be maintained on the ends of the posterior outer row to maintain a maximal lumen in the anastomosis.

L.—The posterior inner row is continued anteriorly to form the anterior inner row of the anastomosis.

M.—The anterior outer row consists of interrupted cotton sutures. These should completely invert the anterior inner row. It is well to protect the suture line with omentum. The poor nutritional state of these patients may delay wound healing, and additional precautions are necessary to minimize leakage from the line of anastomosis.

[First stage *continued on page 316.*]

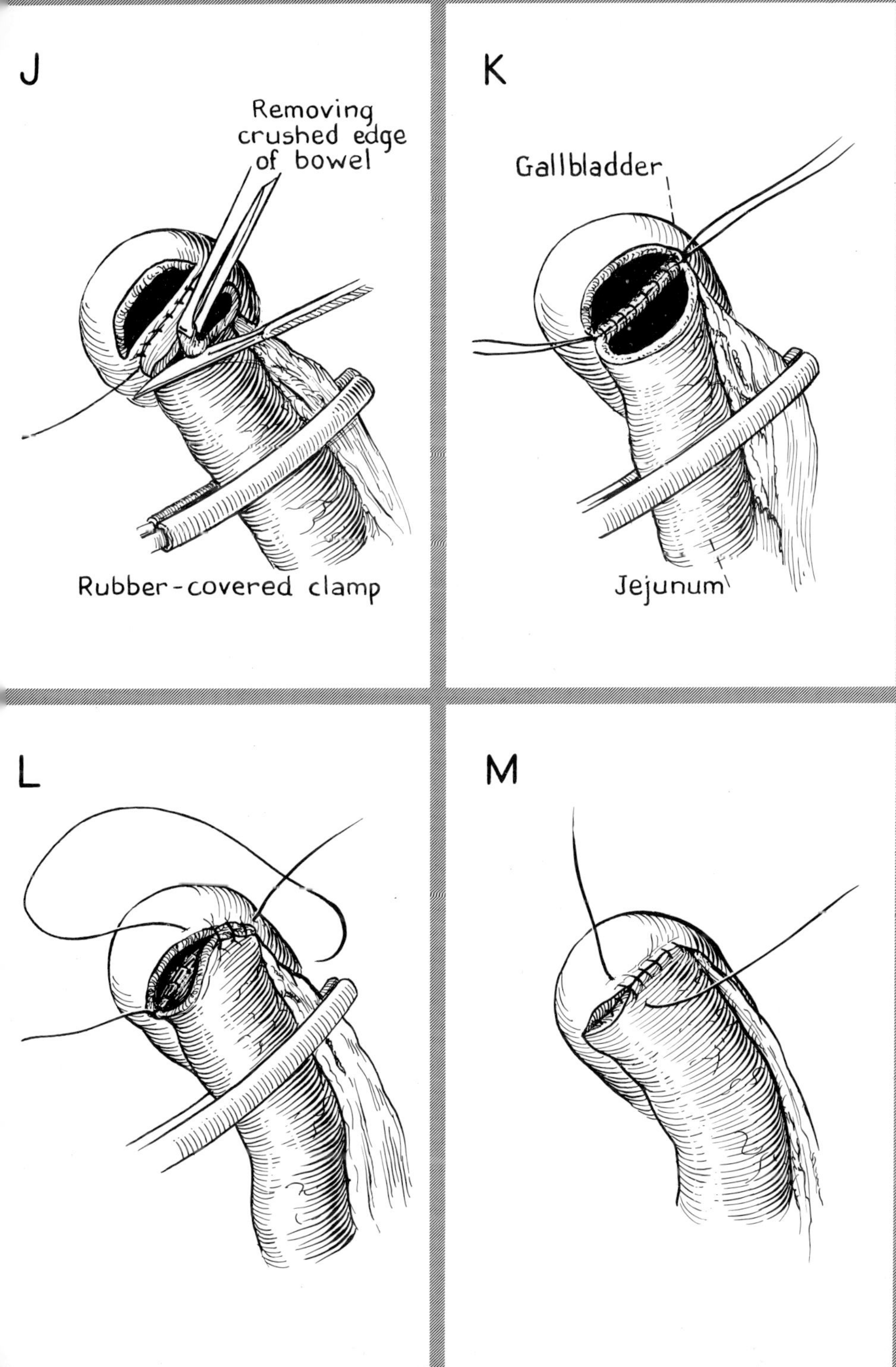
J
Removing crushed edge of bowel
Rubber-covered clamp
K
Gallbladder
Jejunum
L
M

Enteroanastomosis.—N.—The proximal end of the divided jejunum is anastomosed to the distal limb of jejunum about 15 in. below the cholecystojejunostomy, using a technic similar to that for the previous anastomosis. The posterior outer row of sutures consists of a running cotton suture. It is well to oblique this row on the divided end of jejunum to increase the size of the stoma of the anastomosis.

O.—After the posterior outer row of sutures has been placed, an incision is made in the distal limb of jejunum anterior and equal in length to the row of sutures. The opposing surface of proximal jejunum is incised obliquely proximal to the clamp, the incision extending through the opposing wall. The posterior inner row of sutures consists of a continuous over-and-over stitch of catgut and includes all layers of both segments of bowel.

P.—The incision in the proximal jejunum is then continued to the opposite wall, removing a triangular piece of bowel with the clamp. The posterior inner row of catgut is continued to form an anterior inner row. The anastomosis is completed by a row of interrupted cotton sutures which forms the anterior outer row. The free cut edge of mesentery of the proximal jejunum is sutured to the mesentery of the distal limb to obliterate a hole through which a loop of intestine could pass to form an internal hernia with possible strangulation or obstruction.

This Roux-Y type of anastomosis results in an intestinal channel extending from the gallbladder for a distance of 15 in. before coming in contact with gastrointestinal contents. Peristalsis of this limb prevents regurgitation of intestinal contents into the gallbladder and bile ducts and minimizes the danger of an ascending cholangitis.

Q.—The abdominal wall is closed in layers without drainage (Plate 29). Delayed healing is common in these patients and wound closure should be carefully accomplished. It is well to tie the tension sutures over a roll of gauze. The tension and skin sutures may be left for 12–14 days in debilitated patients to assure satisfactory healing.

[Second stage of pancreaticoduodenal resection *on page 318.*]

PLATE 69

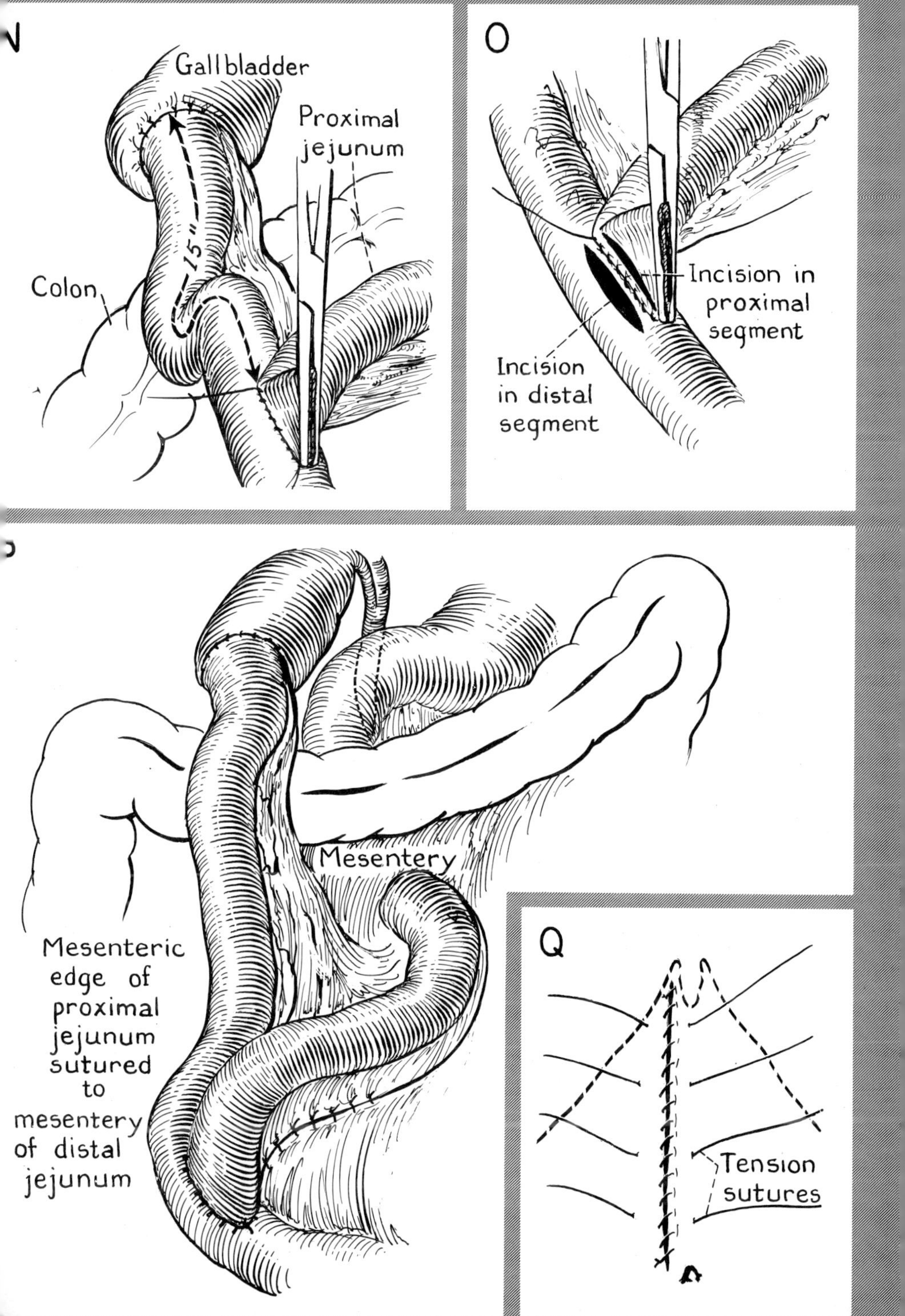

N
Gallbladder
Proximal jejunum
15"
Colon
O
Incision in proximal segment
Incision in distal segment
P
Mesentery
Mesenteric edge of proximal jejunum sutured to mesentery of distal jejunum
Q
Tension sutures

Second Stage

It is well to delay the second stage of the two-stage pancreaticoduodenal resection until the patient's jaundice has subsided and the nutritional state has improved, as indicated by improvement in weight and in results of blood chemistry determinations. Valuable guides include blood protein levels, serum bilirubin and nonprotein nitrogen and liver function tests. Four to six weeks usually are necessary between the first and second stage of this operation to allow optimal improvement without undue delay.

A.—The abdomen is reopened through the scar of the previous upper right rectus incision. The incision may be extended downward if greater exposure is needed. Any adhesions between abdominal contents and the parietal peritoneum should be freed. The gastrocolic omentum is divided between clamps from about the midportion of the greater curvature of the stomach to the pylorus and duodenum. The posterior wall of the stomach is freed from the anterior surface of the pancreas. The peritoneum is divided along the right border of the duodenum, and the second portion of the duodenum is mobilized by freeing its posterior surface. Dissection is continued downward and to the left to free the third portion of the duodenum.

B.—The gastrohepatic omentum in its right portion is divided, including the division and ligation of the gastroduodenal artery. The distal portion of the common bile duct is dissected from adjacent structures and is divided a short distance from the duodenum, leaving a sufficient amount of duct below the cystic duct to permit a careful closure.

C.—The proximal end of the duct is oversewn with a continuous cotton suture and is then inverted with a pursestring suture of cotton.

D.—Small Payr clamps are placed across the stomach above the pylorus, and the stomach is divided between them.

E.—The posterior surface of the head of the pancreas, including the uncinate process, is mobilized and the superior mesenteric vessels and portal vein carefully isolated. The uncinate process may surround these vessels and should be dissected with great care to avoid damaging them.

[Second stage *continued on page 320.*]

PLATE 70

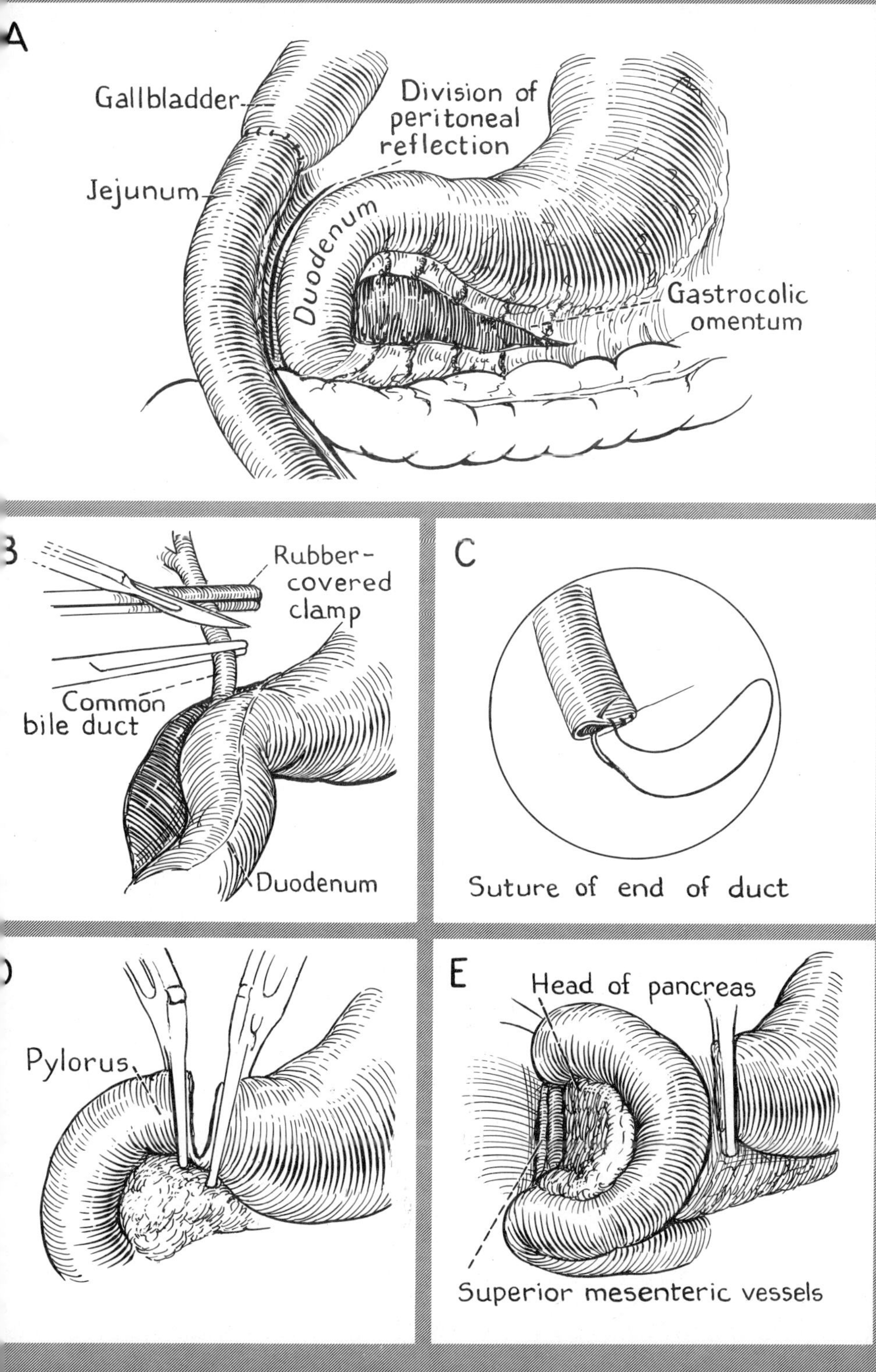
A
Gallbladder
Division of peritoneal reflection
Jejunum
Duodenum
Gastrocolic omentum
B
Rubber-covered clamp
Common bile duct
Duodenum
C
Suture of end of duct
D
Pylorus
E
Head of pancreas
Superior mesenteric vessels

F.—Allis forceps are placed on the body of the pancreas slightly to the left of the desired site of division. The pancreas is transected by sharp dissection. It is well to isolate the main pancreatic duct and to leave a small protruding stump on the left portion of the gland.

G.—The duodenum and head of the pancreas are now fixed only by the fourth portion of the duodenum which is clamped as far to the left as possible while at the same time leaving a stump sufficiently long to permit closure and inversion of the distal end. Two clamps are placed across the duodenum and the bowel divided between them. The proximal duodenum and head of the pancreas are now completely resected.

H.—The distal end of the divided duodenum is closed by an inversion suture placed over the clamp. Use of a continuous cotton suture minimizes the danger of leakage. A second inverting row should be placed over the first.

I.—The advisability or necessity of anastomosing the cut end of the pancreas to the jejunum is debatable. If one decides against this procedure, the pancreatic duct should be carefully ligated and the cut end of the gland well oversewn to prevent leakage of pancreatic juice into the peritoneal cavity. The divided surface of the pancreas is first oversewn by interlocking mattress sutures of cotton. A second continuous over-and-over suture is placed across the end of the gland.

Pancreaticojejunostomy.—*J.*—If an anastomosis is decided upon, it should be made between the cut end of the pancreas and the limb of jejunum extending from the cholecystojejunostomy to the entero-anastomosis. It should be made as close to the cholecystoenterostomy as is possible without placing tension upon the anastomosis. This is usually a distance of 3–4 in. Before anastomosis the cut end of the pancreas should be oversewn with interlocking mattress sutures, with care taken not to ligate the cut end of the duct of Wirsung. This duct should be probed to make sure that it is patent and has not been ligated. A row of interrupted cotton sutures is placed between the posterior surface of the pancreas 3 mm. to the left of the divided edge and the serosal surface of the jejunum in a longitudinal direction. The jejunal wall is incised the length of the first row of sutures and about 5 mm. anterior to it. The incision is carried down to the mucosa.

[Second stage *continued on page 322.*]

PLATE 70

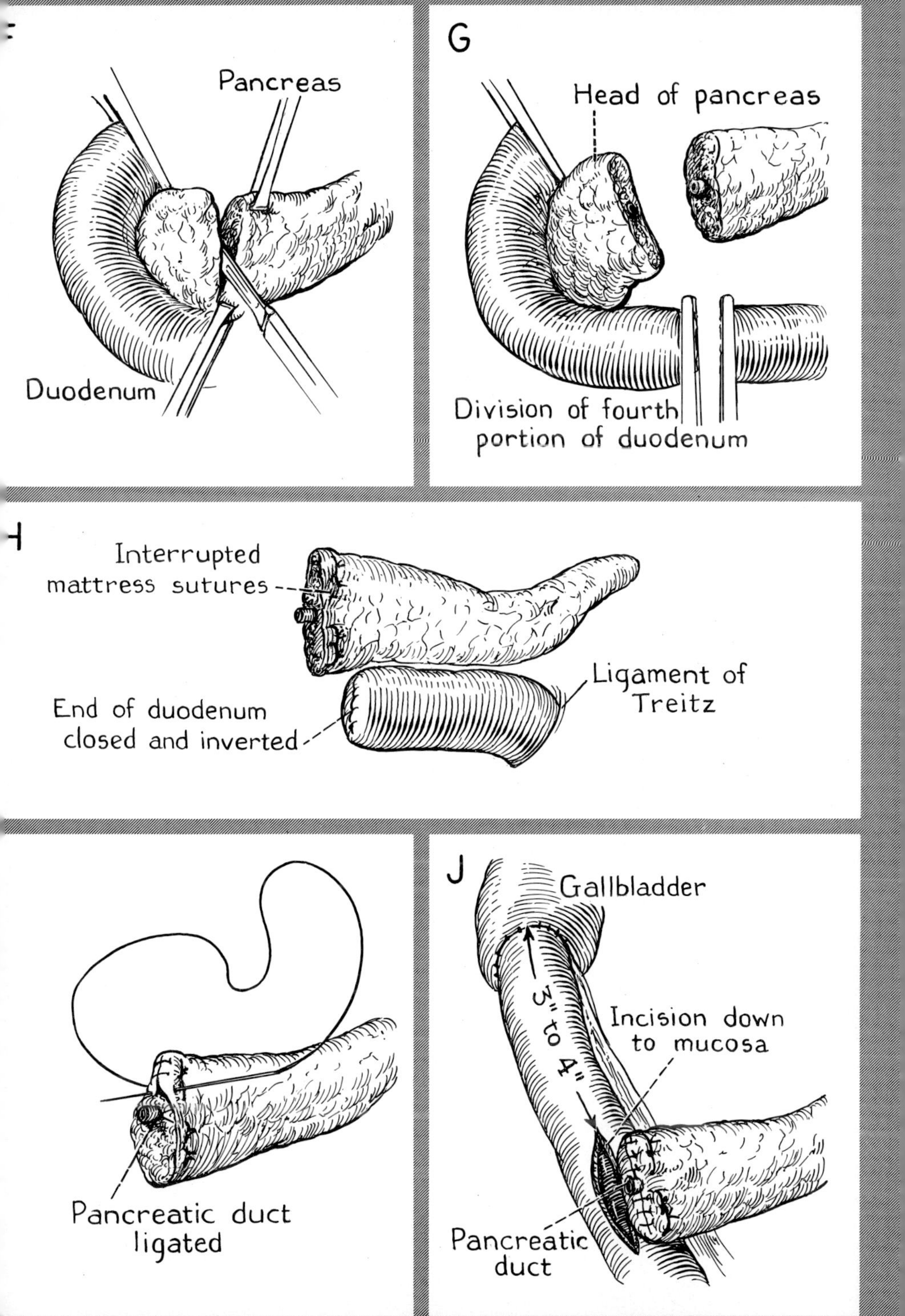

Pancreas
Duodenum
G
Head of pancreas
Division of fourth portion of duodenum
Interrupted mattress sutures
Ligament of Treitz
End of duodenum closed and inverted
Pancreatic duct ligated
J
Gallbladder
3" to 4"
Incision down to mucosa
Pancreatic duct

K.—If the pancreatic duct is dilated, an anastomosis may be made between it and the mucosa of the bowel. An incision is made in the bowel mucosa equal in size to the diameter of the duct. Interrupted cotton sutures are placed between the edge of the duct and the edge of the mucosa of the jejunum on the posterior half.

L.—A piece of rubber tubing as large as can be placed into the duct is inserted into the pancreatic duct with about 2 in. extending into the jejunum. The anterior row of sutures is placed, completing the mucosa-to-mucosa anastomosis of the duct to the jejunal mucosa. Interrupted cotton sutures are placed between the anterior surface of the pancreas and the jejunal wall anterior to the longitudinal incision.

M.—If the pancreatic duct is small, a direct anastomosis of the duct to the mucosa of the jejunum may not be feasible. Under such circumstances, the entire cut end of the pancreas should be anastomosed to the jejunal wall. The incision in the mucosa of the jejunum is made to equal that of the outer layer of sutures. A posterior inner row of catgut sutures is inserted between the cut posterior edge of the pancreas and the full thickness of the posterior edge of the jejunal wall.

N.—This suture is continued around anteriorly to form an anterior inner row. An anterior outer row of interrupted cotton sutures is placed between the anterior surface of the pancreas 3 mm. to the left of the divided surface and the anterior wall of the jejunum close to the line of incision.

[Second stage *continued on page 324.*]

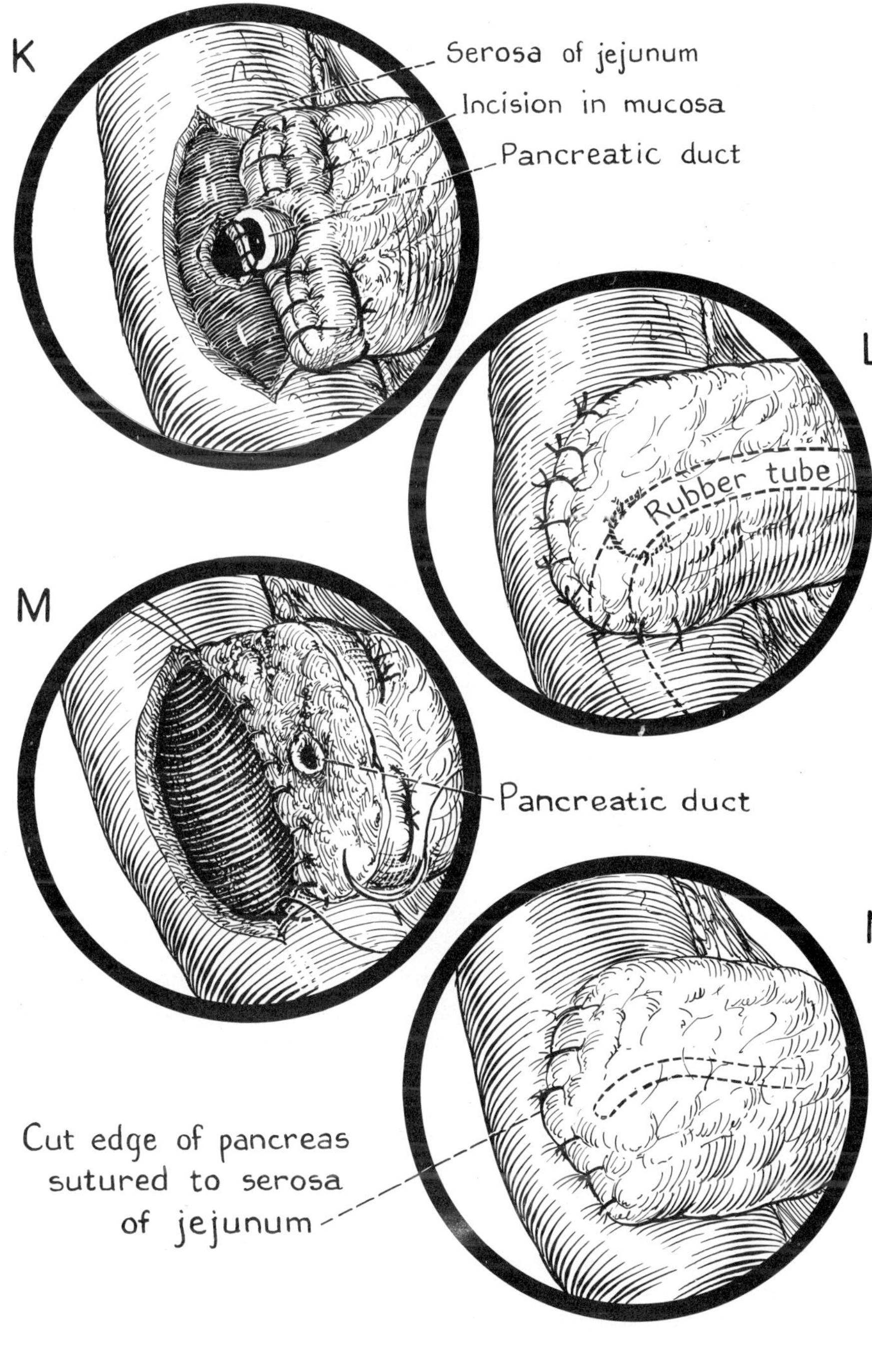
K
Serosa of jejunum
Incision in mucosa
Pancreatic duct
L
Rubber tube
M
Pancreatic duct
N
Cut edge of pancreas sutured to serosa of jejunum

Gastrojejunostomy.–O.–The divided end of the pyloric portion of the stomach should be anastomosed to the jejunum at a site several inches distal to the pancreaticojejunostomy. The anastomosis is made as an end-to-side anastomosis between the end of the stomach and the side of the jejunum longitudinally on its antimesenteric border. The jejunum is grasped with a covered forceps placed longitudinal to the bowel. A second covered clamp is placed across the pyloric end of the stomach parallel to and 2 in. proximal to the Payr clamp at the cut end. The two covered clamps are placed parallel to each other and supported in this position by appropriate clamps. After suitable draping, the anastomosis is made. A posterior outer row of sutures between the posterior wall of the stomach and the jejunum is inserted as a continuous suture, running the full width of the stomach from greater to lesser curvatures.

P.–An incision is made 5 mm. from the suture line through the posterior wall of the stomach to, but not through, the mucosa. The blood vessels encountered should be clamped on their proximal side and ligated. The incision is then carried through the mucosa of the posterior wall of the stomach.

Q.–An incision of equal length, about 5 mm. above the posterior outer suture line, is made through all thicknesses of the jejunum. The posterior inner row consists of a continuous suture of intestinal catgut passing through all layers of both the jejunum and the stomach. After this layer has been placed, the Payr clamp is removed by division of the anterior wall of the stomach.

R.–The posterior inner row is continued around anteriorly, passing through all layers of the jejunum and stomach and everting the edges of both structures. The end of this suture is tied to its beginning, completing the inner rows.

S.–The covered clamps are then removed and the anterior outer row of sutures is placed, inverting the anterior inner row. This completes the anastomosis. Intestinal catgut should be used for the inner rows in all cases. In well nourished patients catgut may be used for the outer rows, but in severely debilitated patients cotton may be preferable. When a nonabsorbable suture is used, the posterior row may be continuous but the anterior row should be of interrupted sutures.

[Second stage *continued on page 326.*]

PLATE 70

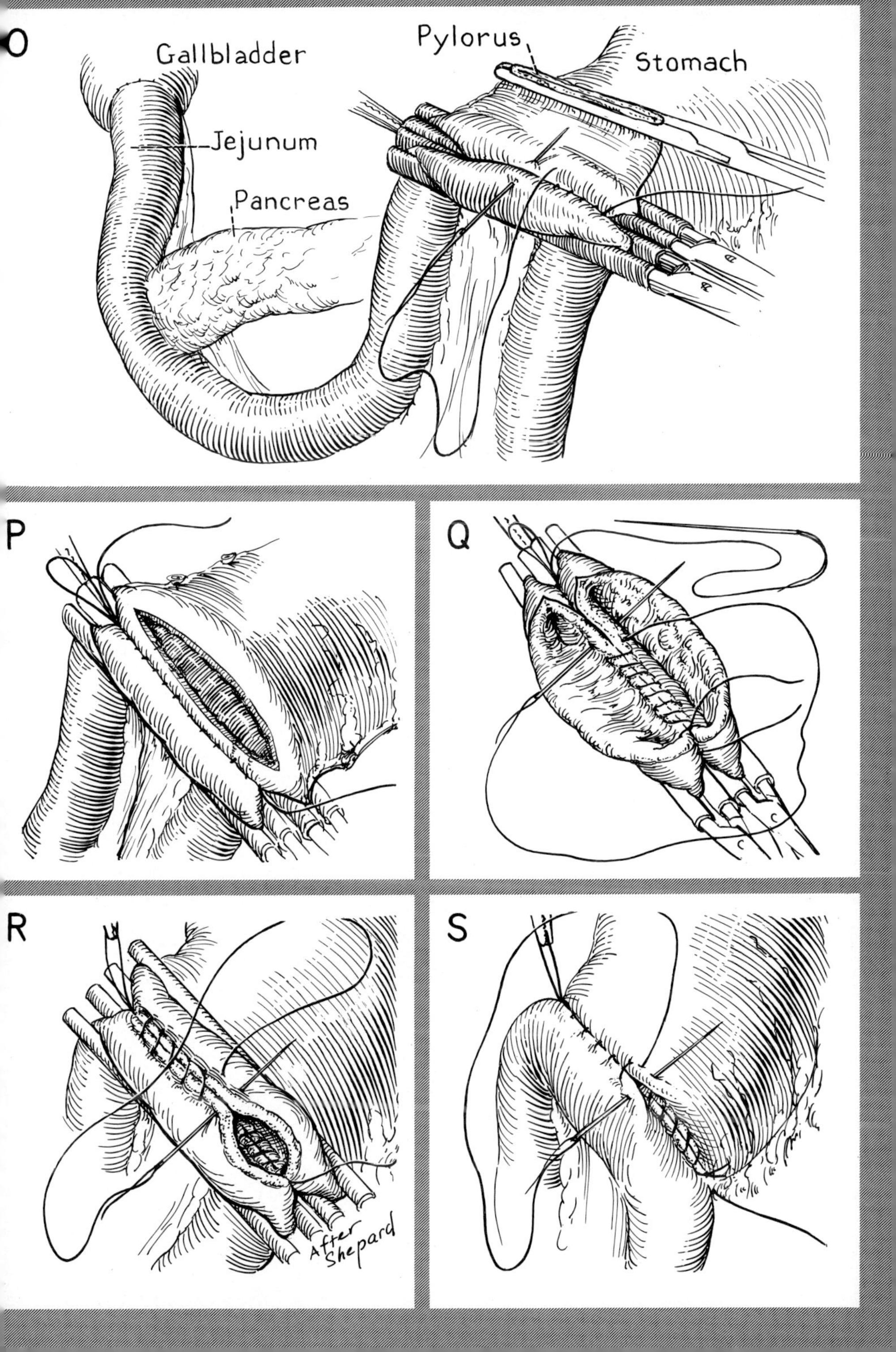
O
Gallbladder
Pylorus
Stomach
Jejunum
Pancreas
P
Q
R
After Shepard
S

T.—The foregoing procedure completes the anastomosis. The end of the divided jejunum is anastomosed to the gallbladder. Distal to this anastomosis, in order, are the pancreaticojejunostomy, the gastrojejunostomy and the jejunojejunostomy below the ligament of Treitz. As peristalsis runs from the gallbladder to the pancreatic anastomosis and then to the stomach anastomosis, there is no tendency for peristalsis to carry gastric contents past and into the biliary ducts and thus encourage cholangitis and hepatitis.

At the conclusion of the second stage of the operation, the abdominal wound is closed in layers with a Penrose drain extending to the subhepatic space.

VARIATIONS.—Many modifications and variations of this technic have been described for pancreaticoduodenectomy. Variations in anatomic and pathologic findings encountered in different patients may make it advisable to vary the type and location of certain anastomoses. However, I think it important that anastomoses be made in such positions that gastric content will not pass over the anastomosis between the extrahepatic biliary tract and the jejunum and thus encourage an ascending biliary tract infection.

U.—This illustrates one type of modification in which the fourth portion of the duodenum is anastomosed to the stomach. A pancreaticojejunostomy has not been made.

V.—Some surgeons prefer to anastomose a loop of jejunum to the gallbladder in the first stage of the operation and then to perform an enteroanastomosis between the two limbs of bowel going to and from the gallbladder. It is argued that gastric contents will pass through the enteroanastomosis and will be unlikely to enter the biliary tree. I believe, however, that this type of anastomosis offers a greater chance for biliary tract infection since gastric contents can continue up the afferent loop and enter the bile ducts.

Occasionally, at the first stage of the operation, the gallbladder may be found to be diseased or unsuitable for anastomosis. Under such circumstances, it is well to open and explore the common duct and insert a T-tube for drainage. The second stage of the operation may then be carried out by a technic similar to the one-stage operation (Plate 71).

T

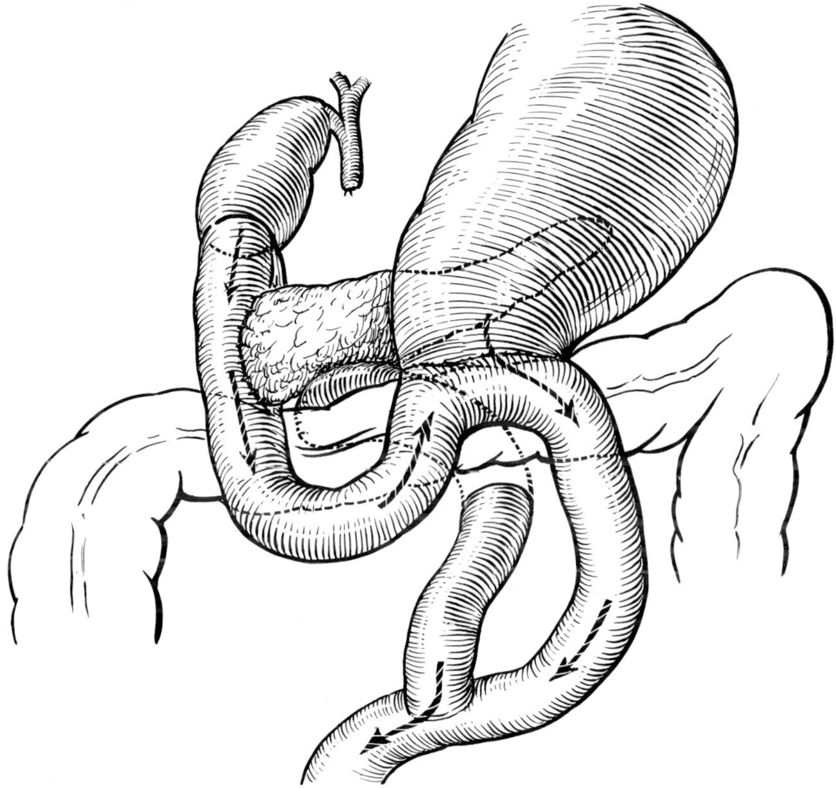

U

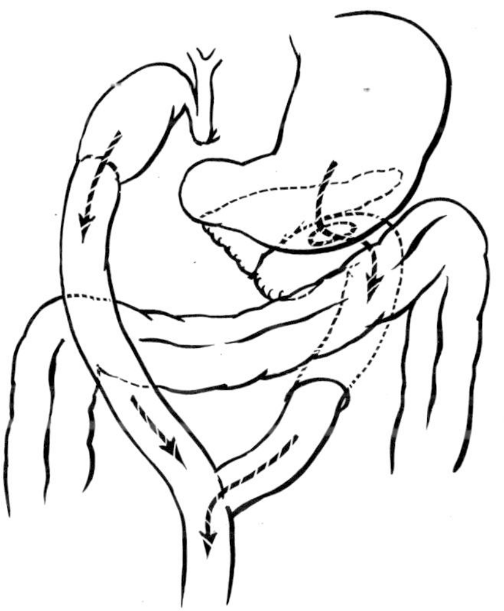

V

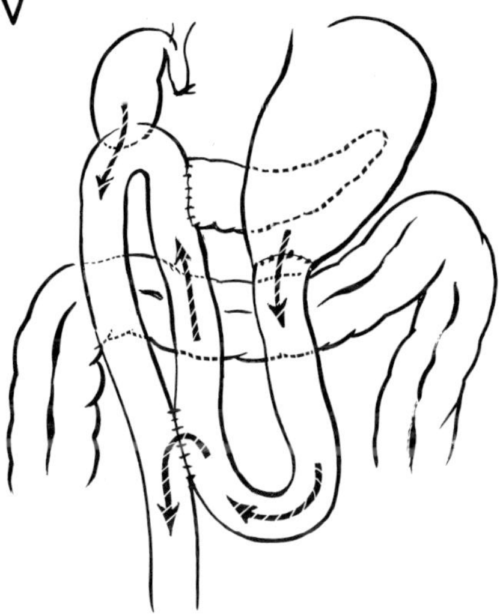

Whipple's Operation

If the nutritional state of the patient will permit, resection of the duodenum and pancreas may be completed in one stage. Many modifications of this operation have been devised but we have found the one recommended by Whipple to be most satisfactory. The technical procedures for the various anastomoses are similar to those described in the two-stage operation. The steps of this operation are as follows. The abdomen is opened through a long, upper right rectus incision. A careful exploration is made for metastases to the liver, adjacent or prevertebral glands or to any structure at a distance from the pancreas. A biopsy of the suspected tumor is made and a frozen-section diagnosis obtained. If this demonstrates the presence of a malignancy, resection may be undertaken if it is technically feasible.

A.—The gastrocolic omentum is divided between clamps along the distal third of the greater curvature of the stomach. The posterior wall of the stomach is freed from the pancreas. The right border of the duodenum is freed by division of the reflecting peritoneum. The second and third portion of the duodenum and the head of the pancreas are mobilized by finger dissection of their posterior surfaces.

B.—The first portion of the duodenum is freed by division of the gastrohepatic omentum at the right and by division of the gastroduodenal artery. The common bile duct is freed from its adjacent structures from the junction of the cystic duct to the duodenum. It is divided close to the duodenum and the distal end ligated. A rubber-covered clamp is placed on the proximal end. The pyloric portion of the stomach is now mobilized and divided between clamps about 2 in. proximal to the pyloric muscles. Dissection of the duodenum is continued distally and along the transverse portion to the ligament of Treitz. The superior mesenteric vessels are carefully elevated from the anterior wall of the fourth portion of the duodenum.

[One-stage pancreaticoduodenal resection *continued on page 330.*]

PLATE 71

A

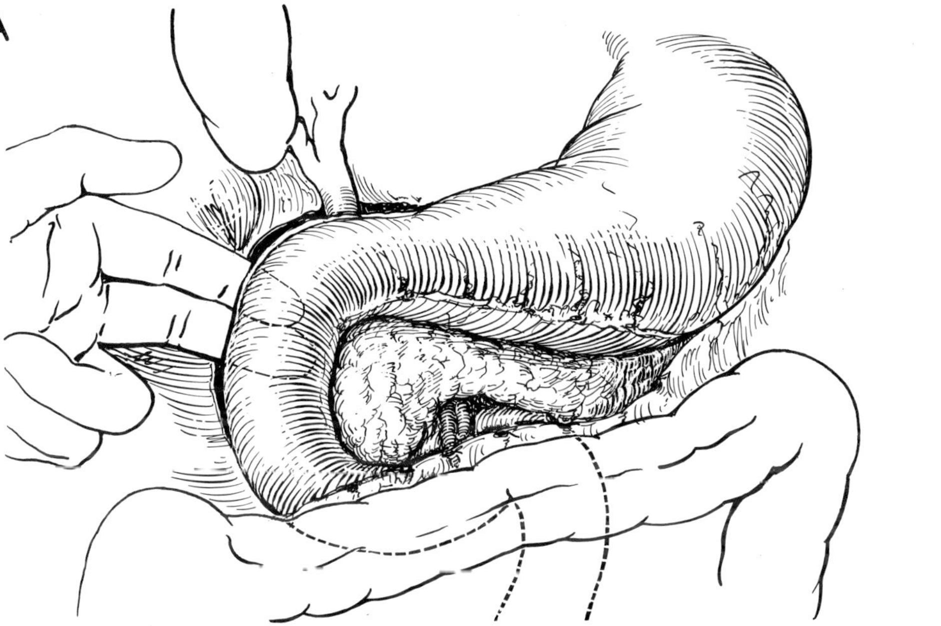

B

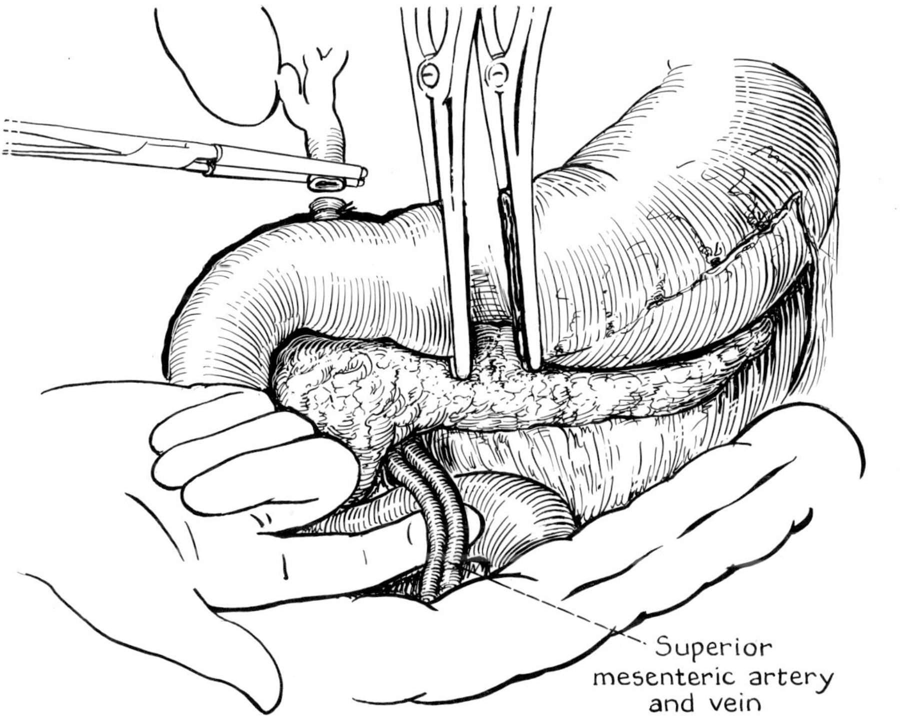

C.—Finger dissection of the fourth portion of the duodenum is continued to the left as far as possible. The transverse colon is then elevated and the proximal jejunum located at the ligament of Treitz. The transverse mesocolon and all existing ligaments and bands between it and the small bowel are separated from the jejunum at the duodenojejunal juncture. This dissection is continued until the entire distal duodenum is freed from all attachments. The jejunum is examined to determine the most proximal point at which it may be divided and at which its mesentery will be of sufficient length to permit elevation of the distal end to the site of the common duct. Such a point can usually be found a few inches below the ligament of Treitz. The jejunum is divided between clamps and its mesentery incised as far as possible. The proximal end of the divided jejunum is closed by an inverting suture. The mesentery to this proximal segment is divided parallel to the bowel, completely mobilizing this segment. At this stage the duodenum and proximal segment of jejunum may be withdrawn from under the mesenteric artery and brought above the transverse mesocolon.

D.—The stomach may now be elevated, exposing the anterior surface of the pancreas. The head of the pancreas is elevated and by careful dissection is freed from the portal vein and superior mesenteric vessels. Great care must be taken not to damage these vessels. Mobilization of the posterior surface of the pancreas is continued to the left for a slight distance beyond the desired site of resection.

[One-stage pancreaticoduodenal resection *continued on page 332.*]

C

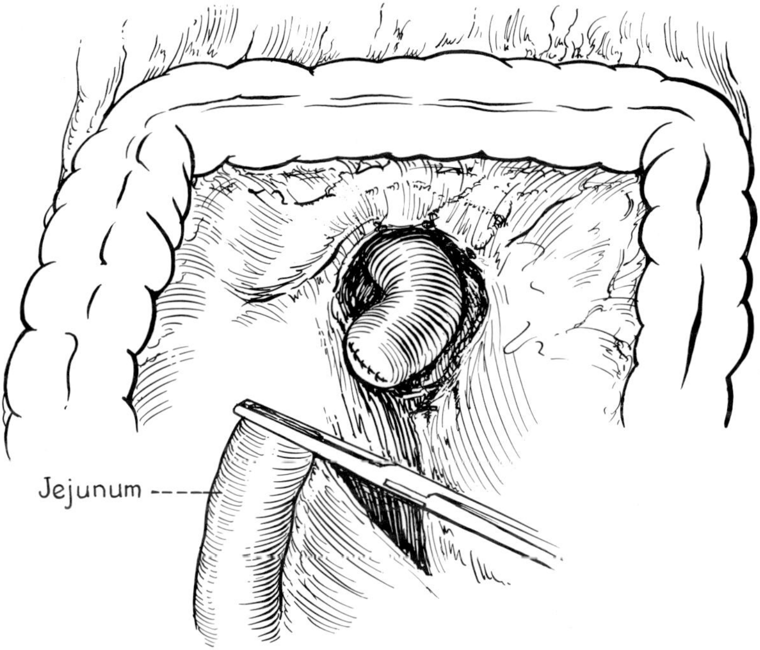
Jejunum

D

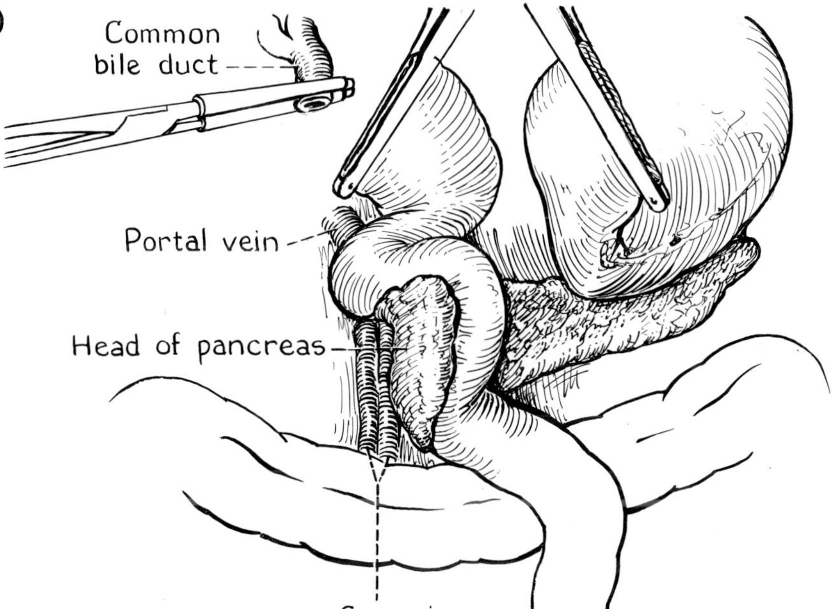
Common bile duct
Portal vein
Head of pancreas
Superior mesenteric vessels

E.—The neck or body of the pancreas is cut across by sharp dissection. This completely frees the head and neck of the pancreas, the entire duodenum and a small segment of pylorus and of jejunum.

F.—The distal end of the jejunum is brought through the opening in the transverse mesocolon and is anastomosed to the cut end of the common bile duct. This is accomplished by an end-to-end anastomosis using an inner row of continuous catgut and an outer row of interrupted cotton.

The end of the pancreas is now anastomosed to the side of the jejunum a short distance distal to the choledochojejunal anastomosis. The site of this anastomosis should be selected so as to avoid traction on the previous anastomosis. The technic of this anastomosis is similar to that employed in the two-stage procedure. The divided end of the stomach should now be anastomosed to the jejunum several inches distal to the pancreaticojejunostomy. This completes the anastomoses since there is no remaining loop of upper small bowel. The gallbladder has been left intact in case it may subsequently be needed for a short-circuiting operation if a stricture should occur. A drain should be placed under the liver and the wound closed in layers.

[One-stage pancreaticoduodenal resection *continued on page 334.*]

E

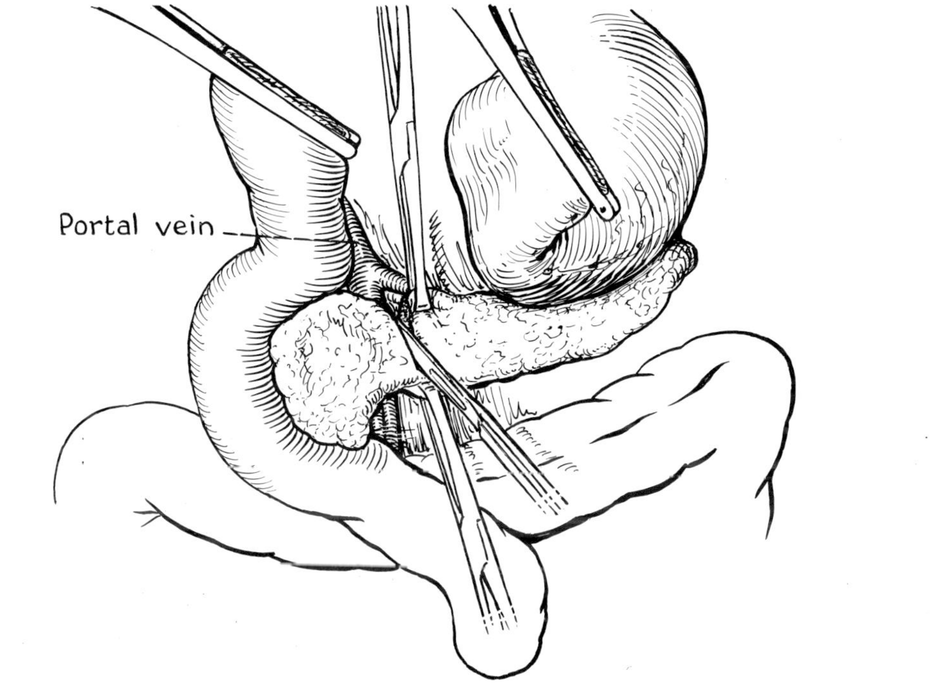
Portal vein

F

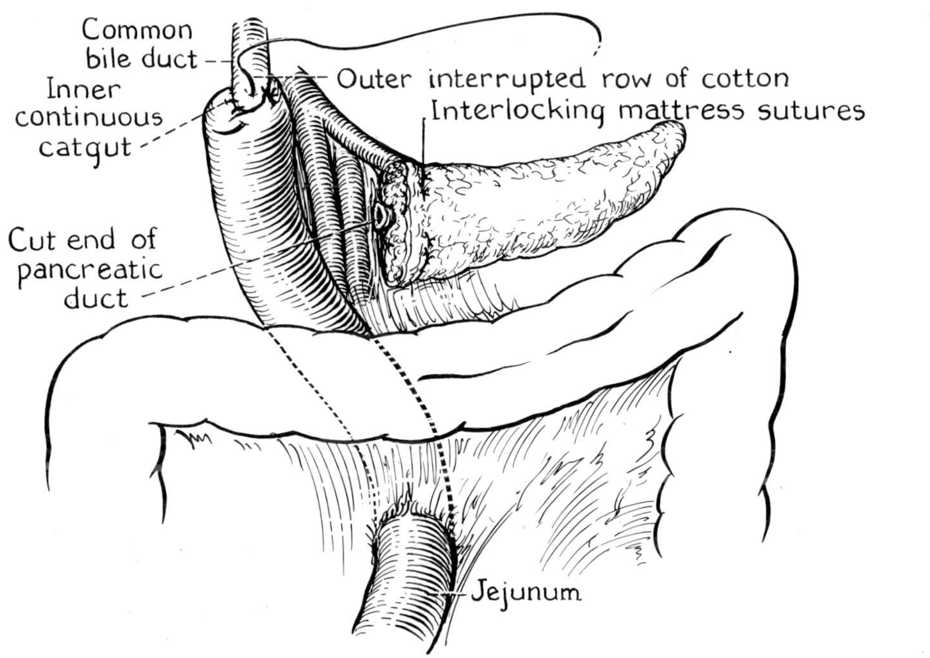
Common
bile duct
Outer interrupted row of cotton
Interlocking mattress sutures
Inner
continuous
catgut
Cut end of
pancreatic
duct
Jejunum

G.—The completed one-stage pancreaticoduodenectomy is shown. The arrows indicate the direction of peristalsis going from the bile duct distalward across the pancreas and past the gastrojejunal anastomosis. This diagram shows the jejunum passing through an opening in the transverse mesocolon. It usually is preferable to have this limb of jejunum retrocolic to minimize traction on the mesentery and to prevent it from causing any obstruction to the passage of contents through the transverse colon. If the mesentery to the jejunum is sufficiently long for the distal end of the divided segment to be brought to the end of the common duct without traction and with ample room for the transverse colon, there is no objection to an antecolic anastomosis.

VARIATIONS.—*H.*—If the carcinoma is confined to the ampulla, there is no indication for removal of the entire duodenum, and modification of the one-stage procedure is satisfactory. The fourth portion of the duodenum is divided and the distal end closed. A loop of jejunum is then brought up anterior to the transverse colon. The common bile duct, pancreas and pyloric end of the stomach are anastomosed to it by end-to-side anastomoses. Care should be exercised to make these anastomoses in the order given.

I.—Another variation in technic is to anastomose the end of the transected pancreas to the open end of the jejunum. The common bile duct is then anastomosed to the jejunum a few inches distal to the pancreaticojejunostomy. The gastrojejunostomy is established several inches distally. Passage of pancreatic juice over the opening into the common bile duct and possible regurgitation into the biliary system does not seem to produce an ascending biliary tract infection or chemical irritation.

In any of these procedures the gallbladder instead of the common duct may be anastomosed to the jejunum if it is not diseased and if the cystic duct is patent. The choice should be governed by the ease with which the anastomosis can be made. Use of the common duct is preferable, keeping the gallbladder in reserve for a subsequent anastomosis if a stricture of the common duct distal to its junction with the cystic duct should occur.

G

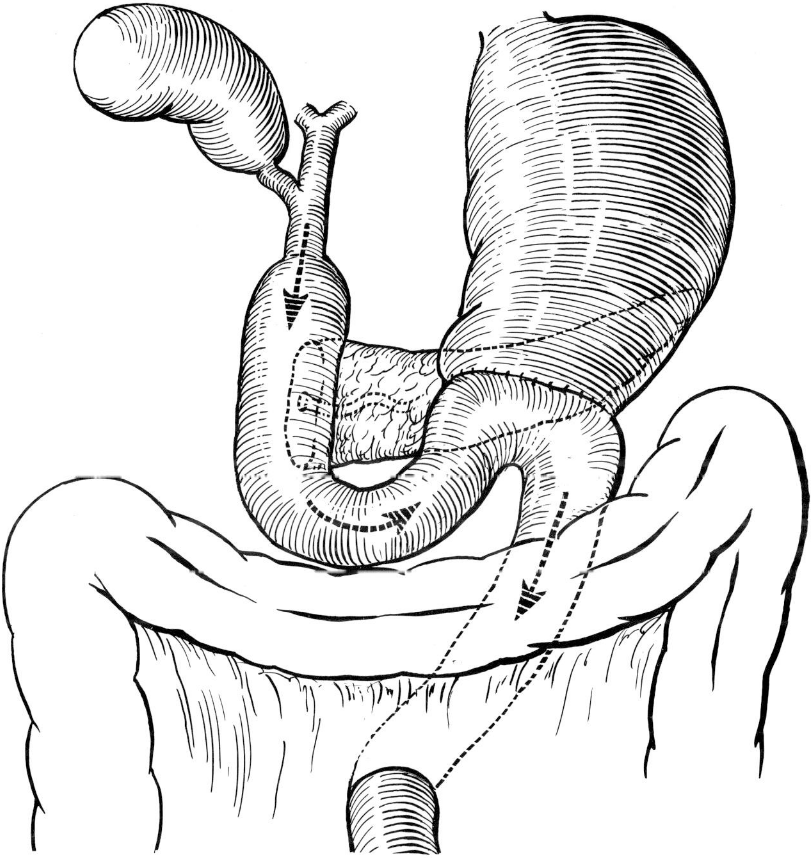

H

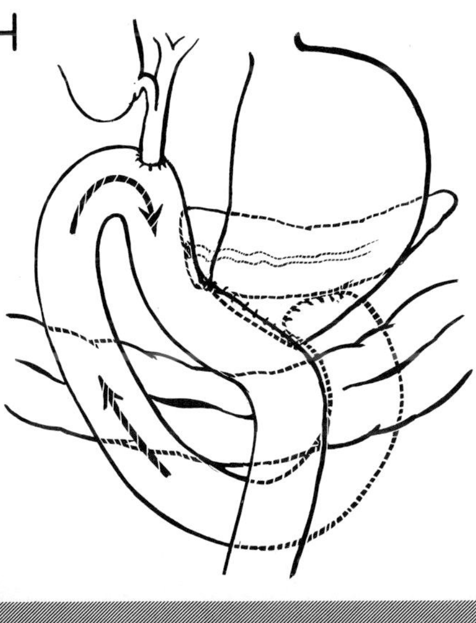

I

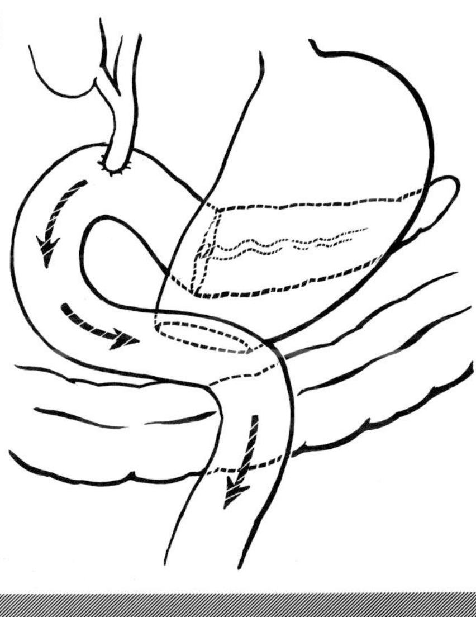

Palliative Procedures for Relief of Biliary Obstruction

When obstructive jaundice exists, the establishment of a functioning anastomosis between the extrahepatic biliary tract and the gastrointestinal tract is preferable to external biliary drainage. Patients improve more rapidly when bile is returned to the gastrointestinal tract than when bile is diverted from the body. If the gallbladder is not diseased and the cystic duct is patent, use of the gallbladder rather than the common duct for the anastomosis usually is preferable. If the gallbladder cannot be used, it may be necessary to anastomose the common bile duct to the most accessible portion of the gastrointestinal tract, usually the duodenum.

If the gallbladder can be used, it is well to anastomose it to the nearest and most easily accessible portion of the gastrointestinal tract. This usually is the stomach, although occasionally the duodenum lends itself more conveniently to this anastomosis. Some surgeons prefer to anastomose the jejunum to the gallbladder by either the loop or Roux-Y technic. The indications and advantages of the various procedures are given below.

Cholecystogastrostomy.—This procedure is described in Plate 58. Cholecystogastrostomy is usually the simplest type of anastomosis to perform and carries with it a minimal risk. It permits bile to flow into the gastrointestinal tract to help improve or maintain the nutritional state of the patient. The operation has been criticized because it permits gastric acids and food to flow into the biliary tract where they may produce inflammatory changes. However, clinical experience has shown that patients who have an inoperable malignancy obstructing the bile ducts seldom show evidences of cholangitis and hepatitis prior to death from the primary disease. When this operation has been performed for obstruction due to pancreatitis, many patients have lived a normal life span without evidence of an ascending biliary tract infection. When the pancreatitis subsides and the common duct becomes patent the anastomosis between the gallbladder and stomach closes in many instances.

Cholecystoduodenostomy.—In some patients, the anatomic proximity of the gallbladder to the duodenum may permit an anastomosis between these two structures with comparative ease. This operation usually is satisfactory, although the digestive action of duodenal contents in a poorly nourished patient increases the risk of leakage from the suture line and the development of a duodenal fistula.

Cholecystojejunostomy.—This procedure is described in Plate 69. The Roux-Y type of anastomosis minimizes the danger of an ascending biliary tract infection. It is technically no more difficult than an anastomosis to a loop of jejunum and an enteroanastomosis. Either has the disadvantage of admitting bile to the jejunum rather than to the duodenum where its presence is important to digestion and in the prevention of the formation of peptic ulcers.

Choledochoduodenostomy.—This procedure is described in Plate 44. The operation is of value in obstruction of the common duct due to pancreatic malignancy when the gallbladder is diseased or the cystic duct obstructed. An anastomosis between the common duct and the gastrointestinal tract is technically more difficult than one between the gallbladder and the bowel. If the surgeon deems it advisable to explore the common duct, he may wish to utilize an incision in it in an anastomosis to the duodenum.

Cholecystostomy.—Cholecystostomy is described in Plate 30. This procedure will permit an escape of bile and the gradual subsidence of jaundice. However, the external drainage of bile prolongs the debility of the patient unless bile can be restored to the gastrointestinal tract. Bile may be returned to the stomach through a nasal tube but this is somewhat distressing to most patients.

Choledochostomy.—Exploration of the common duct as described in Plate 34 may be indicated, particularly when the nature of the obstruction is obscure. In markedly debilitated patients with malignant obstruction of the distal common duct, it may be advisable to suture a T-tube into the common duct and establish external drainage until the patient has sufficiently improved to permit some form of internal drainage.

SECTION IV

The Spleen

CHAPTER 17

Anatomy and Physiology of the Spleen

ANATOMY

THE SPLEEN IS a large lymphoid organ lying in the left upper abdomen under the ninth, tenth and eleventh ribs and resting against the diaphragm. In the normal adult its weight varies between 100 and 200 Gm., with an average weight of 150 Gm. The spleen has three surfaces, the phrenic, gastric and renal. The phrenic surface is convex and lies against the diaphragm. The medial surface is divided into the gastric and renal surfaces by the hilus of the spleen which is a groovelike area through which the vessels, nerves and lymphatics pass. The gastric or anteromedial surface is adjacent to the cardiac end of the stomach and the splenic flexure of the colon. The renal surface, which lies posterior to the hilus, rests upon the anterior portion of the upper pole of the left kidney and the left adrenal gland. The tail of the pancreas lies in contact with the hilus of the spleen in about 8 per cent of adults. In the rest its tip may be from a few millimeters to 13 cm. from the hilus, with an average distance of 3+ cm. between these structures. The anterior border of the spleen usually is notched. In splenomegaly this notching may be palpable through the anterior abdominal wall.

The spleen is covered with peritoneum which reflects from the organ near the hilus to adjacent organs and structures and forms supporting ligaments as well as investments for nerves, vessels and lymphatics.

Plate 72 demonstrates the relationship of the spleen to adjacent organs and the position of the splenic ligaments.

A is a left lateral view of the upper abdominal contents with removal of the lateral chest and abdominal walls and the left portion of the diaphragm.

B shows a cross-section of the body at the level of the splenic pedicle.

The peritoneal reflections to the stomach constitute the gastrosplenic omentum and contain the vasa brevia. The posterior reflection extends from the upper portion of the spleen onto the undersurface of the diaphragm and is termed the splenodiaphragmatic ligament. The lower portion of the posterior reflection extends over the upper pole of the left kidney and is called the splenorenal ligament. The peritoneal reflections which extend down from the spleen to the splenic flexure of the colon are known as the splenocolic ligament.

The ligaments and their contents are of considerable importance in the technic of splenectomy. The anterior peritoneal reflection is in close proximity to the anterior surface of the splenic vessels and pancreas. The splenorenal ligament usually reflects from the posterior edge of the hilus of the spleen a short distance from the posterior surface of the splenic vessels.

The splenic artery arises from the celiac axis and as it runs transversely to the left gives off small branches to the pancreas. Near the hilus of the spleen it gives off numerous branches, including the superior polar, left gastroepiploic, superior terminal and inferior terminal arteries. The vasa brevia arise from the terminal splenic artery or from its terminal branches. Two or more veins from the hilus of the spleen fuse to form the splenic vein. This courses to the right, inferior to the splenic artery. It receives the left gastroepiploic and several pancreatic veins. As it passes anteriorly to the aorta, it becomes fused with the inferior mesenteric vein and then joins the superior mesenteric vein to form the portal vein. Knowledge of the relationship of the splenic vessels to the pancreas is important in minimizing unexpected bleeding during splenectomy. In our studies the splenic vessels were found to course along the posterior superior surface of the pancreas in 90 per cent of dissections. In 5 per cent they were in contact with the superior anterior surface, in 4 per cent

PLATE 72

A

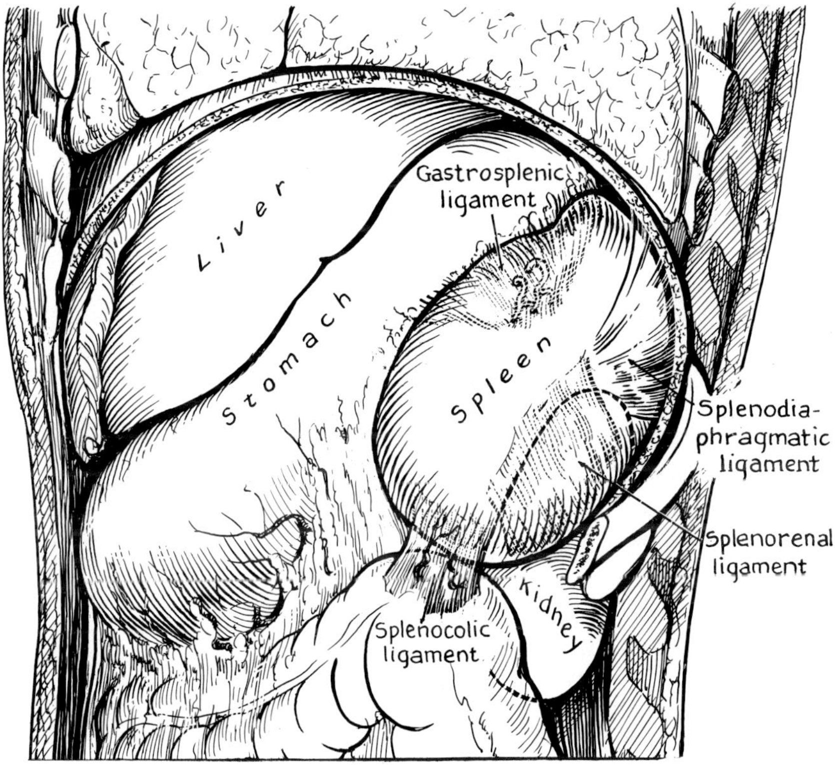
Liver
Stomach
Gastrosplenic ligament
Spleen
Splenodiaphragmatic ligament
Splenorenal ligament
Kidney
Splenocolic ligament

B

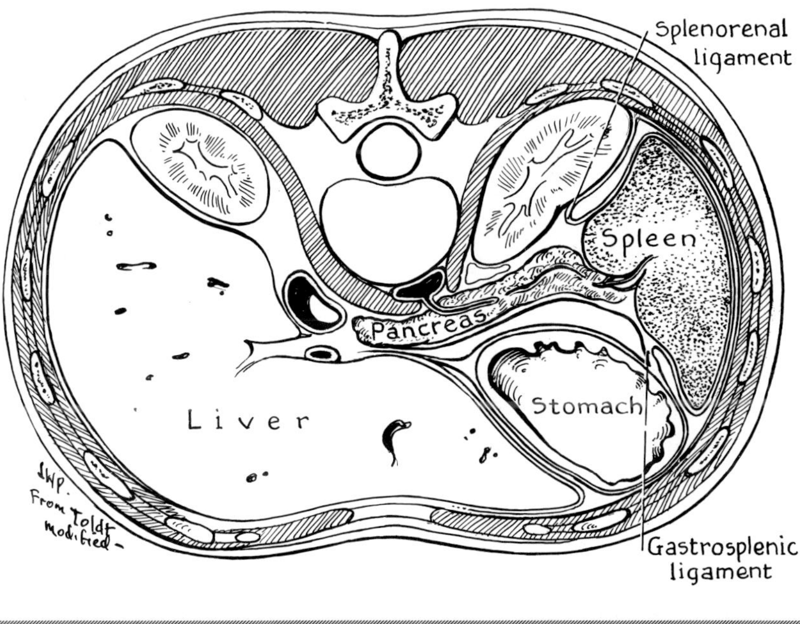
Splenorenal ligament
Spleen
Pancreas
Stomach
Liver
SWP. From Toldt modified-
Gastrosplenic ligament

with the inferior anterior surface and in 1 per cent were posterior and inferior to the pancreas.

Nerves to the spleen originate from the celiac plexus and the right vagus nerve and follow the splenic artery and its branches. The lymphatics of the spleen receive the superficial and deep lymphatics at the hilus and then course through several lymph nodes about the splenic artery to terminate in the celiac glands.

PHYSIOLOGY

The spleen contains the largest collection of lymphoid tissue and the bulk of the reticuloendothelial elements present in the human body. It is intimately concerned with blood destruction and blood formation, although the physiologic mechanism involved in these splenic functions is not known. In fetal life the spleen is active in the formation of all types of blood cells and can revert to this function upon demand at any period of life. In the adult this activity is limited to the production of lymphocytes and monocytes.

The spleen actively participates in the elimination of erythrocytes and products of their disintegration together with bacteria and other foreign matter. This normal process of red blood cell destruction is greatly increased in certain pathologic conditions. In some unknown way, circulating erythrocytes are rendered more fragile by the spleen. By virtue of the reticuloendothelium of the spleen, the hemoglobin from worn-out erythrocytes is converted into bilirubin for passage to the liver. Much of the iron in the body is stored in the spleen and is available for the elaboration of hemoglobin and for the formation of new red blood cells. The spleen, because of its spongy network of pulp, serves as a controllable reservoir system which is of importance in aiding the circulation in volume changes of various kinds. It exerts an inhibitory action on bone marrow hemopoiesis, evidenced by the almost constant occurrence of leukocytosis and thrombocytosis following splenectomy. Other probable functions of the spleen are related to immunity, digestion, metabolism and tumor formation. However, removal of the spleen does not seem to be detrimental to the general well-being of the patient. Certain of its normal functions are shared with other hemopoietic organs and can be quickly taken over after extirpation of the spleen.

CHAPTER 18

Indications and Contraindications for Splenectomy

MOST DISEASES of the spleen are dependent upon disturbances of structure, circulation or other physiologic functions of this organ. Indications for splenectomy are based almost exclusively upon clinical and hematologic evaluation. Splenomegaly is not always an indication for splenectomy. Patients with splenic enlargement may be divided into two groups, in one of which removal of the spleen is alleviative or curative and in the other, is contraindicated.

Splenectomy is indicated in certain hematologic disorders. Torsion and rupture of the spleen frequently demand its removal. In extensive surgical procedures on organs of the left upper abdomen, splenectomy often facilitates the performance of a more complete or more satisfactory operation.

Splenectomy is contraindicated in rapid splenic enlargements from acute infections, splenic metastasis from malignant tumors, parasitic infestations such as trichinosis, filariasis, kala-azar and distomiasis, pernicious anemia and polycythemia. Splenectomy is usually contraindicated in leukemia, lymphoma, hereditary leptocytosis (Mediterranean anemia or Cooley's anemia), hemoglobinopathies, myeloid metaplasia and echinococcus disease. In general, splenectomy may be beneficial in any disease which involves the spleen if a hypersplenic state can be demonstrated. A hypersplenic state is usually present whenever any one or all of the blood cells (erythrocytes, leukocytes and thrombocytes) show a decrease below normal in the peripheral blood and an increase in the bone marrow. The manifestations of hypersplenism are thought to result from a combination of three mechanisms. The spleen, being a large reticuloendothelial organ, may produce antibodies which attach onto blood cells and cause the damaged cells to agglutinate, lyse or be removed more rapidly from the circulation by the reticuloendothelial organs. This mechanism is responsible for most of the acquired hemolytic anemias, thrombocytopenic purpuras and leukopenias which result from certain drug reactions. It is believed that under certain conditions the spleen may remove blood cells from the circulation at a greater than normal rate. The spleen may also release a hormone which is capable of preventing completion of normal hemopoietic maturation in the marrow. This is the explanation usually given for the "maturation arrest" found in the bone marrow in some patients with enlarged spleens.

TABLE 1.—INDICATIONS FOR SPLENECTOMY

1. Splenic trauma
2. Wandering spleen
3. Splenic tumors
4. To facilitate left upper quadrant surgery
5. Splenomegaly producing pressure symptoms
6. Hypersplenism
   a) Idiopathic hypersplenism
   b) Portal hypertension
      *(1) Congestive splenomegaly (Banti's syndrome)
      (2) Splenic vein thrombosis
   **c*) Metastatic malignant tumors
   d) Hypersplenism due to splenic involvement from disorders listed in Table 2
   e) Idiopathic thrombocytopenic purpura
   f) Hereditary spherocytosis (congenital hemolytic jaundice)
   **g*) Acquired hemolytic anemias not controlled by steroid therapy
      (1) Idiopathic
      (2) Secondary to underlying processes listed in Table 2

*In selected cases.

Tables 1 and 2 list those conditions which may be benefited by splenectomy and those for which the operation is contraindicated.

TABLE 2.—CONTRAINDICATIONS AND CONDITIONS NOT AIDED BY SPLENECTOMY

*1. Leukemia
*2. Lymphomas
3. Polycythemia vera (Vaquez-Osler disease)
*4. Myeloid metaplasia of the spleen
*5. Metabolic splenomegalies
*6. Cooley's anemia (thalassemia)
*7. Sickle cell anemia
*8. Idiopathic refractory anemia, hypoplastic anemia, aplastic anemia
9. Cirrhosis of the liver
10. Splenomegalic states due to parasites
11. Acute splenic tumors due to infections

*Splenectomy may be indicated in unusual circumstances associated with pancytopenia or hemolytic anemia.

TRAUMATIC CONDITIONS OF THE SPLEEN

RUPTURE.—Rupture of the spleen must be considered in all patients who have sustained abdominal or chest injuries. Automobile accidents in which the victim is thrown against the steering wheel or against the side of the car, striking the upper abdomen, left flank or the lower left chest frequently cause damage to this organ. Such injuries may also result from falls, blows of varying severity and industrial accidents. Fixation of the spleen by its various ligaments, its close proximity to the ribs and its friable consistency render this organ particularly vulnerable to injury. Diseases such as malaria and syphilis, tumors and splenomegaly of other causes increase the friability of the spleen and make it more susceptible to injury. A large proportion of patients who sustain traumatic rupture of the spleen will die if not treated surgically. The operative mortality will be determined largely by the amount of blood lost and the facilities available for its replacement and by the delay between the time of injury and surgical intervention.

Symptomatology.—The symptoms produced by traumatic rupture of the spleen are largely dependent upon the location and amount of internal hemorrhage. These in turn are dependent on the extent of injury to the organ and the presence or absence of a primary tear in its capsule (Plate 73). Associated injuries to surrounding structures, particularly fractures of the lower left ribs and injuries to the spine or adjacent organs, may mask the symptoms of splenic injury. If the injury does not produce a tear of the splenic capsule, bleeding will occur into the organ or into the adjacent retroperitoneal space through the pedicle. Such injuries permit slow bleeding with little peritoneal reaction. Tenderness may be elicited in the left upper abdomen; it increases with progressive hemorrhage and is accompanied by a gradually enlarging and eventually palpable spleen. When the capsule is torn, symptoms are produced by blood in the adjacent peritoneal cavity. Irritation to the undersurface of the diaphragm produces pain which often radiates to the left shoulder. Peritoneal irritation results in pain in the left upper abdomen or flank which may be severe or dull with gradually increasing intensity. Rigidity of the left upper abdomen will be present. With continued bleeding, pain, tenderness and rigidity extend down along the left abdominal wall and flank to involve the entire side and then may spread to the right and involve the entire abdomen. Large amounts of blood produce flank dulness. Because of the ability of the blood vascular system to accommodate itself to alterations in blood volume, internal bleeding may result in considerable blood loss before changes in blood pressure and pulse rate are produced. If advanced internal hemorrhage occurs and surgical treatment is not instituted early, the typical picture of shock with rapid pulse, low blood pressure, cold, clammy skin, subnormal temperature, air hunger and apprehension will result.

Frequently a period of symptomatic silence follows the initial symptoms of the injury and gives the surgeon a false sense of security. During this period, if there is a suspicion of rupture of the spleen, surgical exploration and splenectomy are indicated. This is a safe procedure and will avoid the dangers incident to subsequent hemorrhage and shock. If rupture of the spleen is suspected and immediate operation is ruled out because of the subsidence of symptoms, the patient should be kept under careful observation so that surgery may be undertaken at once if there are a sudden return and rapid progression of symptoms.

A ruptured spleen occasionally will show little or no immediate evidence of hemorrhage, or there may be an apparent cessation of bleeding for a number of days. Later, sudden symptoms of severe internal hemorrhage will occur. This is due to progressive subcapsular bleeding which may distend the splenic capsule with as much as 1 L. or more of blood. Subcapsular bleeding may be suspected by careful and repeated abdominal examinations. When the capsule finally ruptures, the patient presents symptoms of massive intraperitoneal hemorrhage and shock. Serial blood counts taken during the course of continued subcapsular hemorrhage will reveal progressive secondary anemia and neutrophilic leukocytosis.

Treatment.—The friability of the spleen and the tendency for subcapsular hemorrhage to occur and progress make any attempt to repair splenic injury hazardous. The minimal importance of the spleen and the ability of the body to adjust to its loss with no apparent ill effects are additional reasons for removing the spleen in all cases of trauma.

Early diagnosis, careful observation, the realization that symptomatic silence may follow serious injuries to the spleen and the institution of early splenectomy in suspected cases are essential to successful treatment.

PENETRATING WOUNDS.—Penetrating wounds, inflicted by knives and other sharp objects or by bullets, frequently result in severe splenic hemorrhage. The wound of entrance often is in the chest with the foreign body traversing the lung and diaphragm before striking the spleen. Such wounds demand careful observation and early exploration if there is a suspicion of splenic injury. When the spleen is involved, it should be removed.

TORSION OF THE SPLEEN.—A spleen with loose ligamentous attachment, especially when enlarged, may undergo torsion and, in so doing, strangulation may result. The symptoms depend upon the degree of torsion and secondary strangulation. With pre-existing splenomegaly, if acute left upper abdominal symptoms develop which are consistent with torsion of the spleen, surgical exploration should be considered. Mild degrees of ptosis predispose to torsion of the spleen.

A.—Traumatic rupture of the spleen with tearing of the splenic capsule is illustrated. Bleeding from such injuries produces early and progressive symptoms of peritoneal irritation.

B.—A cross-section of a spleen following injury shows multiple hemorrhages throughout the organ. The capsule has not been torn.

C.—Profuse subcapsular hemorrhage may follow injury in the region of the splenic pedicle without rupture of the capsule of the spleen. In such injuries small, continuous subcapsular bleeding may occur, with progressive distention of the capsule. This may result in delayed rupture of the capsule many days after injury, producing evidences of massive intraperitoneal hemorrhage and shock.

D.—Cross-section of *C* shows a large subcapsular hematoma originating in the region of the splenic pedicle.

E.—A roentgenogram taken after a barium enema shows medial displacement of the splenic flexure and the proximal descending colon by an enlarged spleen. Such studies are of value in demonstrating splenic enlargements due to hemorrhage, tumor or other disease.

F.—In this anteroposterior roentgenogram of the left abdomen, the psoas muscle and an enlarged spleen are seen. When retroperitoneal hemorrhage occurs, the psoas shadow usually is obliterated.

PLATE 73

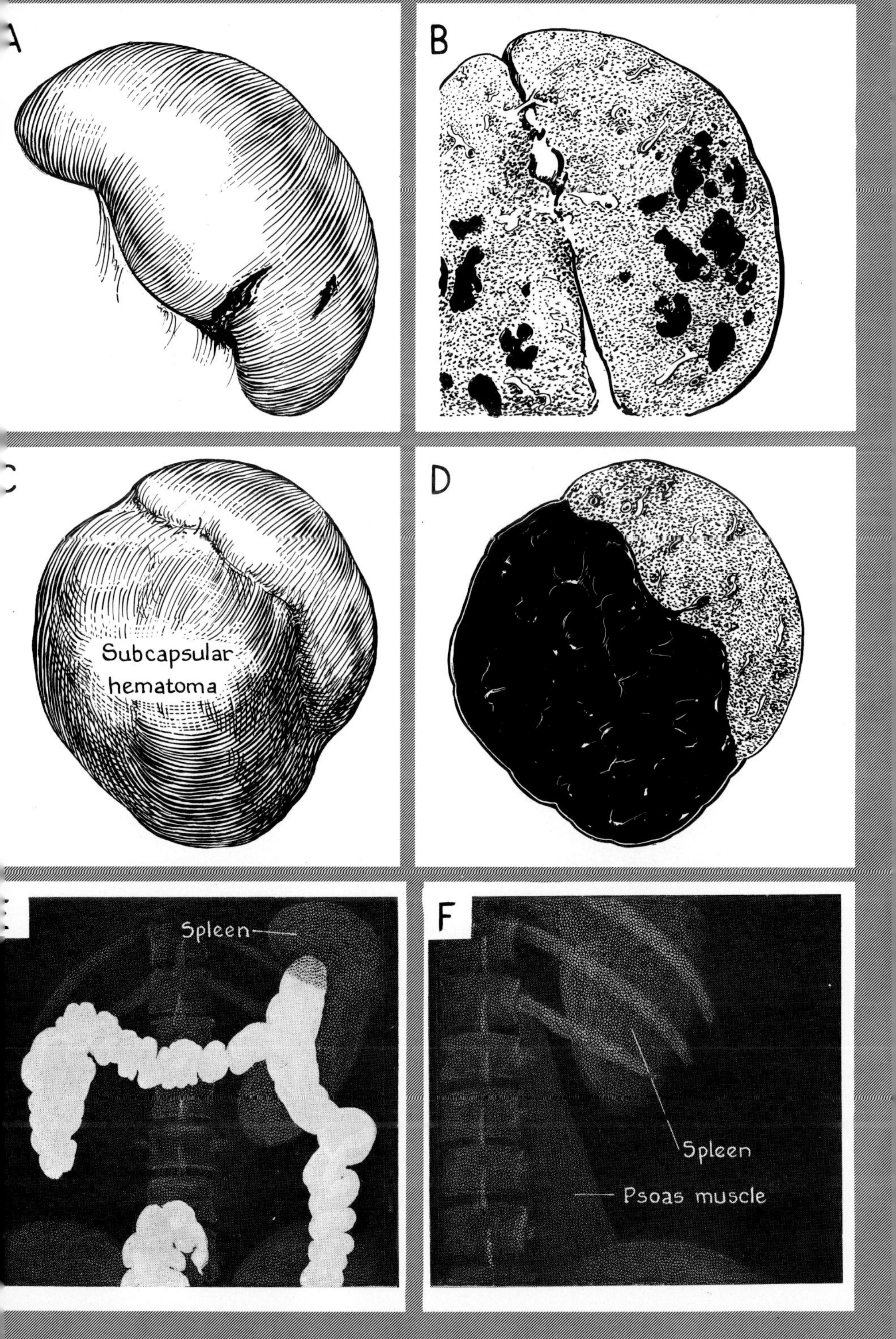

Wandering Spleen

Abnormal positions of the spleen in all parts of the abdomen have been reported. The condition is commoner in females than in males. As is true in ptosis of other organs, displacement of the spleen is due to lax ligamentous attachments. In obese women with flabby abdominal walls and large, roomy pelvic cavities, a wandering spleen may be palpated in the pelvis by rectal or vaginal examination. Prolapse of the spleen into this area may or may not cause symptoms.

Splenopexy or splenectomy may be performed for displacement. Removal of the organ is the procedure of choice because of the functional unimportance of the spleen and the danger incident to attempts at fixation. This is true especially if there has been damage to the spleen secondary to torsion.

Primary Tumors of the Spleen

Primary tumors of the spleen are rare. They may originate from the vascular or supportive elements of the spleen. The sarcomas which have been described include lymphosarcoma, reticulum cell sarcoma and endothelial sarcoma. Leukemias and Hodgkin's disease usually involve the spleen. They cause splenic enlargement with early generalized metastases through the blood stream. Splenectomy would be of little value in these conditions except when a hypersplenic state is present. Various types of angiomas arising from endothelial elements have been reported, ranging from benign lymphangiomas and hemangiomas to the malignant types of hemangioendotheliomas. Cysts of the spleen arising from epithelial and mesothelial elements and dermoids have been described. Splenectomy is the treatment of choice for these primary tumors of the spleen.

Splenectomy as an Aid in Left Upper Abdominal Surgery

Removal of the spleen frequently aids in more adequate exposure of structures in the left upper abdomen and facilitates radical surgical procedures. Many surgeons recommend splenectomy in all total or very high gastric resections. Operations performed through the abdominal approach may be simplified by this procedure. When the transthoracic and transdiaphragmatic approach is used, the spleen frequently is in the way. Its removal can be quickly accomplished with no added danger to the patient. In the surgical extirpation of malignant lesions of organs adjacent to the spleen, more radical resection may be performed by removing the spleen separately or by including it in a block resection, whether or not it is involved by tumor.

Splenomegaly Producing Pressure Symptoms

Occasionally, splenic enlargement may be associated with severe intermittent left upper quadrant pain of sufficient intensity to require narcotics. This symptom is usually alleviated by radiation therapy. In some patients, however, radiation therapy fails to control the distress, so that splenectomy may become necessary.

HYPERSPLENISM

(Splenic Neutropenia and Pancytopenia)

It has been demonstrated that the function of the spleen has an influence on the hemopoiesis in the bone marrow. The exact mechanism by which this "splenic marrow effect" is brought about has not been satisfactorily explained although a hormonal mechanism has been suggested. This hormonal mechanism (hypersplenism) may exercise an inhibitory influence on cell production in the bone marrow or on release of cells to the peripheral blood. When hypersplenism is expressed in the form of an unusual destruction of red blood cells in the spleen, a hemolytic anemia results. Abnormal splenic states may selectively, or in various combinations, exert an unusual effect upon various blood cells and result in certain types of anemia, neutropenia, thrombocytopenia or various combinations of these conditions.

Idiopathic Hypersplenism

Primary splenic neutropenia is characterized by fever, pain over the splenic region and splenic enlargement. The neutropenia is marked. The bone marrow is normal or somewhat hyperplastic. The syndrome may be acute, subacute or chronic. In the primary splenic panhematopenic syndrome there is indiscriminate elimination of all the circulating elements. Leukopenia is the most persistent feature and anemia and thrombocytopenia usually are demonstrable. When the cause for splenomegaly cannot be determined and blood studies show anemia, neutropenia and thrombocytopenia, either singly or in various combinations, the condition may be described as primary hypersplenism. Those syndromes in which the etiology of the splenomegaly can be determined are referred to as secondary splenic neutropenia and panhematopenia. Since they may be associated with many diseases, careful hematologic and bone marrow studies are important in differential diagnosis.

Treatment.—In certain types of anemia, neutropenia or thrombocytopenia and their various combinations, splenectomy is followed by an increase in the number of the previously depleted type of cells in the peripheral blood. In certain cases, splenic pancytopenia associated with a hemolytic component may be corrected by removal of the spleen. Before surgery is undertaken, a careful evaluation and diagnosis should be established by a competent hematologist.

Congestive Splenomegaly

(Banti's Syndrome)

Clinically this syndrome is characterized by signs and symptoms of portal hypertension, anemia, leukopenia and/or thrombocytopenia. Hepatic cirrhosis may or may not be present, depending on the site of obstruction. The pathogenesis of this syndrome is not known. One point of difference seems to be whether portal obstruction is the sole cause or only a contributing factor. The increased portal pressure is followed by congestion in the splenic sinusoids. This is followed by hypertrophy and hyperplasia of the splenic reticulum. A perisplenitis usually occurs and causes peritoneal adhesions which are associated with greatly dilated vasa brevia, making splenectomy a hazardous procedure in the late stages.

Treatment.—Splenectomy is of questionable value in Banti's syndrome. The difficulty in controlling hemorrhage results in a high operative mortality. Furthermore, hemorrhage may recur in one-third to one-half the patients following splenectomy, or the disease may continue to progress, with development of serious hepatic insufficiency. Ligation of the splenic artery has been recommended to cut down the arterial blood supply to the spleen without destroying the venous anastomoses between the portal and systemic systems. This operation is far less hazardous than splenectomy.

If splenectomy is undertaken for Banti's syndrome, the transthoracic and transdiaphragmatic approach makes the spleen more accessible and permits easier control of hemorrhage.

When portal hypertension exists in connection with Banti's syndrome, a portacaval shunt, if feasible, will be of far greater value in reducing the venous pressure in the portal system than other operative procedures.

Splenic Vein Thrombosis

When this phenomenon progresses gradually, the clinical picture is indistinguishable from that of Banti's syndrome. Acute thrombosis is characterized by sudden, acute abdominal pain, pallor and signs of vasomotor collapse. A fatal gastric hemorrhage may follow. When diagnosis can be made, emergency splenectomy should be performed.

Metastatic Malignant Tumors

Tumors arising in distant organs seldom metastasize to the spleen, but involvement from contiguous structures is often noted. Splenectomy occasionally is indicated for metastatic malignancy of the spleen. Because tumors of the proximal stomach may invade the spleen by direct extension or by metastases, wide dissection of all involved structures is desirable. This is particularly important in the transthoracic and transdiaphragmatic approach to gastric neoplasms which have invaded surrounding organs, including the spleen, when mass resection may be of some benefit to the patient. Metastatic malignancy of the spleen which causes symptoms due to pressure or encroachment occasionally is an indication for splenectomy.

Idiopathic Thrombocytopenic Purpura

Thrombocytopenic purpura is a hemorrhagic diathesis resulting from a deficiency in the number of circulating platelets. In the idiopathic variety, the causes for reduced platelets cannot be demonstrated. It is only in this type that splenectomy is beneficial. Clinically, thrombocytopenic purpura is characterized by spontaneous petechiae and/or ecchymoses in the skin, mucous membranes and viscera. Bleeding may occur from the nose, gums, gastrointestinal tract, respiratory tract and genitourinary tract. Intra-cranial bleeding, a serious complication, is a common cause of death, particularly in the adult. The disorder is most common during the first 20 years of life, and females are more frequently affected. Spontaneous remission occurs in 35 per cent of the patients, whereas in 17 per cent the chronic form develops. The chronic form is characterized by cyclic variations in the number of platelets, which may be associated with bleeding episodes. Approximately one third of the patients have enlarged spleens.

The bleeding time is prolonged, and capillary fragility is increased (Rumpel-Leede phenomenon). The coagulation time is normal, but clot retraction is poor. The platelet count is strikingly reduced during bleeding episodes and may be normal during remission. The bone marrow shows a marked increase in immature, mature and degenerated megakaryocytes. Abnormal, free platelets may be seen in blood or in marrow smears. During remission, the morphologic abnormality of the platelets may be the only clue to the patient's disorder, since the other laboratory features may be normal.

Treatment.—Splenectomy is followed by favorable results in 70 per cent or more of patients with idiopathic thrombocytopenic purpura. Relapses are more apt to occur in females than in males. In the acute bleeding phase of the disease, the danger of hemorrhage is great and, if possible, surgery should be delayed until a temporary remission is obtained by the liberal use of blood transfusions. If conservative therapy appears to be ineffective, an emergency splenectomy should be performed to prevent death. The administration of pituitary corticotropin (ACTH) in doses of 50–100 mg. daily or cortisone in doses of 25–100 mg. daily has proved useful in the preparation of the patient for splenectomy. As soon as the rise in the platelet count is sufficient to prevent excessive bleeding, the spleen is removed. A postsplenectomy thrombocytosis may be observed in some patients treated with hormones before the removal of the spleen.

In infants, children and persons over 40, thrombocytopenic purpura usually is mild, undergoes spontaneous remissions induced by blood transfusions and may be completely cured by conservative treatment. In these age brackets splenectomy is only rarely indicated.

Following removal of the spleen, blood platelets may gradually return to a normal level with no reappearance of the bleeding diathesis. Occasionally, the platelet count will fall to the preoperative level without hemorrhagic manifestations. In some patients, however, the platelet count may fall and bleeding recur. This may be due to the presence of an accessory spleen or a splenic tissue rest in other organs. Careful search should be made at the time of operation for such accessory splenic tissue.

Hereditary Spherocytosis (Congenital Hemolytic Jaundice)

This disorder is an erythrocyte (spherocyte) anomaly inherited as a mendelian dominant from either parent. Clinically it is characterized by jaundice, splenomegaly and symptoms of anemia. Cholelithiasis has been reported in as many as 68 per cent of the patients. Leg ulcers are rare. Crises may occur, characterized by symptoms of acute distress and increased anemia. The laboratory findings are diagnostic.

The severity of anemia and of reticulocytosis varies. Diagnosis is based on the erythrocyte morphology, nearly all red cells being spherical instead of the normally biconcave shape. As a result, the patient's erythrocytes have less than normal resistance to solutions of low osmotic pressure (increased osmotic fragility). The bone marrow shows normoblastic hyperplasia (increase in erythrocyte precursors). The indirect serum bilirubin value is increased. Occasionally, stones may pass into the common duct to cause obstructive jaundice. Autoimmune antibodies (positive result of Coombs test) may be found in some patients. They are usually found in patients who have received several transfusions.

Treatment.—Splenectomy is indicated when the diagnosis of congenital hemolytic jaundice is established, and it is advisable at an early age. After removal of the spleen most of the symptoms disappear, although the fundamental defect of the erythrocytes is not entirely abolished.

Blood transfusions administered to patients with congenital hemolytic anemia frequently are followed by severe reactions. For this reason, the administration of blood should be withheld until the spleen has been removed. If the anemia is so severe that splenectomy is hazardous, exceptional care must be used in cross-matching blood and a minimum of blood should be administered. If the patient is in a crisis, an immediate splenectomy should be performed and the administration of blood started after the splenic pedicle has been ligated.

Acquired Hemolytic Anemias Not Controlled by Steroids

Splenectomy is indicated in these disorders whenever steroid therapy fails to induce or to maintain a remission without maintenance therapy. Splenectomy can be expected to produce a remission in from 40 to 60 per cent of the patients with acquired hemolytic anemia.

Miscellaneous Conditions

In some cases of refractory anemia, splenectomy is resorted to on the basis that with removal of the spleen some inhibitory influence upon bone marrow hemopoiesis is removed. In certain selected cases, even when the spleen is normal in size, splenectomy occasionally has resulted in the restoration of a normal or greatly improved cellular blood picture and an unusual and maintained clinical recovery.

Splenectomy also has been performed in sarcoidosis, Hodgkin's disease, tuberculosis, kala-azar, nonlipoid histiocytosis, lymphatic leukemia and related reticuloses and Gaucher's disease. The indications for removal of the spleen in these conditions are pressure symptoms, hemolytic anemia, leukopenia, thrombocytopenia and a leukopenia which forms a bar to effective use of such agents as x-ray, radioactive phosphorus or nitrogen mustard. The operation has been more successful when the bone marrow was normal. Indiscriminate use of this operation is not advocated in these diseases since the proportion of patients in whom the symptoms can be even temporarily relieved by splenectomy will always be small.

In both idiopathic acquired hemolytic anemia and the symptomatic type of acquired hemolytic anemia the results following splenectomy and the administration of corticotropin or cortisone are variable and difficult to predict. In general, hormone therapy followed by splenectomy appears to be the treatment of choice in the more severe cases.

Cysts, primary tumors and abscesses generally are an indication for splenectomy, although a definite diagnosis usually can be made only by exclusion and then not with a high degree of accuracy. About 80 per cent of cysts are false cysts (hemorrhagic type caused by trauma, inflammation or parasites) and the other 20 per cent are true cysts of the dermoid or lymphangiomatous type. Abscess of the spleen is extremely rare and is difficult to diagnose. Most surgeons state that if the spleen is not densely adherent it should be removed. Otherwise, drainage may be the procedure of choice, particularly if it is not necessary to drain across the free peritoneal cavity.

The conditions in which splenectomy is contraindicated have already been mentioned in Table 2 (p. 347). In myeloid metaplasia of the spleen, splenectomy may be beneficial when a hemolytic component is present. The bone marrow is very hypoplastic, and there is histologic evidence of fibrosis of the bone marrow. This disease is often confused with thrombocytopenic purpura, hemolytic anemia and Banti's syndrome.

The selection of cases for splenectomy has been extended in recent years to include several new syndromes. Further, the risks of splenectomy have been greatly reduced by improvement in surgical and anesthetic technics, better pre- and postoperative care and the introduction of massive blood transfusions and antibiotics. With the exception of traumatic rupture and essential thrombocytopenic purpura, splenectomy is not usually indicated in the absence of an enlarged spleen. Still more important is a clear demonstration by sternal puncture that the bone marrow after splenectomy will be capable of responding in the presence of the condition for which splenectomy is used.

CHAPTER 19

Splenectomy

Preoperative Care

Many patients undergoing splenectomy are poor surgical risks because of the general systemic effects of the state of the disease necessitating splenectomy. For this reason a thorough over-all evaluation is important to insure proper management. The replacement of blood loss is particularly important, and blood volume, red blood cell count and hemoglobin must be brought to levels as normal as possible. In certain severe hemorrhagic and traumatic states, it may be impossible to overcome the blood deficit because of continued loss or destruction. Splenectomy may be indicated in patients who have had severe hemorrhage and are in a state of compensated or incipient shock. The patient may manifest tachycardia, an increased respiratory rate or volume and some degree of peripheral vascular constriction or hemoconcentration with diminished blood volume. When such a patient is anesthetized, severe and irreversible shock may develop. Surgery should be delayed if possible until the circulatory state has been improved or returned to as near normal as possible. If such delay would be dangerous, preparation should be made before operation to administer adequate amounts of fluid intravenously during the operation and in the early postoperative period. Two 16 gauge needles or cannulas should be placed in accessible veins and the administration of fluids started before the induction of anesthesia. The blood volume can be temporarily corrected by the use of plasma expanders such as dextran. These solutions are only for volume correction and do not aid in oxygenation of tissues except so far as they increase circulatory efficiency. It is advisable to have equipment available to give intravenous and intra-arterial pressure transfusions if indicated. In hemolytic diseases, blood may be destroyed as rapidly as it can be replaced, and surgery may have to be performed with the blood count remaining dangerously low. The use of fresh blood should be emphasized, because certain essential elements rapidly disintegrate. For example, in thrombocytopenic purpura an attempt to correct the platelet deficiency necessitates the use of fresh blood because the platelets in old blood will have disintegrated.

If the patient has been unable to maintain adequate oral nourishment, deficits secondary to dehydration and starvation must be corrected by use of intravenous solutions containing carbohydrates, proteins and vitamins. The bleeding tendency created by vitamin deficiencies, particularly of vitamins K and C, should be counteracted by administering these vitamins. In certain instances, heparin-protamine titration should be carried out; if an increase of heparin-like substances exists, it can be treated by the use of protamine sulfate or toluidine blue. Careful evaluation of the cardiac system is essential. Kidney function should be studied thoroughly. Incompatible blood transfusions, anoxia, hypotension and many other factors may result in anuria. Antibiotics generally are not used prophylactically but should be administered if there is evidence of infection.

Before surgery, the stomach contents should be effectively aspirated with a Levin-type tube. The tube should be inspected and tested to be sure it is patent and serviceable. Great care should be taken to avoid trauma in passing the tube, especially in patients with hemorrhagic tendencies. Irritation by the tube can cause bleeding into the stomach, esophagus or upper respiratory passages. Blood in the gastrointestinal tract may be regurgitated around the tube during or after operation and pass into the upper respiratory tree. The tube should remain open during the operation to insure adequate decompression, thus avoiding the possibility of vomiting and preventing the spleen from being obscured by a distended stomach. Preanesthetic medication with drugs such as barbiturates, morphine and atropine should be determined by the anesthesiologist and is dependent upon the patient's physical state as well as the anesthetic agent to be employed.

Anesthesia

In determining the anesthetic agent to be used for splenectomy, not only the factors of anesthesia and relaxation but the effect of the anesthetic agent on the size of the spleen must be considered. Relaxation of the abdominal wall is important to permit exposure of the spleen, which lies in a high posterolateral position under the left diaphragm. Dilatation of the spleen will result in an increased loss of blood into the organ. Spinal anesthesia produces definite splenic dilatation, often to two or three times the previous size. The high anesthesia level necessary for splenectomy, often as high as the fourth thoracic segment, may in itself cause shock, thus making spinal anesthesia undesirable. Cyclopropane also may cause slight increase in the size of the spleen. If anesthetic agents producing splenic dilatation are administered to patients with severe anemia, the loss of systemic blood into the spleen may be sufficient to produce shock. Ether is the only known anesthetic agent which causes constriction of the spleen. It may cause sufficient contraction of this organ for it to lose one-third to one-half its total volume and thus to return a considerable amount of blood to the systemic circulation. In poor risk patients with severe anemia or in patients with diseases which have hemorrhagic tendencies, anesthetic agents and technics which tend to increase bleeding should be avoided.

The regurgitation of blood and other contents from the gastrointestinal tract into the upper respiratory tree during operation is a real hazard. The maintenance of a free airway and the prevention of such regurgitation may be accomplished by the use of an endotracheal tube. In patients with bleeding tendency, the endotracheal tube should be avoided when possible for fear of bleeding into mucosa with resultant glottic or subglottic obstruction. As a general rule, ether anesthesia is probably the safest for this group of patients although adequate skill may make other anesthetic technics work as well.

Incisions.—Numerous incisions have been recommended for the abdominal approach to the spleen. These include a left paramedian, left rectus, left subcostal, various modifications of the left transverse and the hockey-stick incision which begins as a high, left rectus incision and curves out and down across the rectus muscle. The hockey-stick, the left subcostal and modifications of the left transverse incision give good exposure of the left upper abdomen if the medial end of the incision is carried as high as possible near the midline of the abdomen. These incisions have the disadvantage of being accompanied by considerable bleeding because of the necessary transection of the rectus muscle and often of the left transversalis and oblique muscles. The opening and closing of these wounds prolong the operation and this increases the mortality and morbidity in some of the poor risk patients.

A.—Except when dense vascular adhesions are likely to exist, as in Banti's disease, a long, high, left paramedian or muscle-splitting left rectus incision gives excellent exposure with a minimal amount of bleeding and loss of time. The incision must extend as high as possible between the ensiform process and the left costal margin and should extend down about 2 in. below the umbilicus. The length of the incision should be proportionate to the size of the spleen.

B.—This incision when combined with good relaxation permits wide retraction of the left abdominal wall. A C. W. Mayo retractor placed in the left side of the incision under the left costal margin gives excellent exposure of the spleen and permits rapid, safe and simplified removal. If additional exposure is needed, a transverse or oblique extension of this incision may be made across the abdominal muscles.

C.—The splenic ligaments are next isolated, doubly clamped, divided and the ends ligated. The order of this division depends upon the ease of access. This diagram shows the splenocolic ligament being divided first.

[Splenectomy *continued on page 366.*]

PLATE 74

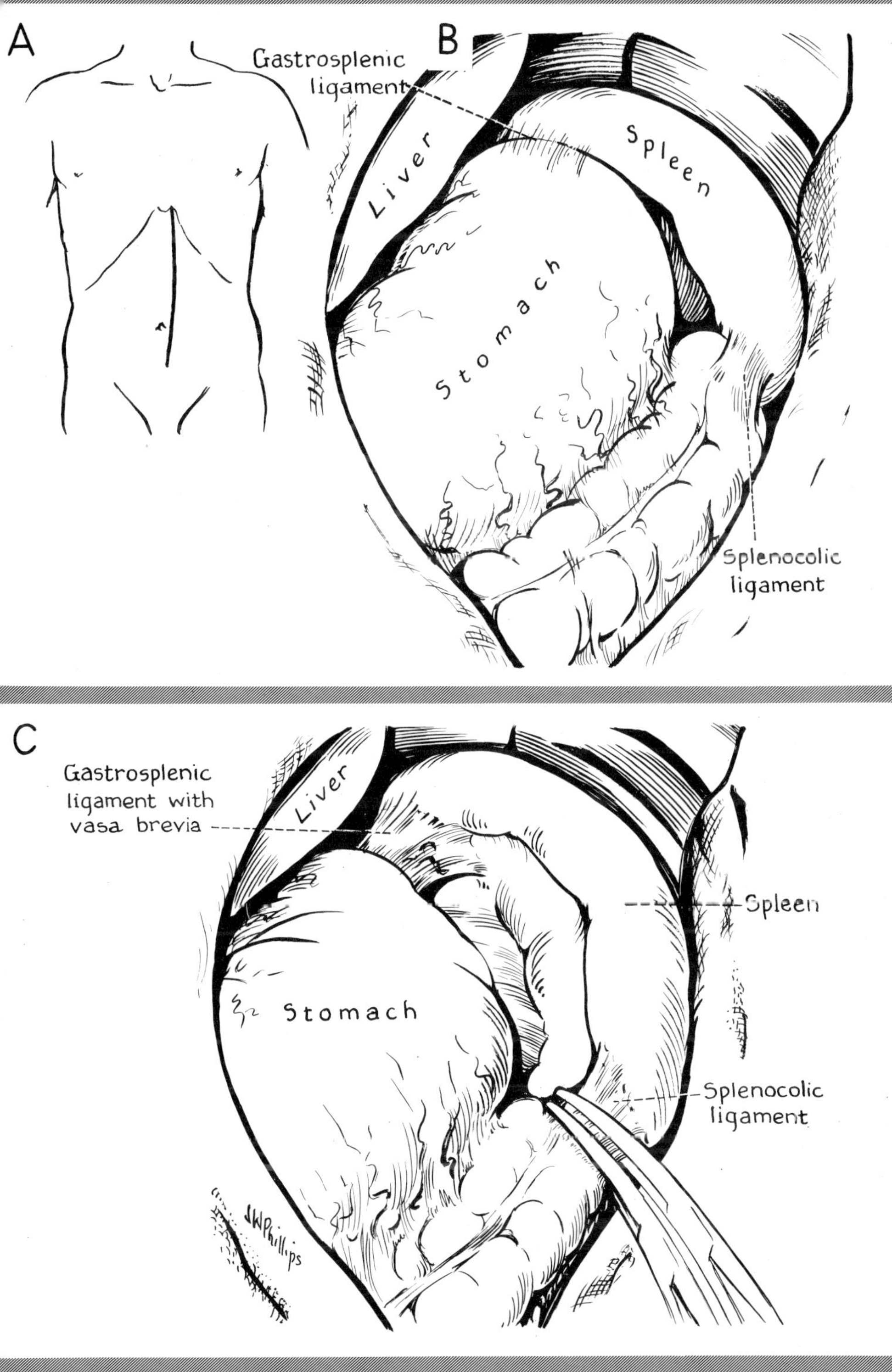
A
B
Gastrosplenic ligament
Liver
Spleen
Stomach
Splenocolic ligament
C
Gastrosplenic ligament with vasa brevia
Liver
Spleen
Stomach
Splenocolic ligament
JWPhillips

D.—The spleen is fixed in its high, posterior position chiefly by the splenodiaphragmatic and splenorenal ligaments. This peritoneal fold contains few blood vessels. When the spleen is grasped and retracted forward and toward the midline, the posterolateral ligaments can be divided either by sharp or finger dissection without danger of damaging the splenic vessels.

E.—As soon as these ligaments are divided, the spleen can be elevated into the wound. If not initially divided, the two main remaining supporting ligaments, the gastrosplenic and splenocolic, are readily accessible and can be clamped, divided and ligated. Occasionally mobility may be facilitated by dividing these ligaments before dividing the posterolateral peritoneal fold. The division of these ligaments permits the spleen to be hinged medially without tension upon the splenic vessels because they enter the organ on its medial surface and extend directly medially from it. The tail of the pancreas occasionally lies against the hilar surface of the spleen. It may have any possible relation to the splenic vessels but is most frequently found anterior and slightly inferior to them. It should be carefully dissected from the spleen and its vessels. At this stage, the splenic artery may be identified and ligated separately before ligation of the veins although in most instances this is of little value. The anterior peritoneal reflection may be dissected from the anterior surface of the splenic vessels if desired.

[Splenectomy *continued on page 368.*]

D

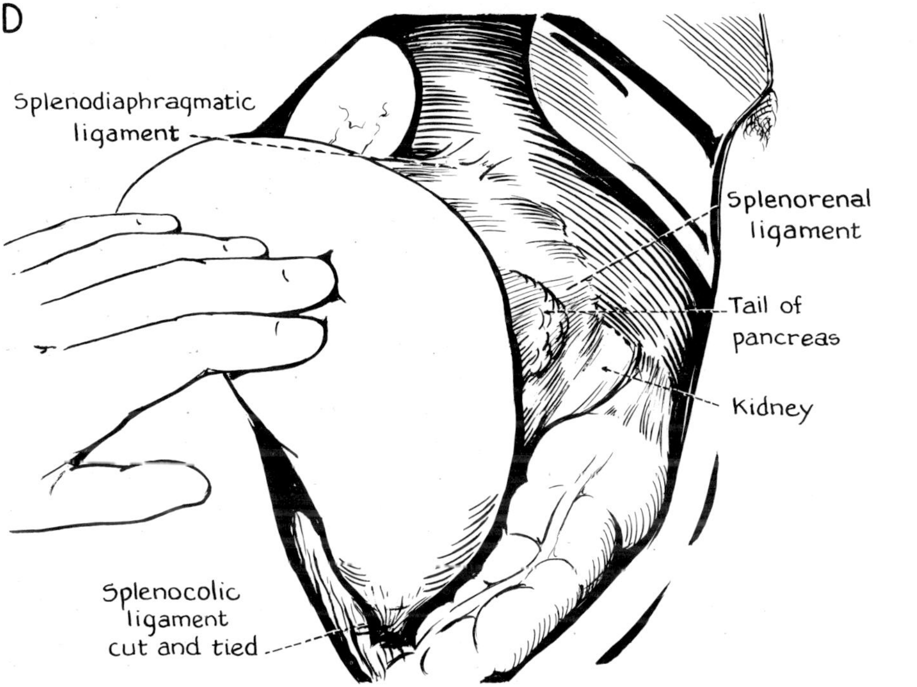
Splenodiaphragmatic ligament
Splenorenal ligament
Tail of pancreas
Kidney
Splenocolic ligament cut and tied

E

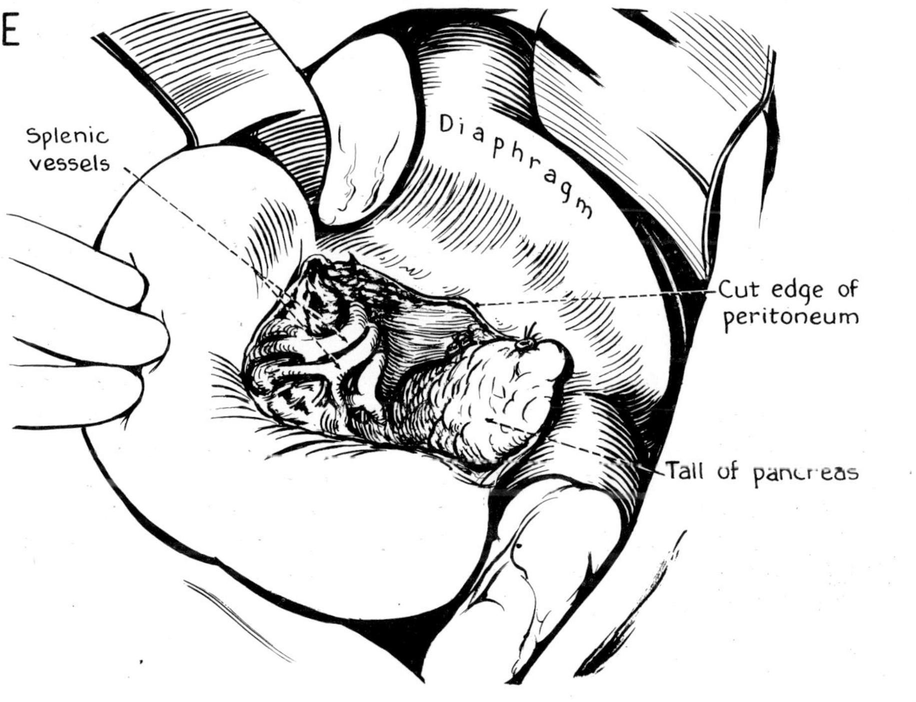
Splenic vessels
Diaphragm
Cut edge of peritoneum
Tail of pancreas

F.—The splenic artery and veins are then securely clamped, usually with three strong Kocher clamps, and are divided between the distal two clamps. This leaves two clamps on the proximal side of the vessels to minimize the danger of their escape which could result in profuse bleeding. The pedicle should be doubly ligated. It is often advisable to separate the ends of the individual vessels and ligate them separately.

If oozing occurs posterior to the spleen after division of the splenodiaphragmatic and splenorenal ligaments, a large, moist pack placed behind the spleen will minimize blood loss. Bleeding vessels in this area should be individually ligated after the spleen is removed. A careful search should be made for accessory spleen in those diseases in which such structures may cause a persistence of symptoms. They are most often found in the region of the splenic pedicle but may lie anywhere within the abdomen.

G and *H.*—Preliminary ligation of the splenic artery has been recommended to check arterial blood flow into the organ and to permit the spleen to return some blood to the systemic circulation. To expose the artery for ligation, it is necessary to enter the lesser gastric cavity through the gastrohepatic or gastrocolic omentum. The peritoneum covering the posterior wall of the lesser gastric cavity must be incised over the artery and the vessel isolated. The dissection, especially in patients with hemorrhagic tendencies or with engorgement of venous channels, may be tedious and time consuming and blood loss may be greater than the amount recovered from the spleen. Preliminary ligation of the splenic artery, if desired, can be accomplished more simply and satisfactorily after the organ has been mobilized. It may be of value when dense adhesions containing numerous venous channels are found between the spleen and diaphragm and when the spleen is fixed and difficult to mobilize. This is rarely encountered when accepted indications for splenectomy are followed.

Wound closure.—The wound is closed in layers, ligating all bleeding points. Tension sutures are placed at fairly close intervals well back from the skin edges and extend through the skin, subcutaneous tissue and external rectus fascia. After closure of the skin they are tied over a gauze roll to exert pressure upon the incision. This minimizes the danger of bleeding from the skin edges and the formation of hematomas within the wound.

PLATE 74

F

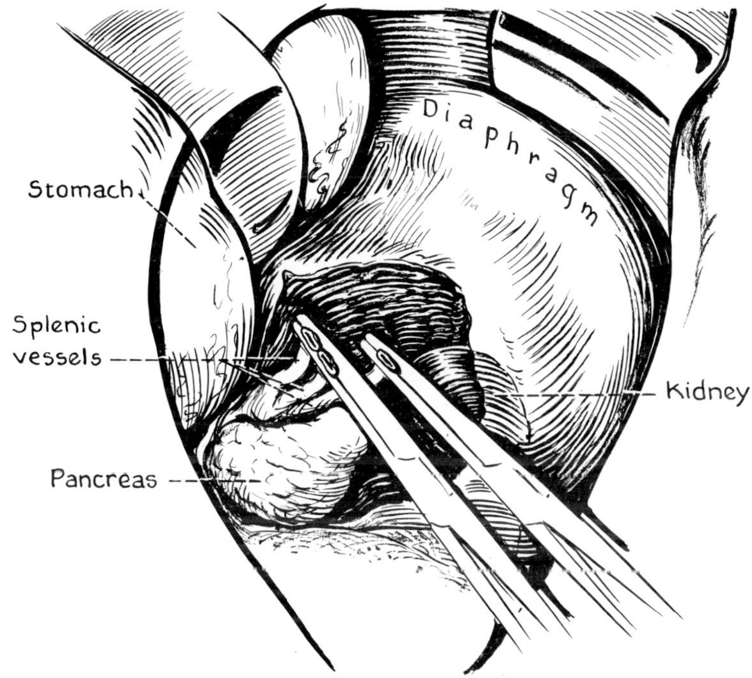

G

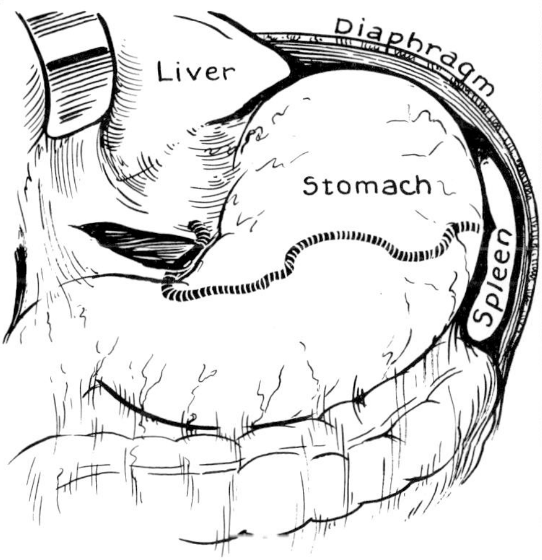

Approach to splenic artery through gastrohepatic ligament

H

Approach to splenic artery through gastrocolic ligament

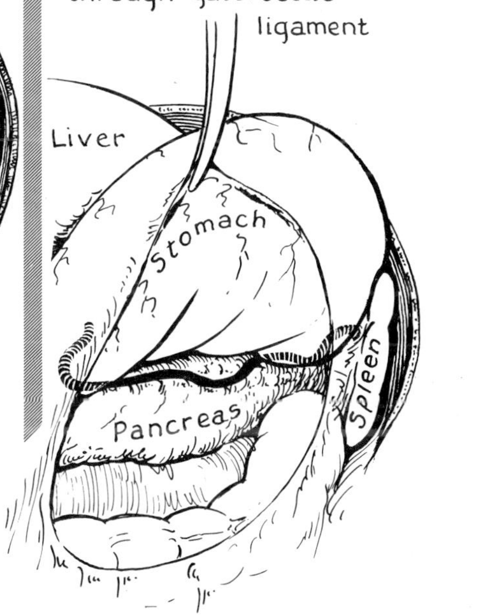

It may be advisable to expose the spleen through a transthoracic approach if dense and vascular adhesions are believed to exist between the spleen and the undersurface of the diaphragm, as in Banti's disease or after previous left upper abdominal surgery or infection. The patient should be anesthetized intratracheally and placed on the right side. The chest may be opened through the eighth or ninth left intercostal space or through the bed of the ninth rib. The latter incision is preferable if the spleen is very large since better exposure can be obtained.

A.—The skin incision is made over the entire length of the ninth rib. It should begin close to the spinous process and extend downward and forward beyond the costal cartilage. (The dotted line shows the extension for a combined thoracoabdominal approach; see p. 374.) The muscles and periosteum overlying the ninth rib are divided and the periosteum elevated from the rib surface. It is important to remove as much as the rib as possible to secure good exposure.

B.—The parietal pleura then is incised through the rib bed and the ribs separated by a rib spreader. The diaphragm is opened from its costal insertion in the mid or anterior axillary line to a point slightly to the left of the esophageal hiatus.

C.—Retraction of the diaphragm exposes the spleen with its ligaments and adhesions. Division and ligation of the ligaments and adhesions may be carried out under direct vision in the order most suitable to each case. Primary division of the gastrosplenic and splenocolic ligaments may partially diminish the blood supply to the spleen and the amount of oozing incident to division of adhesions to the diaphragm.

[Transthoracic splenectomy *continued on page 372.*]

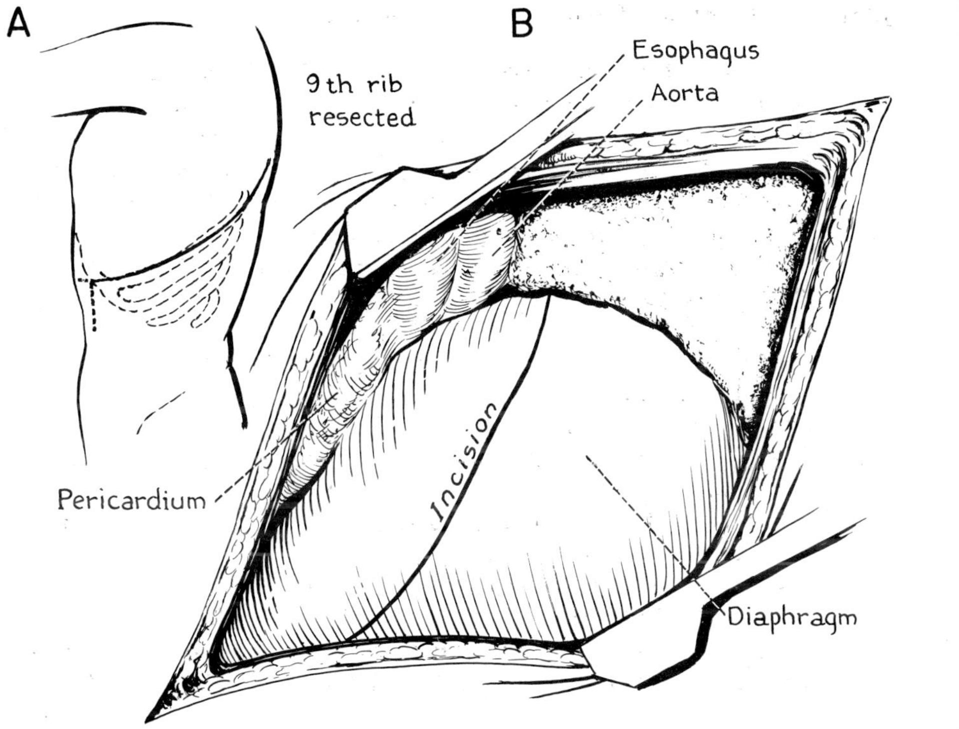
A
9th rib
resected
B
Esophagus
Aorta
Pericardium
Incision
Diaphragm

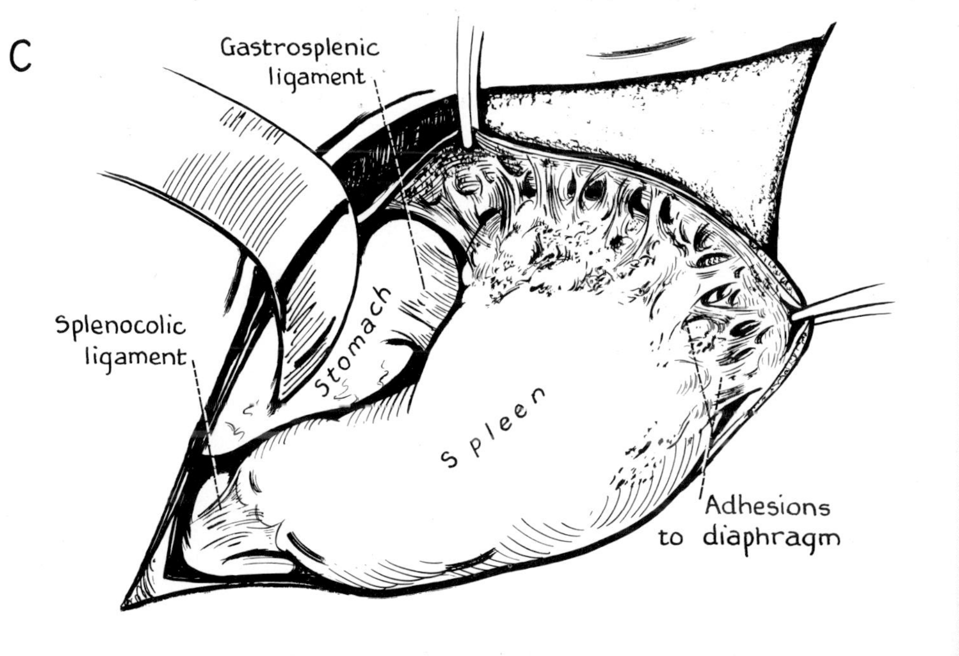
C
Gastrosplenic
ligament
Splenocolic
ligament
Stomach
Spleen
Adhesions
to diaphragm

D.—If the splenic artery is accessible, primary ligation of it at this time may be advisable. Adhesions between the spleen and the diaphragm are clamped, divided and ligated, following which splenodiaphragmatic and splenorenal ligaments are sectioned. This sufficiently mobilizes the spleen so that it may be brought anteriorly and medially and the pedicle exposed posteriorly.

E.—The tail of the pancreas is carefully dissected from the pedicle and the splenic vessels securely clamped and divided.

Closure.—After all bleeding is controlled, the diaphragm is closed with a continuous chromic catgut suture reinforced with interrupted sutures if desired. The ribs are approximated and the thoracic cavity is closed in layers with continuous chromic catgut. A catheter drain is placed in the pleural cavity through the wound or through a stab wound at a more dependent level, and the thoracic muscles are closed around it. After completing the muscle closure, the anesthetist should re-expand the lung to express all air from the pleural cavity, at which time the catheter may be removed and the skin closed. If desired, the catheter may be left in the thoracic cavity for 24 hours to insure expansion of the lung. The catheter must be attached to a water-seal bottle or some form of constant suction.

Combined Abdominothoracic Approach

F.—If the abdomen is opened through an abdominal approach and unexpected adhesions are encountered which will increase the difficulty and hazards of splenectomy, the incision may be extended into the chest through the ninth interspace and the diaphragm divided according to the aforementioned technic. The indication for such an approach should be rare.

PLATE 75

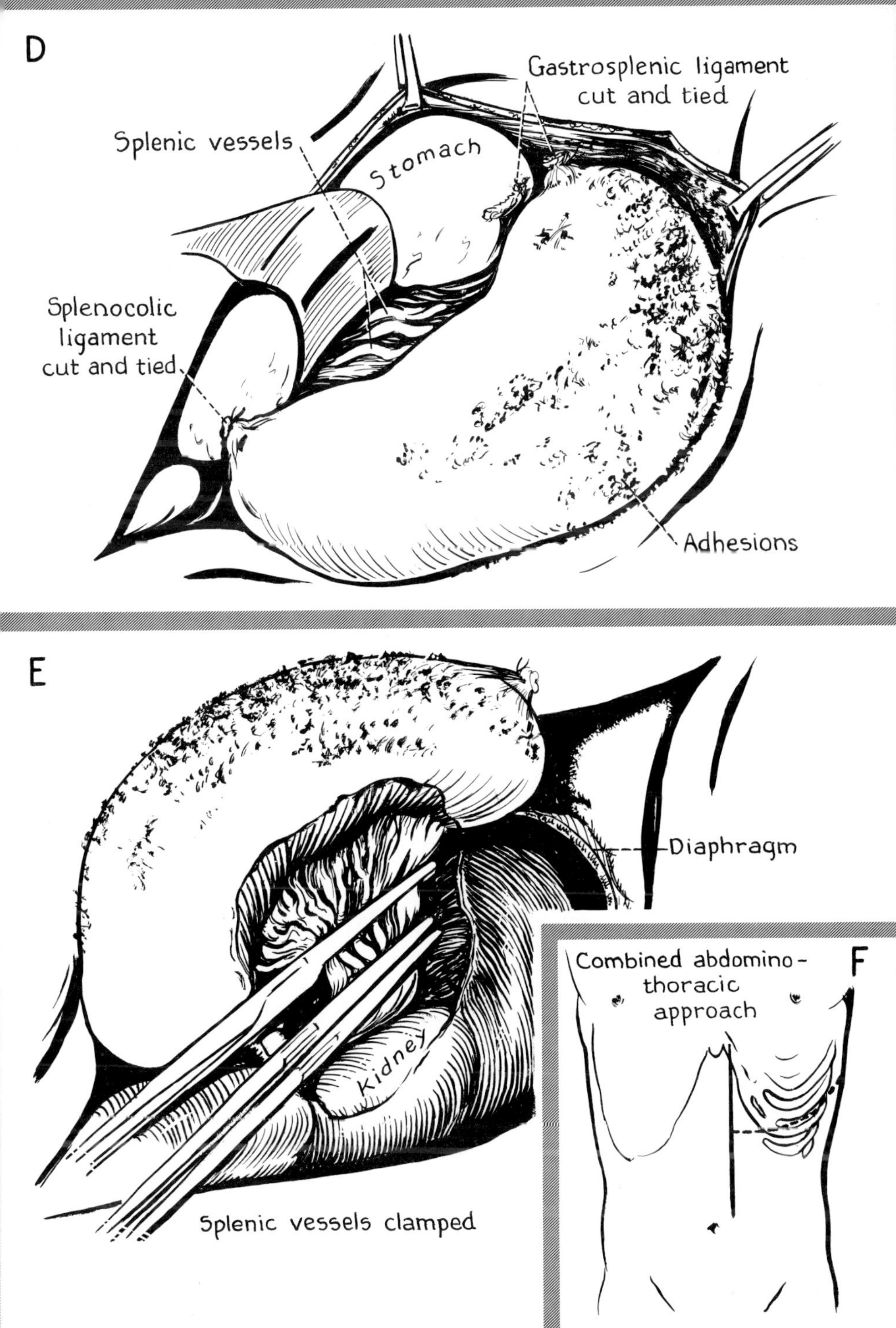

D
Gastrosplenic ligament cut and tied
Splenic vessels
Stomach
Splenocolic ligament cut and tied
Adhesions
E
Diaphragm
Kidney
Splenic vessels clamped
Combined abdomino-thoracic approach
F

Some surgeons prefer to expose the spleen through a combined thoracoabdominal approach, as indicated in Plate 75, A. This gives greater access to the contents of the left upper abdomen. The thoracic cavity may be opened by an incision made through the eighth left intercostal space. The incision should begin close to the spinous process and extend downward and forward beyond the costal cartilage. It may be continued onto the abdomen transversely across the rectus muscle, downward at its lateral border or downward as a muscle-splitting incision through any desired portion of the left rectus muscle.

The intercostal muscles are divided down to the pleura which is then incised through the entire length of the exposed intercostal space. The ninth costal cartilage is sectioned and the rectus muscle split longitudinally or divided transversely according to the desires of the surgeon. The diaphragm is opened from its insertion directly beneath the divided costal cartilage to a point slightly to the left of the esophageal hiatus. The peritoneum is opened directly beneath the rectus muscle incision. The ribs on each side of the intercostal incision now can be widely separated by a rib spreader. Splenectomy can then be carried out by a technic similar to that described in the transthoracic approach (Plate 75).

After the spleen has been removed and all bleeding controlled, the diaphragm is closed, following which the abdominal wall is closed without drainage. The divided ends of the costal cartilage should be approximated with strong, nonabsorbable sutures to minimize separation and friction. The thoracic cavity is closed in layers (p. 372). The increased magnitude of the thoracoabdominal incision results in increased postoperative morbidity. Division of the costal cartilage is followed by more pain and by tenderness at the site of division. For these reasons, the transthoracic approach is preferable when it is adequate.

Postoperative Care

The amount of blood lost during the operation should be estimated and adequate replacement made. If anoxia is present, oxygen should be administered, preferably by nasal catheter or mask. Careful attention must be given to the circulatory, respiratory and genitourinary systems. It is important to keep the lungs well aerated. To avoid atelectasis, a "stir up" regime consisting of frequent turning, coughing, deep breathing, carbon-dioxide inhalations and tracheobronchial toilet, if indicated, should be carried out. Circulatory depression in most instances can be adequately treated by the maintenance of circulatory volume with intravenous infusions. Vasopressors are indicated only to maintain an adequate circulation until such time as blood and other fluids are administered intravenously in adequate amounts. A careful record of renal function should be maintained. If large amounts of blood are given, calcium should be administered intravenously to overcome the effects of the citrate and excess potassium. It should be remembered that the use of fresh whole blood is advisable in the presence of hemorrhagic disease. To aid in the excretion of blood by-products, alkalinization of the urine is helpful.

Generally, it is possible to administer oral feedings early in the postoperative period. If ileus develops, nutrition must be maintained by administration of intravenous solutions of glucose, aminoacids and vitamins. Ileus may become quite severe, especially following splenectomy for rupture of the spleen in which there has been extensive intra-abdominal hemorrhage or when there is an associated spinal injury. The accompanying distention of the abdomen may, by pressure upon the diaphragm, produce incomplete expansion of the lower lung fields and increase the danger of postoperative atelectasis or pneumonia. It may also increase the possibility of evisceration or wound disruption. Intestinal decompression by the use of a Levin, Harris or similar type of gastrointestinal tube is important. These tubes demand constant attention to prevent blockage and subsequent increased distention. When the motor activity of the intestine begins to return, it may be stimulated by drugs such as neostigmine. Although morphine is an excellent small bowel stimulant, it should be used cautiously because of its depressing action on the respiratory and circulatory systems. The administration of vitamins K and C should be continued. Antibiotics are used when indicated.

Early ambulation ordinarily is possible. Precautions should be taken against the development of phlebitis. Symptomatic thrombosis of the splenic vein may develop. Thrombophlebitis is commoner after splenectomy than after most surgical procedures. Careful assessment of the elements of the blood immediately after surgery and during the first postoperative days should be made to ascertain the effects of the splenectomy. Postoperative hemorrhage is counteracted by the use of fresh blood, adequate vitamins, protamine sulfate and other measures when indicated. When hemorrhagic tendencies exist and are difficult to correct, it is well not to remove the sutures until the tenth or twelfth postoperative day because of delayed wound healing in the presence of hematoma formation, anemia or impaired nutrition. When specific indications have existed for splenectomy, the postoperative course is usually without incident, but the aforementioned complications should be anticipated and prevented.

Factors Increasing Morbidity and Mortality

The most important factor complicating splenectomy is hemorrhage and resultant shock. Bleeding may occur into the gastrointestinal tract or the tissues or from the wound. It should be combated by the use of appropriate intravenous solutions, whole blood and vitamins C and K. During the operation, the stomach, intestine and other organs should be handled as gently as possible to minimize trauma which may produce bleeding.

Pulmonary complications likewise may prove serious. The danger of atelectasis and pneumonia can be minimized by the prevention of aspiration into the upper respiratory tree, avoidance of lung compression from distention and the minimal use of drugs which are respiratory depressants. The patient should be urged to cough up any secretions within the lungs. Tracheobronchial suction by endoscopic procedures or even by catheters should be avoided or used to a minimum in hemorrhagic diseases because of the danger of producing bleeding. Morphine, Demerol and other depressing drugs should be used in minimal doses. The use of local anesthesia for regional block is advisable to relieve pain so that the patient may be stimulated to breathe more deeply and to cough more readily.

Index

D

E

F